W9-DJE-174

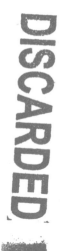

Human Reasoning and Cognitive Science

Human Reasoning and Cognitive Science

Keith Stenning and Michiel van Lambalgen

A Bradford Book
The MIT Press
Cambridge, Massachusetts
London, England

MIT Press books may be purchased at special quantity discounts for business or sales promotional use. For information, please email special_sales@mitpress.mit.edu or write to Special Sales Department, The MIT Press, 55 Hayward Street, Cambridge, MA 02142.

This book was set in latex by the authors. Printed and bound in the United States of America.

Library of Congress Cataloging-in-Publication Data

Stenning, Keith.
  Human reasoning and cognitive science / Keith Stenning and Michiel van Lambalgen.
       p. cm. – (A Bradford book)
  Includes bibliographical references and index.
  ISBN 978-0-262-19583-6 (hardcover : alk. paper) 1. Cognitive science. 2. Reasoning. 3. Logic. I. Lambalgen, Michiel van, 1954- II. Title.
BF311.S67773 2008
153.4–dc22

                                                    2007046686

10 9 8 7 6 5 4 3 2 1

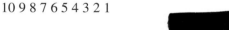

To Nye (KS)
To Stijn (MvL)

Contents

Preface

In the late summer of 1998, the authors, a cognitive scientist and a logician, started talking about the relevance of modern mathematical logic to the study of human reasoning, and we have been talking ever since. This book is an interim report of that conversation. It argues that results such as those on the Wason selection task, purportedly showing the irrelevance of formal logic to actual human reasoning, have been widely misinterpreted, mainly because the picture of logic current in psychology and cognitive science is completely mistaken. We aim to give the reader a more accurate picture of mathematical logic and, in doing so, hope to show that logic, properly conceived, is still a very helpful tool in cognitive science. The main thrust of the book is therefore constructive. We give a number of examples in which logical theorizing helps in understanding and modeling observed behavior in reasoning tasks, deviations of that behavior in a psychiatric disorder (autism), and even the roots of that behavior in the evolution of the brain.

The manuscript was tried out by us in many courses over the past five years, and has been much improved as a result of the insightful questions of our students. Rineke Verbrugge and Bart Verheij also taught a course from a draft and we thank them and their students for much insightful feedback. We also thank the colleagues who commented on individual chapters or their precursors: Theodora Achourioti, Jonathan Adler, Marian Counihan, Richard Cox, Hartmut Fitz, Jim Greeno, Fritz Hamm, Wilfrid Hodges, Tikitu de Jager, Phil Johnson-Laird, Hans Kamp, Alex Korzec, Max Roberts, Lance Rips, Heleen Smid, and Martin Stokhof. Special thanks go to Bob Kowalski, who read and commented on the entire manuscript. The mistakes are, of course, our own.

We dedicate this book to our children.

PART I

Groundwork

1 Introduction: Logic and Psychology

The purpose of this book is twofold. Our first aim is to see to what extent the psychology of reasoning and logic (more generally, semantics) are relevant to each other. After all, the psychology of reasoning and logic are in a sense about the same subject, even though in the past century a rift has opened up between them. Very superficially speaking, logic appears to be normative, whereas the psychology of reasoning is descriptive and concerned with processing. The first question then is: what is the relation between these two fields of inquiry?

The psychology of reasoning as a field currently adopts a particular view of this relation: we propose a quite different one. The book therefore should be relevant to students of logic who are interested in applications of logic to cognition. But the book should also be relevant to any psychologist who is interested in reasoning or communication, or any other cognitive capacity where a cognitive account has to be founded on an informational analysis of a cognitive capacity. These two groups come to the topic with very different methodological equipment. The logic student interested in cognition comes with an understanding of the level of abstraction that modern logical theories operate at, but with possibly sparse knowledge of psychological observations of reasoning. Students of psychology come with knowledge of the experimental literatures, but those literatures are strongly formed by a different conception of logic – a conception, current in the nineteenth century,[1] in which logic is thought of as a *mechanism* for reasoning, and a universal, normatively valid mechanism at that.

This presents us with an educational dilemma. The logical analyses presented here are couched at a level which is intended to be comprehensible to nonlogicians with sufficient patience to digest logical formulas.[2] From experience, the problems encountered are not so much problems about the technicalities of the systems (which are often not the main point here) but background assumptions about what logic is about and what such systems do and do not attempt to provide. So our message to the psychology student venturing here would

---

1. Although already at that time more refined conceptions existed; compare section 1.3 on Husserl.
2. Chapter 2 does duty as an introduction to those aspects of logic most important for our purposes.

be that we promise to show that these analyses can make a real difference to how empirical investigations are designed, so venturing is well worthwhile. But understanding requires that many routine assumptions about logic are left at the door. Modern logical theories provide a conceptual and mathematical framework for analyzing information systems such as people's reasoning and communication. They do not settle mechanisms or processes of reasoning, but without their conceptualization, it is impossible to know what are empirical and what are conceptual questions.

To the student venturing from logic our message is that we obviously cannot provide more than the very bare outlines of a few empirical results, along with some pointers to the literature. So we need to warn against assuming that the empirical phenomena are as simple or separable as they are bound to appear. The immense contribution that psychology has made to understanding the mind largely consists of bodies of empirical knowledge about what phenomena are replicable under what range of conditions. Much of this knowledge is implicit in the literature.

This educational dilemma leads naturally to our second wider aim, to discuss some of the theories offered in the literature from the point of view of the philosophy and methodology of science. For instance, both mental models theory and evolutionary psychology, which take their starting points in observations about the psychology of reasoning, have become hugely popular explanatory paradigms in psychology. We will see that the experiments claimed to support these theories are marred by conceptual confusions and attendant methodological errors, and that the theories themselves show little awareness of the subtleties of logic. Part of our purpose is therefore to propose a different methodology for this field, which takes Marr's idea of "levels of analysis" seriously.

1.1 Forms of Rationality

Traditionally, rationality is taken to be a defining characteristic of human nature: "man is a rational animal," apparently capable of deliberate thought, planning, problemsolving, scientific theorizing and prediction, moral reasoning, and so forth. If we ask what "rational" means here, we can read such things as: "In rational discourse one strives to arrive at justified true belief," a definition of rationality from an era oriented toward theory. Our more pragmatically oriented age has extended this concept of rationality to actions. For instance, in the MIT *Encyclopedia of Cognitive Science*, "rational agency" is defined as a coherence requirement:

> [T]he agent must have a means-end competence to fit its actions or decisions, according to its beliefs or knowledge representations, to its desires or goal-structure.

Without such coherence there is no agent. The onus here is on the term *fit* which seems to have a logical component. If an action is performed which is not part of a plan derived to achieve a given goal, there is no fit. In this sense checking my horoscope before mounting the bike to go to work is not rational, and neither is first puncturing the tires.

Philosophy, then, studies the question: are there optimal rules for conducting such activities? Various logics, scientific methodology, heuristics, probability, decision theory, all have claims to normative status here, where normativity means that everybody should obey the rules of these systems in all circumstances. As a consequence, there exists an absolute distinction between valid arguments and fallacies. Judged by these standards, human reasoning in the laboratory is very poor indeed (as shown by the seminal experiments of Wason [295] for logic and Kahneman and Tversky [150] for probability), and it has therefore been said that humans are actually not rational in the sense defined above.

It is usually assumed that the results obtained in the psychology of reasoning tell us something about the *rationality*, or rather the absence thereof, of human reasoning. The following extended quotation from Peter Wason, one of the founding fathers of the field whose "selection task" will serve as our entrypoint below, exemplifies this attitude to perfection. He writes, concluding an overview of his selection task paradigm for *The Oxford Companion to the Mind*,

> Our basic paradigm has the enormous advantage of being artificial and novel; in these studies we are not interested in everyday thought, but in the kind of thinking which occurs when there is minimal meaning in the things around us. On a much smaller scale, what do our students' remarks remind us of in real life? They are like saying "Of course, the earth is flat," "Of course, we are descended from Adam and Eve," "Of course, space has nothing to do with time." The old ways of seeing things now look like absurd prejudices, but our highly intelligent student volunteers display analogous miniature prejudices when their premature conclusions are challenged by the facts. As Kuhn has shown, old paradigms do not die in the face of a few counterexamples. In the same way, our volunteers do not often accommodate their thought to new observations, even those governed by logical necessity, in a deceptive problem situation. They will frequently deny the facts, or contradict themselves, rather than shift their frame of reference.
>
> Other treatments and interpretations of problem solving could have been cited. For instance, most problems studied by psychologists create a sense of perplexity rather than a specious answer. But the present interpretation, in terms of the development of dogma and its resistance to truth, reveals the interest and excitement generated by research in this area. (Wason [300,p. 644])

What lies behind remarks such as Wason's is the view that reasoning, whether logical or probabilistic, can be judged to be rational if certain reasoning *rules* from a fixed, given set are followed. If these rules are not followed, dire consequences may result. A good example of this attitude is furnished by Stanovich's book *Who is Rational?* [254]. The following quotation gives some idea of the

passions that infuse this approach. Stanovich considers irrationality to lead to
the occurrence of

> wars, economic busts, technological accidents, pyramid sales schemes, telemarketing
> fraud, religious fanaticism, psychic scams, environmental degradation, broken marriages,
> and savings and loan scandals [254,p. 9]

and believes teaching good reasoning, that is, normatively correct rules, will go
some way toward improving this distressing situation.

Stanovich's discussion of rules governing reasoning introduces a distinction
between *normative*, *descriptive*, and *prescriptive* rules. We give brief characterizations of the three kinds, followed by representative examples.

- *Normative* rules: reasoning as it should be, ideally

    - Modus tollens: $\neg q, p \rightarrow q/\neg p$,
    - Bayes' theorem: $P(D \mid S) = \frac{P(S|D)P(D)}{P(S)}$.

- *Descriptive* rules: reasoning as it is actually practiced

    - Many people do not endorse modus tollens and believe that from $\neg q, p \rightarrow q$ nothing can be derived.

    - In doing probabilistic calculations of the probability of a disease given a cluster of symptoms, even experts sometimes neglect the "base rate" and put $P(D \mid S) = P(S \mid D)$.

- *Prescriptive*[3] rules: these are norms that result from taking into account our bounded rationality, i.e., computational limitations (due to the computational complexity of classical logic, and the even higher complexity of probability theory) and storage limitations (the impossibility of simultaneously representing all factors relevant to a computation, say, of a plan to achieve a given goal).

    - The classically invalid principle $\neg q, p \wedge r \rightarrow q/\neg p \wedge \neg r$ is correct according to *closed–world reasoning*, which is computationally much less complex than classical propositional logic, and ameliorates storage problems.

    - Chater and Oaksford's "heuristic rules" for solving syllogisms. [36]

In terms of these three kinds of rules, Stanovich then distinguishes the following
positions on the relationship between reasoning and rationality [254,pp.4–9]:

- *Panglossian.* Human reasoning competence and performance is actually normatively correct. What appears to be incorrect reasoning can be explained

---

3. The term is not very apt, but we will stick to Stanovich's terminology.

by such maneuvers as different task construal, a different interpretation of logical terms, etc. (A famous defense of his point of view can be found in Henlé [122].) As a consequence, no education in "critical thinking" is necessary.

- *Apologist.* Actual human performance follows prescriptive rules, but the latter are in general (and necessarily) subnormal, because of the heavy computational demands of normatively correct reasoning. This point of view was defended by Oaksford and Chater [205, 36]. As a consequence, education in "critical thinking" is unlikely to be helpful.

- *Meliorist.* Actual human reasoning falls short of prescriptive standards, which are themselves subnormal; there is therefore much room for improvement by suitable education (Stanovich's own position).

- *Eliminativist.*[4] Reasoning rarely happens in real life, and mainly in institutional contexts such as schools. By contrast, true rationality is adaptiveness: we have developed "fast and frugal algorithms" which allow us to take quick decisions which are optimal given constraints of time and energy. This position is defended by evolutionary psychologists such as Cosmides and Tooby[47, 48] and, in more constructive detail, by Gigerenzer [95].

It will be helpful for the reader if we situate our own position with respect to this scheme. We are definitely not in the eliminativist camp, since we take the view that reasoning is everywhere, most prominently in discourse comprehension. This prime example is often overlooked because of the association of reasoning with conscious processing, but this association is wrong: some reasoning is automatic.[5] The same example leads us to think that human reasoning may not be so flawed after all, since it operates rather competently in this domain. We are not Panglossians either, although we emphasize that interpretation is of paramount importance in reasoning. But even if interpretation is important, and interpretations may differ, people may reason in ways which are inconsistent with their chosen interpretation. From a methodological point of view this means that if one uses a particular interpretation to explain performance, one must have evidence for the interpretation which is independent of the performance. The apologist and meliorist positions introduce the distinction between normative and prescriptive rules. Here it becomes clear that Stanovich's scheme is predicated on the assumption that reasoning is about following rules from a fixed, given set, say classical logic, rules which should apply always and everywhere. For if there is no given set of rules which constitutes the norm, and the norm is instead relative to a "domain," then the domain may well include the

---

4. Actually, this category does not occur in [254], but we have added it due to its increased prominence.
5. Chapter 5 has more on this.

cognitive constraints that gave rise to the notion of prescriptive rules, thus promoting the latter to the rank of norm. This is what we will argue for in several places in the book, in particular in chapter 11.

In the next section we briefly look at the role logic once played in cognitive science, and the reasons for its demise.

1.2   How Logic and Cognition Got Divorced

The cognitive sciences really got off the ground after they adopted the information-processing metaphor (Craik [52]):

1. Cognitive explanations must refer to models, conceived of as representational mechanisms

2. which function "in the same way" as the phenomena being represented

3. and which are capable of generating behavior and thoughts of various kinds.

The role of logic in this scheme was twofold: on the one hand as a formal, symbolic, representation language (which is very expressive!), on the other hand as an inference mechanism generating behavior and thoughts. It was furthermore believed that these inference mechanisms are continuous with overt reasoning; that is, the same processes can be applied both reflectively and automatically.

An extreme form of this attitude is of course Piaget's "logicism" [216], which maintains that the acquisition of formal-deductive operations is the crown of cognitive development. Piaget did the first studies to show that preschool children do not yet master simple classical predicate logic; but he also assumed that everyone gets there in the end. This proved to be the Achilles heel of this form of logicism. Indeed, Wason's selection task was inter alia directed against this assumption, and its apparent outcome – a striking deviation from classical logical reasoning – seemingly undermined the role of logic as an inference mechanism. A further criticism concerned the alleged slowness of logical inference mechanisms, especially when search is involved, for example when backtracking from a given goal. Thus, Newell and Simon style "production systems"[199], of which Anderson and Lebiere's ACT-R [2], is the most famous example, keep only the inference rule of modus ponens, allowing fast forward processing, at the cost of considerable complications elsewhere.

Lastly, the advent of neural network theory brought to the fore criticisms of the symbolic representational format given by logic: it would be tied to brittle, all-or-none representations, uncharacteristic of actual cognitive representations with their inherently fuzzy boundaries. As a further consequence of this brittleness, learning symbolic representations would be unrealistically hard. As a result, from the position of being absolutely central in the cognitive revolution, which was founded on conceptions of reasoning, computation, and the analysis of language, the psychology of deduction has gone to being the deadbeat of cognitive psychology, pursued in a ghetto, surrounded by widespread skepticism as to whether human reasoning really happens outside the academy. "Isn't what we *really* do decision?" we increasingly often hear. Many eminent psychology departments do not teach courses on reasoning. Imagine such a psychology department (or indeed any psychology department) not teaching any courses on perception. Even where they do teach reasoning they are more likely to be focused on analogical reasoning, thought of as a kind of reasoning at the opposite end from deduction on some dimension of certainty.

We will argue that logic and reasoning have ended up in this ghetto because of a series of unwarranted assumptions. One of the tasks of this book is to examine these assumptions, and show that they do not bear scrutiny. As a prelude, we consider the vexed issue of the normative status of logic, through some of the history of present day conceptualizations.

1.3   Two Philosophers on the Certainty of Logic: Frege and Husserl

Famously, Aristotle provided the first rules for reasoning with quantifiers of the form "All A are B," "Some A are B," "No A are B" and "Some A are not B," starting centuries of work on how to provide principled explanations for the validity of some syllogisms, and the invalidity of others. This search for an explanation turned to the notion of validity itself (*überhaupt*, we are tempted to say), and Kant opined in the *Critique of Pure Reason* that logical laws constitute the very fabric of thought: thinking which does not proceed according to these laws is not properly thinking.[6]

In the nineteenth century, this "transcendental" doctrine of logic was watered down to a naturalistic version called *psychologism*, which holds that all of thinking and knowledge are psychological phenomena and that *therefore* logical laws are psychological laws. To take an example from John Stuart Mill, the law of noncontradiction $\neg(A \wedge \neg A)$ represents the impossibility of thinking contradictory thoughts at the same time. Thus, normative and descriptive rules coincide. What came after, a strong emphasis on normativity, can to a large extent be seen as a reaction to this view. Gottlob Frege was the driving force behind the reaction, and his views still exert their influence on the textbooks.

---

6. It is impossible to do justice here to Kant's thinking on logic. It is still common to think of Kant's logic as primitive, and its role in the *Critique of Pure Reason* as an instance of Kant's architectonic mania. This is very far from the truth, and Kant's thinking on, for instance, logical consequence remains relevant to this day. In fact, our concluding chapter 11 has many affinities with Kant, although it would require another book to explain why. Béatrice Longuenesse's *Kant and the Capacity to Judge* [175] is an excellent guide to the wider significance of Kant's logic. The reader may also consult Patricia Kitcher's *Kant's Transcendental Psychology* [159] for an exposition of Kant's relevance to cognitive science. Kitcher's remarks on the similarities between Kant's first *Critique* and Marr's program in cognitive science [183] have influenced chapter 11. We thank Theodora Achourioti for pointing out these connections.

1.3.1 Frege's Idealism in Logic

Frege did not hesitate to point out the weak empirical basis of psychologism: is it really true that we cannot simultaneously think contradictory thoughts? Wish it were so! His chief argument, however, was theoretical, and consisted of two main reservations about a naturalistic treatment of logic (and mathematics):

1. Psychologism makes logic pertain to ideas only, and as a consequence it lacks resources to explain why logic is applicable to the real world.

2. Logical and mathematical knowledge are objective, and this objectivity cannot be safeguarded if logical laws are properties of individual minds.

We now present a few extracts from Frege's writings to illustrate his views on psychologism.

As regards 1 we read:

> Psychological treatments of logic ... lead then necessarily to psychological idealism. Since all knowledge is judgmental, every bridge to the objective is now broken off. (G. Frege, *Nachgelassene Schriften*; see [85])

> Neither logic nor mathematics has the task of investigating minds and the contents of consciousness whose bearer is an individual person. (G. Frege, *Kleine Schriften*; see [85])

> The logicians ... are too much caught up in psychology ... Logic is in no way a part of psychology. The Pythagorean theorem expresses the same thought for all men, while each person has its own representations, feelings and resolutions that are different from those of every other person. Thoughts are not psychic structures, and thinking is not an inner producing and forming, but an apprehension of thoughts which are already objectively given. (G. Frege, letter to Husserl; see 6, p. 113 of [135])

The last sentence is especially interesting: if "thinking is not an inner producing and forming," cognitive science has no business investigating thinking, logical reasoning in particular. What the psychologist finds interesting in reasoning is precisely what steps the mind executes in drawing an inference, i.e., in the process more than the result. The quotation just given suggests that logic itself has little to contribute to this inquiry, and indeed psychologists have generally heeded Frege's message, either by designing logics which are supposedly cognitively more relevant (e.g., Johnson-Laird's 'mental models' [145]. See Chapter 10, especially 10.6.3), or by ignoring the contributions that formal logic can make to theories of processing. This is a pity, since, as will be shown in the body of the book, the technical apparatus of logic has much to offer to the psychologist.

Here is an excerpt relevant to 2:

> If we could grasp nothing but what is in ourselves, then a [genuine] conflict of opinions, [as well as] a reciprocity of understanding, would be impossible, since there would be

no common ground, and no idea in the psychological sense can be such a ground. There would be no logic that can be appealed to as an arbiter in the conflict of opinions. (G. Frege, *Grundgesetze der Arithmetik*; the relevant part is reprinted in [85])

From the last quotation we gather that it is apparently highly desirable that logic "can be appealed to as an arbiter in the conflict of opinions," and that therefore there must be a single, objectively valid logic. The second quotation (from the letter to Husserl) provides a reason to believe there is one: logic is as it were the physics of the realm of thought, since it studies the structure of the "objectively given" thoughts. Psychologism is a threat to this normative character of logic, and since a logic worthy of the name must give rise to norms for thinking, psychologism is not a possible theory of logical validity. But, as we have seen, Frege must invoke an objectively given realm of thought to buttress the normative pretensions of logic, and this assumption seems hard to justify. However, if one is skeptical about this objective realm of thought, the specter of relativism rises again. At first sight, the normativity of logic seems to be bound up with the uniqueness of logic; and what better way to safeguard that uniqueness than by positing some underlying reality which the logical laws describe?

This is indeed a serious problem, and to solve it requires rethinking the sense in which logic can be considered to be normative. In a nutshell, our answer will be that norms apply to instances of reasoning only after the interpretation of the (logical and nonlogical) expressions in the argument has been fixed, and, furthermore, that there are in general multiple natural options for such interpretations, even for interpreting the logical expressions. Thus, the reasoning process inevitably involves also steps aimed at fixing an interpretation; once this has been achieved, the norms governing logical reasoning are also determined. It will not have escaped the reader's attention that the view of reasoning just outlined[7] is very different from the one implicitly assumed by the standard paradigms in the psychology of reasoning. As this book goes to press, a special issue on logical views of psychologism covering a range of contemporary positions is published [171].

One aim of this book is to present a view of reasoning as consisting of reasoning *to* and reasoning *from* an interpretation, and to apply this view to experimental studies on reasoning. In philosophy, our precursor here is Husserl, who is playing Aristotle (the metaphysician, not the logician) to Frege's Plato. Husserl's views on logic never made the logic textbooks (at least explicitly), but we nonetheless believe that one can find in him the germs of a semantic conception of logic, which comes much closer than Frege's to how logic functions in actual reasoning.

---

7. The outline is very rough indeed. For instance, the phrase "once this has been achieved" suggests that the two stages are successive. As we will see in the experimental chapters, however, it is much closer to the truth to view these stages as interactive.

1.3.2   Husserl as a Forerunner of Semantics

It was Frege who converted Husserl to antipsychologism. When we read Husserl's criticism of psychologism in *Logische Untersuchungen* [134], we at first seem to be on familiar ground. If logical laws were empirical laws about psychological events, they would have to be approximative and provisional, like all empirical laws. But logical laws are exact and unassailable, hence they cannot be empirical.[8] Psychologism about logical laws also leads to skeptical relativism: it is in principle possible that different people reason according to different logical laws,[9] so that what is true for one person may not be true for another – truth, however, is absolute, not indexed to a person.

So far these arguments are question begging: we may have a strong desire for logical laws to be exact and unassailable and objective, but we need a justification for assuming that they are. In trying to provide one, Husserl develops a strikingly modern view of logic, and one that is much more conducive to playing a role in cognitive science than Frege's. Husserl's *Logische Untersuchungen* brings the important innovation that logic must be viewed, not as a normative, but as a theoretical, or as we would now say, mathematical, discipline. Logic as a theoretical discipline is concerned with "truth," "judgment," and similar concepts. Husserl grounds the normative status of logic via a combination of the theoretical statement "only such and such arguments preserve truth" and the normative statement "truth is good," to conclude: "only such and such arguments are good." Splitting off the normative from the mathematical component of logic is potentially beneficial, since it focuses attention on what exactly justifies the normative statement "truth is good," and thus opens up space for a relativized version such as "(this kind of) truth is good (for that purpose)."

In slightly more detail,[10] Husserl introduces an essentially modern division of logic as concerned with

1. "the pure forms of judgments" (i.e., the syntax of a formal language, but here implying a Kantian delineation of what can be said at all);

2. "the formal categories of meaning" (i.e., the semantic study of concepts such as "variable," "reference," "truth," "proposition," "consequence"[11]);

---

8. Husserl remarks correctly that even if logical laws are considered empirical, psychologism is under the obligation to explain how we can acquire them, and that no account of how logical laws are learned has been forthcoming.

9. In modern times this is occasionally cheerfully accepted. The logician Dov Gabbay once said in an interview: "Everybody his own logic!"

10. Here we are much indebted to David Bell's *Husserl* [17], in particular pp. 85 –100. The quotes from Husserl are taken from Bell's monograph.

11. It is of some interest to observe here that for Frege, semantics, although intuitively given, was not a proper field of scientific study, since it involves stepping outside the system which is given a semantic interpretation. See also footnote 12. We agree with Husserl that it is both possible and necessary to reflect on semantic interpretation.

3. "the formal categories of objects" – that is, what is known as "formal on-
   tology," the study of such concepts as "object," "state of affairs," "continuum," "moment." This can be read as saying that part of logic must be
   the characterization of the structures on which the chosen formal language
   is interpreted; the next quotation calls these structures "possible fields of
   knowledge":

   > The objective correlate of the concept of a possible theory, determined exclusively in
   > terms of its form, is the concept of a possible field of knowledge over which a the-
   > ory of this form will preside. [This field] is characterized by the fact that its objects
   > are capable of certain relations that fall under certain basic laws of such-and-such a
   > determinate form ... the objects remain entirely indeterminate as regards their mat-
   > ter... (*[17,p. 90-1]*)

4. Lastly, rational thinking also involves *systematization*, and therefore pure
   logic must also comprise a study of formal theories, not only of propositions
   and their inferential relationships; in Husserl's words

   > The earlier level of logic had taken for its theme the pure forms of all significant
   > formations that can occur within a science. Now however, judgment systems in their
   > entirety become the theme (*Formale und transzendentale Logik* [17,p. 90-1]).

Modern logic has followed this last injunction, and studies what is known as
"metaproperties" of a logical system such as consistency, the impossibility of
deriving a contradiction in the system. Among the most important metaproperties are metatheorems of the form "only such-and-such argument patterns preserve truth," which depend on a preliminary characterization of the notion of
truth in the "possible field of knowledge" studied. Normativity comes in only
via a principle of the form "in this particular field of knowledge, truth of such-
and-such a form is good, therefore only such-and-such arguments are good."
This means that logical laws are unassailable in the sense that they are mathematical *consequences* of the structure of the domain studied, but by the same
token these laws are relative to that domain. The reader will see in the body of
the book that this view of logic, as not providing absolutely valid norms but as
giving norms valid relative to a particular domain, sheds new light on results
in the psychology of reasoning which have traditionally been taken to show the
incompatibility of logic and actual reasoning.[12]

---

12. The preceding paragraphs are not intended as an exegesis of Husserl's thought; our intention is only
to identify some strands in Husserl which we consider to be fruitful for thinking about logic. The contrast
drawn here between Frege and Husserl is a particular case of the more general distinction, first proposed by
Jean van Heijenoort [281], between "logic as a universal language" and "logic as a calculus." On the former
conception of logic, whose main champion is Frege, logic is concerned with a single universe of discourse,
and the semantic relation between logical language and that universe is ineffable. On the latter conception
(which ultimately gave rise to the modern "model–theoretic logics" [15]), there are many possible universes
of discourse, logical languages are reinterpretable to fit these universes, and semantics is a legitimate object
of scientific study. Van Heijenoort's contrast has been called "a fundamental opposition in twentieth century
philosophy" by Hintikka [125] and has been applied to Frege and Husserl in Kusch [165].

For the mathematically inclined reader we include an example of Husserl's views as applied to the domain of arithmetic. If this domain is given a classical, Platonistic interpretation, that is, as concerned with objects which exist independently of the human mind, then the following is *not* a logical law:

(1)   (†) if *A or B* is provable (in system *S*), then *A* is provable (in system *S*) or *B* is provable (in system *S*)

because on the one hand Gödel's incompleteness theorem has shown that there is a sentence *A* such that neither *A* nor $\neg A$ is provable in classical arithmetic, whereas on the other hand the "law of excluded middle" $A \vee \neg A$ is a logical law in classical arithmetic. If, however, the domain of arithmetic is conceptualized as being about particular mental constructions, as mathematicians of the intuitionistic persuasion claim, then it is a mathematical fact that (†) is a logical law (and that therefore the law of excluded middle is not). Normative issues arise, not at the level of logical laws (e.g., the law of excluded middle), but at the level of what description to choose for the domain of interest. Changing one's logical laws then becomes tantamount to changing the description of the domain.

Husserl's view has the value of focusing attention on the relation between mathematics and empirical phenomena in general, as one source of difficulty in understanding the relation between logic and human reasoning. The relation between mathematics and empirical phenomena is problematical in any domain, but it may be more problematical in this domain than most. Appreciating the continuity of these problems, and identifying their source is one way forward. Seeing logic as the mathematics of information systems, of which people are one kind, is quite a good first approximation to the view we develop here. This view helps in that it makes clear from the start that one's choice is never between "doing psychology" and "doing logic." Understanding reasoning is always going to require doing both, simply because science does not proceed far without mathematical, or at least conceptual apparatus.

So we see history turning circle, though not full circle. Like Mill and Husserl, we see logic and psychology as very closely linked. Frege rejected this view. Husserl developed a much more sophisticated view of the relation, which foreshadows our own in its emphasis on semantics. Later, Frege's view of logic foundered on Russell's paradoxes which showed that logic couldn't be universal and homogeneous. In response logic developed the possibility of explicitly studying semantics, and still later, developed a multiplicity of logics. Much of the technical development necessary for studying semantics took place in the context of the foundations of mathematics which took logic very far from psychology. In mid-twentieth century, Montague reapplied the much transformed technical apparatus of logical semantics to the descriptive analysis of natural languages. We now apply the availability of a multiplicity of logics back onto the subject matter of discourse and psychology. Of course psychology too has changed out of all recognition since Mill – the whole apparatus of psychological experiment postdates Mill's view. So our "psychologism" is very different from Mill's, but the closeness of psychology and logic is something shared. Our psychologism clearly requires an account of how logic in its modern guise as mathematical system is related to psychology in its modern guise as experimental science.

1.4 What the Reader May Expect

The remainder of the book is structured as follows. Chapter 2 is a somewhat unorthodox introduction to logic, which tries to break the hold of classical logic by showing it results from contingent assumptions on syntax and semantics. Systematic variation of these assumptions gives rise to several logics that have applications in actual human reasoning. This chapter in particular introduces closed–world reasoning, a form of reasoning that will be very important in part II of the book. In chapters 3 and 4 we study the Wason selection task from the vantage point developed in this introduction and in chapter 2: as a task in which subjects are mostly struggling to impose an interpretation on the experimental materials instead of engaging with the materials as the experimenter intends them to do. Chapter 3 contains many examples of tutorial dialogues with subjects which show what interpretational difficulties they experience, and chapter 4 reports on experiments establishing that alleviating these difficulties by modifying the task instructions leads to a vast increase in correct performance, when measured against the classical competence model.

The selection task has played a major role in debates on evolutionary psychology, with Cosmides [47] claiming that her results on facilitation of the task with social contract materials show that the only abilities humans have in logical reasoning are due to an innate module for "cheater detection." We believe that this highly influential point of view is mistaken, for two reasons: a faulty view of logic, and a faulty view of evolution. chapter 5 considers the influence this faulty logical paradigm has had on the psychology of reasoning, and chapter 6 is a lengthy discussion of the evolution of human cognition. The latter chapter introduces a hypothesis that will play an important role in part II: that the origin of the human ability for logical reasoning must be sought in the planning capacity, and that closed–world reasoning (which governs planning) is therefore a very fundamental form of reasoning, stretching across many domains.

Chapter 7 applies this idea to the analysis of the suppression task (Byrne [28]), which is standardly interpreted as providing evidence for "mental models" and against "mental rules." We show that the data from this task can be explained on the assumption that subjects assimilate the task to a discourse–processing task, using closed–world reasoning, by presenting a rigorously formal model of subjects' reasoning in a logical system called "logic programming," which we consider to be the most appealing form of closed–world reasoning. We also present data from tutorial dialogues corroborating our interpretation of what subjects are doing. In chapter 8, it is shown that closed–world reasoning has a revealing neural implementation and that there need not be an opposition between logical and connectionist modeling. Chapter 9 applies the ideas of chapters 7 and 8 to autism. We analyse several tasks on which autistic people are known to fail, such as the false belief task and the box task, and find that these tasks have a common logical structure which is identical to that of the suppression task discussed in chapter 7. This leads to a prediction for autistic people's behavior on the suppression task, which has been verified. This latter result is analysed in terms of the neural implementation developed in chapter 8, which then allows us to make a connection to the genetics of autism. Chapter 10 discusses syllogisms. These are, of course, the first reasoning patterns studied in psychology, but for us their interest lies in the necessity to apply substantial interpretational theories from linguistics and philosophy to explain the data. This explains why syllogisms only occur near the end of the book: the reader must first be familiar with both interpretation processes of reasoning to an interpretation and derivational processes of reasoning from the interpretation imposed.

Lastly, chapter 11 makes explicit our view of logic and its relevance to actual reasoning. The role of logic is to aid in "going beyond the information given" when processing information. Just as in visual information processing, mathematical structure (edges etc.) must be *imposed* upon the retinal array, because this structure is not literally present in the data, so some logical form must first be imposed on a problem requiring reasoning before the actual reasoning can take place.

In the end, we aim to convince the reader that using the formal machinery of modern logic leads to a much more insightful explanation of existing data, and a much more promising research agenda for generating further data. If we succeed, then there are general morals to be drawn about what philosophy of science is appropriate for the psychology of "higher" cognitive functions.

At present, experimental psychology is much influenced by a Popperian philosophy which sees hypothesis testing as the central activity in science. We will see that Wason himself was much influenced by this account of science in explaining his subjects' responses. But Popper's account, important as it is, in the intervening years has been shown to be a very partial account. If science is hypothesis testing, where do hypotheses come from? Why test this one rather than that? A great deal of science is exploration and observation which don't fall easily under the umbrella of hypothesis testing. Highly developed sciences such as physics, which are overwhelmingly the cases studied by philosophers of science, have powerful abstract bodies of theory which guide exploration and observation, and through them the selection of hypotheses, when the time comes to test hypotheses. Psychology lacks such bodies of abstract theory, and so one sees implicit theories playing important roles in choosing what hypotheses to test. "Surprisingness" of a phenomenon as compared to some implicit theory of that phenomenon is a crucial quality indicating when hypothesis testing is worth the effort. If Wason's observations of failures of rationality in the selection task hadn't been so counterintuitive, then we (and you) would never have heard of them. We will expend considerable effort in chapter 3 in making explicit Wason's (implicit) background theory against which the results are so surprising, and in showing how logic can provide explicit background abstractions which change the way hypotheses can be chosen and experiments designed.

A corollary of the lack of background abstract theories in psychology is the use of direct operationalization of abstract concepts in experimental procedures: data categories are assumed to be very closely related to their theoretical categories. As a consequence, the data observed are supposed to have a direct bearing on the theoretical hypotheses. In mature sciences this doesn't happen. There are always 'bridging' inferences required between observation and theory, and an apparent falsification may direct attention to unwarranted auxiliary assumptions. Especially in chapter 10, though also throughout, we will illustrate how logic can open up space for observation and exploration between data and theory. Young sciences like psychology require lots of observation and exploration, so a methodology which opens up space for these activities is vital.

In the study of human cognition, this space between data and theory or hypothesis is particularly broad because of our human capacity for multiple interpretation. Indeed, some resistance to taking interpretation seriously in studying reasoning comes from the belief that this space is too broad to be bridged. Once we acknowledge the possibility of full human interpretive capacities, then, so the argument goes, the possibility of science goes out the window. In particular it is often felt that the scientific study of reasoning is impossible once it is allowed that the logical expressions are subject to the possibility of multiple interpretations. Rejecting the possibility of multiple interpretation because it is held to make science impossible is truly the logic of the drunk searching beneath the lamppost who prefers the illuminated circle to the dark space where he knows he lost his keys. We take the general human capacity for multiple interpretation to be as close to fact as it is possible to get in cognitive science, and prefer to follow it where it leads in choosing our methods of investigation. In fact, one sees this battle fought repeatedly in each area of human cognition. It remains under control to some extent in perception, because there the experimenter has "stimulus control" – she can twiddle the display, and observe what the subject reports seeing.[13] But in, for example, memory, the problem has been

---

13. In fact this is something of an illusion, because the subject brings preexisting knowledge to bear in

recognized ever since Ebbinghaus [68] invented nonsense syllables in order to eliminate the interpretive effects of subjects' long-term knowledge which is beyond experimental control. In memory, the problem leads to a split between the Ebbinghaus tradition of laboratory experimentation on abstracted materials, and the Bartlettian tradition of studying, for example, autobiographical memory [12]. Both have contributions to make, but both require an understanding of their distinctive approaches to assimilate those contributions.

The problem of treating "content" or "general knowledge" or "experience prior to the experiment" is endemic in psychology, and the life of the psychological researcher is much taken up with getting around the barriers it throws up. The psychology of reasoning's adoption of "abstract tasks" can be seen as following in the Ebbinghausian tradition, and reaction against those tasks as Bartlettian rejection of that tradition. Logic itself is interpreted by psychologists as the most extreme form of the Ebbinghausian approach in which content is banished entirely. However, our argument is that this is no longer true in modern logic. The default logics we present here are actually interpretable as modeling the relation between a working memory holding the experimental input materials and a long-term memory holding "general knowledge." So these logics present a formalization of "content." They thus attack psychology's central problem head-on. Of course, they do not offer a model of the long-term memory of some actual adult human being (nor even an idealized adult human being at standard temperature and pressure). But they do offer precise formal models of how large databases of default conditionals can control the interpretation of richly meaningful input texts. Essentially similar computer architectures are the basis for implementing real-world useful databases of general knowledge in practical applications. Of course the philosophical problems of "symbol grounding" remain. But nevertheless, here is the first plausible head-on approach to the formal modeling of content which offers to reconcile Ebbinghaus with Bartlett.

It should be evident that these issues are close to the heart of problems about the relations between the humanities and the sciences, and it is entirely fitting that they should come up when trying to do scientific research into the nature of the human mind. It is interesting that representatives of more conservative approaches to both sciences and the humanities have felt it important to try to defeat the very possibility of cognitive science's computational model of the mind. We hope to explain just why that model is felt to be so threatening, to defuse some of the concerns arising, and to show that one can avoid both misplaced scientific reductionism and postmodern hyperrelativism by engaging in a logically based and experimentally informed study of human interpretive capacities.

---

making perceptual interpretations, but it is an illusion persistent enough to allow progress.

2 The Anatomy of Logic

We have seen that logic was once thought relevant to the study of cognition both as a representational format and as an inference mechanism, and that developments in psychology (Wason, increasing prominence of neural network modeling, decision theory) and in philosophy (concerns with normativity, antipsychologism) have led to the widely shared view that logic is irrelevant to cognition. We have sketched a new view of logical reasoning, following Husserl, in which reasoning is simultaneously formal and relative to a domain. On this view, cognitive science needs to be much more attentive to *semantics* – because meaning is often not given but constructed. Indeed, we will see that subjects' behavior in reasoning tasks (e.g., Wason's selection task) is much less irrational than is commonly thought, once one takes into account that these subjects are struggling to impose a meaning on the task. It is by no means obvious to the subject that her reasoning must be based on the classical interpretation of the conditional as material implication. In fact, the interest of the standard reasoning tasks lies precisely in the window it offers on subjects' efforts to impose meaning. As a first step toward weaning the reader away from the idea that the semantics of logical expressions is given by classical logic, this chapter presents the reader with an overview of the semantic possibilities.

This chapter is organized as follows. We start from a popular conception of logical reasoning according to which, to see whether an argument is valid, one translates it into the formal language of classical logic and checks the resulting pattern for classical validity. We argue that this conception is inadequate, and oppose it to a formal version of Husserl's view, in which one distinguishes reasoning *from* an interpretation and reasoning *to* an interpretation.[1] We conceive of the latter as a form of parameter setting. To illustrate the idea, we start from the four parameter choices defining classical logic, which is appropriate for the

---

1. We will use the verb "to interpret" in this book in its *Oxford English Dictionary* sense of "to make out the meaning of," and the noun "interpretation" as the result of that activity, or occasionally as the process itself. This is not saying much if we do not explain what "to make out" and "meaning" mean. In fact, most of this book is concerned with explaining what is involved in "making out the meaning of," and no simple explanation can be given at this stage.

domain of classical mathematics, and by systematic variation of the parameters obtain logics which are appropriate for other domains.

2.1   How Not to Think about Logical Reasoning

In the psychology of reasoning literature one commonly finds a picture of reasoning as proceeding according to preestablished logical laws, which can be applied by anybody in any circumstances whatsoever.

It would not do to blame the psychologists for this, because it is a picture frequently promulgated in the philosophical literature. To take just one example, we see Ryle [239] characterizing logical constants (for example, *all, some, not, and, or, if*) as being indifferent to subjectmatter, or as it is sometimes callled, *topic neutral*. Characterizations such as this are related to a superficial reading of the classical definition of validity, say for a syllogism such as

> All A are B.
> All B are C.
> Therefore, all A are C.

The validity of this schema is taken to mean something like "whatever you substitute for A, B and C, if the premises are true for the substitution, then so is the conclusion." Analyzing an argument thus consists of finding the topic-neutral expressions (the logical constants), replacing the topic-dependent expressions by variables, and checking whether a substitution that verifies the premises also verifies the conclusion. If so, one knows that the argument is correct for the particular substitution one is interested in.

This *schematic* character of inference patterns is identified with the "domain-independence" or "topic neutrality" of logic generally, and many take it to be the principal interest of logic that its laws seem independent of subject matter. In fact, however, logic is very much domaindependent in the sense that the valid schemata depend on the domain in which one reasons, *with what purpose*. We therefore view reasoning as consisting of two stages: first one has to establish the domain about which one reasons and its formal properties (what we will call "reasoning *to* an interpretation") and only after this initial step has been taken can one's reasoning be guided by formal laws (what we will call "reasoning *from* an interpretation").

2.2   Reasoning to an Interpretation as Parameter Setting

We should start with an informal illustration of what the process of interpretation involves, which falls into at least two questions – what things are actually in the domain? and also: what kinds of reasoning will be done about them? We start with the former question, which has been extensively studied in the formal semantics of natural languages. We illustrate the general distinction between the two questions with some homely examples of discourse understanding, which will then introduce a particular distinction that will figure centrally in the rest of the book.

> Once upon a time there was a butcher, a baker, and a candlestick maker. One fine morning, a body was discovered on the village green, a dagger protruding from its chest. The murderer's footprints were clearly registered in the mud. ...

Well, what follows from this discourse? For example, how many people are there? If we take the most likely approach to interpreting this discourse outside of logic class, we will assume that there are at least three people – a butcher, a baker, and a candlestick maker. There are, of course also the corpse and the murderer, but it is an active question whether these are identical with any of the former three, and who else may there be in this dire place? These questions are questions about what things, or people, or other entities are in the domain of interpretation. Mundane as these questions are, they are absolutely central to how natural language functions in progressively constructing interpretations as discourse proceeds.

It should be made clear from the outset that discourse interpretation is not at all exhausted by composing the meanings of the lexical items (as given by the dictionary) in the way dictated by the syntax of the sentences. Contextual information plays a crucial role. For instance, the question, what are the characters in this discourse? is a question about what is in the current domain of interpretation, and the answer to this question may well depend on discourse context, as we shall see. Clearly our knowledge of the dictionary plays a role in our answer to this question, but does not by itself provide the answer. Domains of natural language interpretation are often very local, as they are here. They often change sentence by sentence as the discourse proceeds. It is this sense of interpretation, rather than the dictionary-level sense, which generally occupies us here.

Suppose now we have instead a discourse that runs as follows:

> Some woman is a baker. Some woman is a butcher. Some woman is a candlestickmaker. Some person is a murderer. Some person is a corpse. All women are men.[2, 3, 4]

Now we are much more likely to entertain considerably more possibilities about how many people there are, cued perhaps by the "logical puzzle" style of the discourse. Now it becomes entirely possible that the butcher may turn out to be the baker, or one person might pursue all three professions, even before we

---

2. NB. The *Oxford English Dictionary* defines, under its first sense for *man*, "a human being irrespective of gender."

3. "Oh *man!*, these guys' language is archaic!" addressed to a female human is an example of the *Oxford English Dictionary*'s archaic usage hidden in modern oral vernacular English.

4. The previous two footnotes are irrelevant if this discourse is processed from a skeptical stance.

start on the problem about who is dead and who has been nasty, and just who else is in this village, if there is one.

The first discourse is likely to be understood with what we will call a *credulous* stance. As we interpret the discourse, we take our task to be to construct a model of the story which is the same as the speaker's "intended model," and we assume that we are to use whatever general and specific knowledge we have, including the assumption that the speaker is being cooperative in constructing her discourse, to help us guess which model this is. The second discourse is likely to be understood with what we will call a *skeptical* stance in which we do not use any information save the explicitly stated premises, and we are to entertain all possible arrangements of the entities that make these statements true. This stance explains already why the footnotes are completely irrelevant to this interpretation and merely designed to lead us astray.

First note that these different stances lead to quite different numbers of people in the domains of interpretations of the two texts. In the first discourse we know[5] that there is no policeman although we also know, from general knowledge, that this is likely to change rather soon. In the second we do not know whether there is a policeman, but unless we are explicitly told that there isn't (or told something which explicitly rules it out) then we still do not know, even though no policeman is ever mentioned. These "number-of-things" questions are only the most tangible tip of the iceberg of differences between the domains we get when we process with these two different stances, but they suffice for our present illustrative purposes.

Credulous and skeptical stances are good examples of the second kind of issue about interpretations – what kinds of reasoning will we do about the things in the domain? Credulous reasoning is aimed at finding ideally a single interpretation which makes the speaker's utterances true, generally at the expense of importing all sorts of stuff from our assumed mutual general knowledge. Skeptical reasoning is aimed at finding only conclusions which are true in *all* interpretations of the explicit premises. These are very different goals and require very different logics, with, for example, different syntactic structures and different concepts of validity. The differences in goals are socially important differences. In credulous understanding we accept (at least for the purposes of the discourse) the authority of the speaker for the truth of what is said. We are only at an impasse when there appears to be a contradiction which leaves us with no model of the discourse, and when this happens we try to repair our interpretation in order to restore a model. In skeptical understanding, we consider ourselves as on allfours with the speaker as regards authority for inferences, and we may well challenge what is said on the basis that a conclusion doesn't follow because we can find a single interpretation of the premises in which that conclusion is false.

---

5. By what is known as "closed–world reasoning," for which see section 2.3.

A good illustration of the distinction between credulous and skeptical reasoning is furnished by legal reasoning in the courtroom, of which the following is a concrete example (simplified from a case which recently gained notoriety in the Netherlands). A nurse is indicted for murdering several terminally ill patients, who all died during her shifts. No forensic evidence of foul play is found, but the public prosecutor argues that the nurse must have caused the deaths, because she was the only one present at the time of death. This is an example of "plausible" or "credulous" reasoning: an inference is drawn on the basis of data gathered and plausible causal relationships.[6]

The defense countered the prosecutor's argument with an instance of 'skeptical' reasoning, by arguing that the cause of death might as well have been malfunctioning of the morphine pumps, and contacted the manufacturer to see whether morphine pumps had had to be recalled because of malfunctioning – which indeed turned out be the case (although in the end it did not help the defendant). The move of the defence can be viewed as enlarging the class of models considered, thus getting closer to the standard notion of logical consequence where one considers all models of the premises instead of a restricted class. Here is Ryle [239,p.116] again, this time with a very pertinent remark:

> There arises, I suppose, a special pressure upon language to provide idioms of the [logical] kind, when a society reaches the stage where many matters of interest and importance to everyone have to be settled or decided by special kinds of talk. I mean, for example, when offenders have to be tried and convicted or acquitted; when treaties and contracts have to be entered into and observed or enforced; when witnesses have to be cross-examined; when legislators have to draft practicable measures and defend them against critics; when private rights and public duties have to be precisely fixed; when complicated commercial arrangements have to be made; when teachers have to set tests to their pupils; and ... when theorists have to consider in detail the strengths and weaknesses of their own and one another's theories.

We have chosen to illustrate the kinds of issues that go into deciding what domain is adopted in an interpretation with this particular distinction because it is the one that is at the center of many of the misunderstandings between experimenter and subject in the psychology of reasoning experiments. The *what things are in the domain?* question is always present in any process of interpretation. The *what kind of reasoning are we doing?* question is rather different for different distinctions.

So far we have been talking about domain in a rather loose manner, as roughly synonymous with universe of discourse. For logical purposes it is important to make a type-token distinction here. The domain mentally constructed while interpreting a discourse is a concrete instance – a token – of a general kind –

---

6. A note for the logically minded reader: this can be viewed as an inference where the premises are interpreted on a very restricted class of models, namely models in which no "mysterious" events happen, neither divine intervention nor unknown intruders.

the type – which determines the logical properties of the token. It is very hard to completely pin down this general notion of a type of domain itself; we will try to do so in a later chapter on evolutionary approaches to reasoning, where the notion of "domain specificity" of reasoning plays an important role. But we can at least list some examples that will be treated in this book: actions, plans and causality; contracts; norms; other people's beliefs; mathematical objects; natural laws. Slightly more formally, a domain is characterized by a set of mathematical representations, called *structures*, of the main ingredients of the domain (e.g., the objects in the domain, their relations, the events in which they participate), together with a formal language to talk and reason about these structures. The connection between structures and formal language is given by what is technically known as a definition of satisfaction: a characterization of how the formal language is interpreted on the relevant set of structures. This notion of domain is extremely general, and instead of being more precise at this point, we refer the reader to the different examples that will be given below.

The reader may wonder why language and logic should be relative to a domain: isn't there a single language – one's mother tongue – which we use to talk and reason about everything? Much of the progress in mathematical logic in the last century shows, however, that it is not useful to have a single language (with a single semantics) for talking about everything. For instance, the vague predicates that we will meet when discussing diagnostic reasoning in medicine can perhaps be represented by fuzzy logic with its continuum of truth–values (see section 2.2.3), but it would make no sense to use this semantics for classical mathematics. For another example, consider two radically different ways of doing mathematics: classical and constructive mathematics. Very roughly speaking, the difference is that the former tradition, unlike the latter, accepts the principle of bivalence: a sentence is either true or false (see section 2.2.3 for an explanation of why this principle is sometimes unwarranted). Constructive mathematics is often useful in computer science, because the results it yields have algorithmic significance, while this is not guaranteed of results in classical mathematics. It occasionally happens that the same mathematician may apply both methods, depending on the domain she is working in. So does she believe in bivalence, or doesn't she? The answer is that sometimes she does, and sometimes she doesn't, whatever is most appropriate to the domain of interest. In this sense logics are local. One might want to argue that in such cases one should adopt the weakest logic (in this case the one without bivalence) as one's generally valid logic; after all, how can a principle such as bivalence be called logical at all if it is considered to be false in some domains? One quick answer to this argument is that this "weakest logic" soon trivializes when including more domains, for example when considering also uncertain information instead of just truth and proof. One may conclude from this that logic as a system of generally valid inference principles has no role to play in actual reasoning. Another option, and the one advocated here, is to give up the idea that logic must be such a system. Clearly, however, if logic is not given, the question becomes how one comes to reason in a particular logic. The answer argued for in the book, and made explicit in chapter 11, is that mastering a particular domain essentially involves mastering its logical laws. These brief indications must suffice at this stage, and we will return to the wider issues in the concluding chapter.

We are now ready to delve into the technicalities. The approach to logic which we would like to advocate views logics from the point of view of possible syntactic and semantic choices, or what we will call parameter settings. This metaphor should not be taken too literally: we do not claim that a logic can be seen as a point in a well-behaved many-dimensional space. The use of the term parameter here is analogous to that in generative linguistics, where universal grammar is thought to give rise to concrete grammars by fixing parameters such as word order.[7] The set of parameters characterizing a logic can be divided in three subsets

1. Choice of a formal language

2. Choice of a semantics for the formal language

3. Choice of a definition of valid arguments in the language

As we shall see, different choices for the parameters may be appropriate in different domains – each domain gives rise to a notion of structure, and in principle each domain comes with its own language.[8]

To familiarize the reader with this idea, we first present classical propositional logic as resulting from four contingent assumptions, which are sometimes appropriate, sometimes not. We will then vary these assumptions to obtain a host of different logics, all useful in some context.

2.2.1 Classical Propositional Logic

The purpose of this section is to show that classical logic is inevitable once one adopts a number of parameter settings concerning syntax, meaning and truth, and logical consequence; and furthermore that these settings are open to debate. The relevant parameter settings are:

1. [*syntax*] fully recursive language: if φ, ψ are formulas, then so are $\neg\varphi$, $\varphi \to \psi$, $\varphi \vee \psi$, $\varphi \wedge \psi$, ...[9];

---

7. This is just an analogy; we are not committed to anything like UG.
8. This approach to logic was pursued in the 1980s under the heading of "model theoretic logics"; see [14].
9. This definition generates formulas like $(\varphi \to \theta) \to \psi$. The iteration of a conditional inside the antecedent of another conditional illustrated by this last formula will turn out to be a distinctive property of this language, which sets it off from the language we use to model credulous interpretation.

2. [*semantics*] truth–functionality: the truth–value of a sentence is a function of the truth–values of its components only;

(2′. as a consequence: evaluation of the truth–value can be determined in the given model (the semantics is *extensional*));

3. [*semantics*] bivalence: sentences are either true or false, with nothing in between;

4. [*consequence*] the Bolzano–Tarski notion of logical consequence[10]:

$$\alpha_1 \ldots \alpha_n / \beta \text{ is valid iff } \beta \text{ is true on all models of } \alpha_1 \ldots \alpha_n.$$

These assumptions force a unique formalization of the logical connectives *not, and, or, if … then*, as given by the familiar truth–tables in figure 2.1.

p	$\neg p$
1	0
0	1

p	q	$p \wedge q$
1	1	1
0	0	0
1	0	0
0	1	0

p	q	$p \vee q$
1	1	1
0	0	0
1	0	1
0	1	1

p	q	$p \rightarrow q$
1	1	1
0	0	1
1	0	0
0	1	1

Figure 2.1   Truth–tables for classical logic.

It is instructive to see how our four assumptions (in conjunction with intuitive judgments about meaning) lead to the formalization of the conditional "if … then" as the "material implication" $\rightarrow$ defined by the above truth–table.

Truth–functionality requires that if the truth–values of p, q are given, so is that of $p \rightarrow q$, and bivalence forces these to be either 0 or 1. We can see from this that if p is true and q is false, then $p \rightarrow q$ must be false; for if it were true then modus ponens ($p, p \rightarrow q \models q$) would fail. Furthermore an application of the definition of validity shows that the following argument patterns are valid : $p, q \models q$ and $p, \neg p \models q$. From this it follows from the intuitive meaning of the conditional that $q \models p \rightarrow q$ and $\neg p \models p \rightarrow q$. Indeed, one may argue for an implication $p \rightarrow q$ by assuming p and inferring from this (and given premises) that q. But this reduces $q \models p \rightarrow q$ to $p, q \models q$. The validity of $\neg p \models p \rightarrow q$ is established similarly.

The classical definition of validity is *monotonic*, that is, if $\alpha_1 \ldots \alpha_n \models \beta$, then also $\delta, \alpha_1 \ldots \alpha_n \models \beta$. It follows that the valid argument $q \models p \rightarrow q$ forces $p \rightarrow q$ to be true if p, q are true and if $\neg p, q$ are true; in addition, $\neg p \models p \rightarrow q$ forces $p \rightarrow q$ to be true if $\neg p, \neg q$ are true. We have now justified all the lines of the truth–table.

---

10. Whether this historical attribution is correct is debatable; see [71], also for elaborate discussion of the flaws of this particular definition of validity.

Domains to which classical logic is applicable must satisfy the four assumptions. Classical mathematics is a case in point. Here it is assumed that all statements are true or false – together with truth–functionality this gives the celebrated principle of excluded middle $p \lor \neg p$, which we will see in action later. The definition of logical consequence is a very important feature of modern mathematics: it implies that a counterexample to a theorem makes it false. Trivial as this may seem nowadays, this has not always been the case; in the eighteenth and nineteenth centuries it was not uncommon to conclude that a purported counterexample did not belong to the "domain" of the theorem, thus effectively restricting the class of models. One may consult the work of Lakatos, in particular [167], for instructive examples.[11]

Are these four assumptions in general always fulfilled? The next sections provide example domains in which various combinations of the assumptions obviously fail, and we will indicate what logics are appropriate to these domains instead.

2.2.2 Truth–Functionality without Bivalence

Why would every statement be either true or false? This depends of course very much on what you want to mean by "true" and "false." One could stipulate that "not true" is the same as false, but such a stipulation is definitely inappropriate if we consider "true" to mean "known to be true." One example of where this occurs in practice is a computerized primality test which checks whether the input $2^{1257787} - 1$ is a prime number. One could say that, while the program is running, the statement "$2^{1257787} - 1$ is a prime number" is undecided; but a decision may follow in the end, if the program halts.[12]

One possibility to formalise this idea, originated by [160] is to add a third truth–value u for "undecided" or "not known to be true and not known to be false"; u can (but need not) "evolve" toward "known to be true" or "known to be false" when more information comes in. This uniquely determines the truth–tables as given in figure 2.2.

The other three assumptions characterizing classical logic are still in force here. The resulting logic is appropriate to the domain of computable functions, and also to paradoxical sentences such as "I am false," and more generally to languages which contain their own truth predicate (such as natural language).

---

11. A note for the logically minded reader. In principle the language of classical mathematics is fully recursive. In practice, restrictions apply, so that particular structures, for example the reals, are described in a restricted language. One of the triumphs of mathematical logic is the use of these restrictions in language to prove positive results about the structures that the language describes.

12. It does, and the number is prime.

p	¬p
1	0
0	1
u	u

p	q	$p \wedge q$	p	q	$p \vee q$	p	q	$p \to q$
1	1	1	1	1	1	1	1	1
0	0	0	0	0	0	0	0	1
u	u	u	u	u	u	u	u	u
1	0	0	1	0	1	1	0	0
1	u	u	1	u	1	1	u	u
0	1	0	0	1	1	0	1	1
0	u	0	0	u	u	0	u	1
u	1	u	u	1	1	u	1	1
u	0	0	u	0	u	u	0	u

Figure 2.2   Truth–tables for Kleene three-valued logic.

2.2.3   A Domain in which Bivalence is Truly Ridiculous

Here is an excerpt from a textbook on cancer, in a section on differential diagnosis. The reader should realise that this is the kind of text that guides a physician in her decision making. We have distinguished typographically two classes of expressions: in **boldface** vague expressions like "small," "painful," "entire," "changes," "diffuse without sharp demarcation," "feels like a tumour," ...; and in *italic* qualitative-probabilistic adverbs like "usually," "often," "approximately 15% of the cases," "if *A* maybe *B*," "infrequently – more often."

> **Chronic** cystic disease is *often* confused with carcinoma of the breast. It *usually* occurs in parous women with **small** breasts. It is present *most commonly* in the **upper outer quadrant** but *may* occur in other parts and eventually involve the **entire** breast. It is *often* **painful**, particularly in the pre-menstrual period, and accompanying **menstrual disturbances** are *common*. Nipple discharge, *usually* **servous**, occurs in *approximately 15% of the cases*, but there are no **changes** in the nipple itself. The lesion is **diffuse without sharp demarcation** and without fixation to the overlying skin. Multiple cysts are **firm, round and fluctuant** and *may* transilluminate *if* they contain a **clear** fluid. A **large** cyst in an area of chronic cystic disease **feels like a tumour**, but is *usually* **smoother and well-delimited**. The axillary lymph nodes are *usually* not **enlarged**. **Chronic** cystic disease *infrequently* shows **large bluish** cysts. *More often*, the cysts are multiple and **small**. (J.A. del Regato. Diagnosis, treatment and prognosis. Pages 860–861. In L.V. Ackerman (editor) *Cancer* 1970.

To find logical regularities in this domain is challenging, to put it mildly. Vague predicates have sometimes been formalized using many-valued logics, and there have been attempts to model frequency adverbs using probability theory. The reader is urged to compare the preceding piece of text with the formal systems that follow, to see whether they add to her understanding.

It is also important to be aware that in real life vagueness may be treated by being avoided. Consider the locus classicus for the rejection of logic in cognitive science: Rosch and Mervis's arguments for its inapplicability to human classificatory behavior in [233]. Classical logic represents the extension of a predicate by a set, to which things either belong or they don't. No half measures. But people classify things by shades. They represent typical members of extensions. Red is typified by the color of blood and the color of red hair is a peripheral red. There is cognitive structure here which there is not in a set. And so, argue Rosch and Mervis, logic is inapplicable.

This is a good example of a levels confusion. Rosch and Mervis are concerned with the dictionary meanings of vague words such as *red*. Logic is concerned with meaning as it occurs at the discourse level and has very little to say about the dictionary level; but the point is that it need not. Suppose we start a conversation which includes the word *red*. It is unlikely that the vagueness of this term will become critical to our mutual interpretation – we may be happy that we know how to classify all the relevant objects (perhaps three traffic lights) with regard to this term perfectly crisply. If it does become a problem then we may resort to increased precision – "by red I mean crimson lake as manufactured by Pigment Corp." – which may or may not replace the word red entirely. Practically all natural language words are vague, and they would be useless if they weren't, but if we design our discourse well, their vagueness will be well tailored to the local communicative situation.

Another way to make the same point is with reference to Marr's methodology as outlined in [183,p. 357ff], in particular chapter 7, where he conducts a dialogue with himself and asks

> *What do you feel are the most promising approaches to semantics?*

The answer is

> Probably what I call the problem of multiple descriptions of objects and the resolution of the problems of reference that multiple descriptions introduce. . . . I expect that at the heart of our understanding of intelligence will lie at least one and probably several important principles about organizing and representing knowledge that in some sense capture what is important about our intellectual capabilities, [namely:]
>
> 1. The perception of an event or object must include the simultaneous computation of several different descriptions of it, that capture diverse aspects of the use, purpose, or circumstances of the event or object.
>
> 2. That the various descriptions referred to in 1. include coarse versions as well as fine ones. These coarse descriptions are a vital link in choosing the appropriate overall scenarios . . . and in establishing correctly the roles played by the objects and actions that caused those scenarios to be chosen.

A coarse description of a vague predicate, using classical logic, may well be able to model the avoidance of the vagueness which is endemic in discourse.

Alternatively, we may move to a finer description, meet vagueness head-on, and change our logic. We give two examples.

Dealing with Vagueness: Łukasiewicz Logic

This logic also differs from classical logic in that it has a third truth–value ($\frac{1}{2}$), but this value now means "intermediate between true and false," and not "undecided, but possibly decided at some later time." The reader may verify that the truth–tables in figure 2.3 have been calculated according to the following formulas: $\neg p$ corresponds to $1 - p$, $p \wedge q$ to $\min(p, q)$, $p \vee q$ to $\max(p, q)$, and $p \to q$ to $\min(1, 1 + q - p)$. Once one has seen that the tables are calculated

p	$\neg p$
1	0
0	1
$\frac{1}{2}$	$\frac{1}{2}$

p	q	$p \wedge q$	p	q	$p \vee q$	p	q	$p \to q$
1	1	1	1	1	1	1	1	1
0	0	0	0	0	0	0	0	1
$\frac{1}{2}$	$\frac{1}{2}$	$\frac{1}{2}$	$\frac{1}{2}$	$\frac{1}{2}$	$\frac{1}{2}$	$\frac{1}{2}$	$\frac{1}{2}$	1
1	0	0	1	0	1	1	0	0
1	$\frac{1}{2}$	$\frac{1}{2}$	1	$\frac{1}{2}$	1	1	$\frac{1}{2}$	$\frac{1}{2}$
0	1	0	0	1	1	0	1	1
0	$\frac{1}{2}$	0	0	$\frac{1}{2}$	$\frac{1}{2}$	0	$\frac{1}{2}$	1
$\frac{1}{2}$	1	$\frac{1}{2}$	$\frac{1}{2}$	1	1	$\frac{1}{2}$	1	1
$\frac{1}{2}$	0	0	$\frac{1}{2}$	0	$\frac{1}{2}$	$\frac{1}{2}$	0	$\frac{1}{2}$

Figure 2.3   Łukasciewicz logic

using the above formulas, there is no reason to stop at three truth–values; one might as well take a continuum of truth–values in $[0, 1]$. This system is called *fuzzy logic*. The important point to remember is that fuzzy logic is still truth–functional; in this respect it differs from our next example, probability theory, which is not.

Probability: a Many-Valued, Non-truth–Functional Semantics

One could try to represent frequency adverbs like "usually," "often" by means of probabilities. For instance, if p is the proposition that "The axillary lymph nodes are not enlarged," then 'usually(p)' could mean "the probability of p is greater than 60%," where probability is here taken in the sense of relative frequency. This idea leads to the following definition.[13]

A *probability* on a propositional language $\mathcal{L}$ is a function $P : \mathcal{L} \longrightarrow [0, 1]$ satisfying

1. $P(\varphi) = 0$ if φ is a contradiction;

2. if φ and ψ are logically equivalent, $P(\varphi) = P(\psi)$;

3. if φ logically implies $\neg\psi$, then $P(\varphi \vee \psi) = P(\varphi) + P(\psi)$.

---

13. Note that probability is used as a semantics only. One could also try to develop "probability logics" where "the probability of p is c" is a statement of the object language.[113]

The implicit assumption underlying this definition is that the formulas in $\mathcal{L}$ satisfy the classical logical laws, so that "equivalence," "contradiction" etc. are uniquely defined. It is in fact not so easy to define probability on nonclassical logics. This will be one of criticisms when discussing recent attempts to explain logical reasoning by assuming underlying probabilistic reasoning processes: probabilistic reasoning is too much tied to classical logic to be able to encompass the wide variety of reasoning that actually occurs.

The reader may wish to show that this semantics is *not* truth–functional: the only restriction on the values of $P(\varphi \wedge \psi)$, $P(\varphi)$ and $P(\psi)$ is the a priori restriction $P(\varphi \wedge \psi) \le P(\varphi), P(\psi)$.

Non-Truth–Functional Semantics: Intuitionistic Logic

In classical mathematics one often finds proofs which appeal to the principle of excluded middle, the syntactic analogue of bivalence. Mathematicians in the constructivist or intuitionistic tradition have pointed out that the use of this principle leads to proofs which are completely uninformative. Here is a toy example of this phenomenon.

Definition 1 *A* rational *number is one which can be written as $\frac{p}{q}$ for natural numbers p, q; an* irrational *number is one which cannot be so written.*

Suppose you want to prove:

Theorem 1 *There are irrational numbers a, b such that a^b is rational.*

PROOF. It is known that $\sqrt{2}$ is irrational. Consider $\sqrt{2}^{\sqrt{2}}$.

- If $\sqrt{2}^{\sqrt{2}}$ is rational, put $a = b = \sqrt{2}$ and we are done.

- If $\sqrt{2}^{\sqrt{2}}$ is irrational, put $a = \sqrt{2}^{\sqrt{2}}$, $b = \sqrt{2}$, then $a^b = (\sqrt{2}^{\sqrt{2}})^{\sqrt{2}} = \sqrt{2}^2 = 2$.

Either way you have the requisite a and b. $\qquad\square$

But what have you proved? Do you now *know* how to construct irrational a, b are such that a^b is rational? Such uninformative proofs, which do not yield concrete constructions, are typical of the use of the principle of excluded middle, which some therefore reject. If one characterises *intuitionistic logic* syntactically as classical logic *minus* the schema $\varphi \vee \neg\varphi$ (for all φ), then one can indeed show that proofs of existential statements in intuitionistic logic invariably yield concrete witnesses.

The semantics of intuitionistic logic is very different from what we have seen so far, where propositions took numbers as truth–values. The failure of the principle of excluded middle does not mean truth–functionally adding a third truth–value, one reason being that $\varphi \wedge \neg\varphi$ is still a contradiction, and inspection of the truth–tables for Kleene logic or Łukasciewicz logic shows that this is not the case there.[14] Instead we have the non-truth–functional "provability interpretation of truth," of which the following are examples

1. e.g., $\varphi \wedge \psi$ means: "I have a proof of both φ and ψ."

2. $\varphi \vee \psi$ means: "I have a proof of φ or a proof of ψ."

3. $\varphi \rightarrow \psi$ means: "I have a construction which transforms any given proof of φ into a proof of ψ."

4. special case of the previous: $\neg\varphi$ means "any attempted proof of φ leads to a contradiction."

Clearly, $\varphi \vee \neg\varphi$ is not valid on this interpretation, because it would require us to come up with a proof that φ or a proof that φ leads to a contradiction; and often one has neither.

An Intensional Logic: Deontic Logic

Deontic logic is concerned with reasoning about *norms*, i.e., what one *ought* to do; e.g., "if a person is innocent, he ought not to be convicted." We shall see in our discussion of the Wason selection task, however, that its scope extends much wider. At the syntactic level, (propositional) deontic logic consists of classical propositional logic plus the operator O, governed by the clause that if φ is a formula, so is $O\varphi$. The intuitive meaning of $O\varphi$ is "it ought to be the case that φ." Note that O cannot be a truth function, such as $\neg$; the truth of Op depends on the meaning, not the truth–value, of p. That is, both the propositions "my bike is grey" and "I don't steal" are true, but the latter ought to be the case, unlike the first.

The *intensional* semantics for deontic logic computes 'compliance'–values of formulas in a given model by referring to other models. One assumes that every model w has a "normatively perfect counterpart v"; this is formally represented by a relation: $R(w, v)$. In such a "normatively perfect" world v only what is permissible is the case; e.g., in w an innocent person may be convicted, but in v with $R(w, v)$ this same innocent person will not be convicted. We may now put $w \models Op$ if and only if for all v satisfying $R(w, v)$: $v \models p$.

To see the difference with classical logic, compare the conditionals $p \rightarrow q$ and $p \rightarrow Oq$. If in a given world, p is true and q is false, then $p \rightarrow q$ is simply false, whereas $p \rightarrow Oq$ can be true, in which case the given world is not "normatively perfect."

---

14. Another reason is that one would also like to get rid of the principle of double negation elimination $\neg\neg\varphi \rightarrow \varphi$.

Our last example, closed–world reasoning, is one in which the consequence relation is the main focus. Since closed–world reasoning will occupy us much throughout, it warrants a new section.

2.3   The Many Faces of Closed–World Reasoning

As we have seen above, the classical definition of validity considers *all* models of the premises. This type of validity is useful in mathematics, where the discovery of a single counterexample to a theorem is taken to imply that its derivation is flawed. But there are many examples of reasoning in daily life where one considers only a subset of the set of all models of the premises. In this section we review some examples of closed–world reasoning and their formalization.

One example is furnished by train schedules. In principle a schedule lists only positive information, and the world would still be a model of the schedule if there were more trains running than listed on the schedule. But the proper interpretation of a schedule is as a closed world – trains not listed are inferred not to exist. This is like our example of the butcher, baker, and candlestickmaker on page 21. Note that there is a difference here with the superficially similar case of a telephone directory. If a telephone number is not listed, we do not therefore conclude that the person does not have a telephone – she might after all have an unlisted number. In fact a moment's reflection suggests that such examples can be found within the "train schedule" domain. From the point of view of a prospective passenger, the inference that there is no train between two adjacently listed trains may be valid, but for a train spotter interested in trains passing through on the track, trains "not in service" may well occur between listed services. Thus, world knowledge is necessary to decide which logic is applicable.

2.3.1   Closed–World Reasoning, More Formally

Consider the Dutch database for public transportation www.9292ov.nl, which you consult for planning a trip from Amsterdam to Muiden. The database contains *facts* about trains and buses leaving at specific times, and also *rules* of the form

1. if bus 136 leaves Naarden-Bussum at 10:06, it will arrive in Muiden at 10:30

2. if train from Amsterdam CS in direction Naarden-Bussum leaves at 9:39, it will reach Naarden-Bussum at 10:00.

Backward chaining of the rules then generates a *plan* for getting from Amsterdam to Muiden.

Now suppose that www.9292ov.nl says that there is no trip that starts in Amsterdam at 9:10 and brings you to Muiden at 9:45. Then we will act as if there *is* no such trip, but why? This is an example of *closed–world reasoning*, which is appropriate if one may assume that the database lists all available positive information.

Formally, closed–world reasoning (in the version we prefer) differs from classical logic in the syntactic, semantic, and consequence parameters.

Syntactically, the occurrence of $\rightarrow$ is restricted to formulas of the form $p_1 \wedge \ldots \wedge p_n \rightarrow q$. This amounts to changing the recursive definition of the propositional language; iteration of implication is not allowed, and neither are occurrences of negation in antecedent and consequent.

Semantically, $\wedge$, $\vee$ have their customary classical interpretation, but $\rightarrow$ has a special closed–world interpretation given by

1. if all of $p_1, \ldots, p_n$ are true, then so is q;

2. if one of $p_1, \ldots, p_n$ is false and there is no other implication with q as a consequent, q is false;

3. more generally: if for $i \leq k$, $p_1^i \wedge \ldots \wedge p_{n_i}^i \rightarrow q$ are all the formulas with q in the consequent, and if for each $i \leq k$ one of $p_1^i, \ldots, p_n^i$ is false, then q is also false.

The most important technical feature of closed–world reasoning is that the associated consequence relation is *nonmonotonic*. We have encountered the monotonicity property of classical logical consequence when discussing the material implication; we repeat it here for convenience. As we have seen, the Bolzano–Tarski definition of validity of an argument $\varphi_1, \ldots, \varphi_n / \psi$ is: for all models $\mathcal{M}$ such that $\mathcal{M} \models \varphi_1, \ldots, \varphi_n$, also $\mathcal{M} \models \psi$. Given this definition, $\models$ is *monotone* in the sense that $\varphi_1, \ldots, \varphi_n \models \psi$ implies $\varphi_1, \ldots, \varphi_n, \theta \models \psi$ for any sentence θ. closed–world reasoning, however, is not monotonic in this sense: the inference from the database

> there is no trip which starts in Amsterdam CS at 9:10 and ends in Muiden before 9.45,"

licensed by closed–world reasoning, may be destroyed by additions to the database (e.g., a fast Interliner bus).

2.3.2   Unknown Preconditions

Real-world actions come with scores of preconditions which often go unnoticed. My action of switching on the light is successful only if the switch is functioning properly, the house is not cut off from electricity, the laws of electromagnetism still apply. It would be impossible to verify all those preconditions; we generally do not even check the light bulb although its failure occurs all too often. We thus have a conditional "if *turn switch* then *light on*" which does not become false the moment we turn the switch only to find that the light does not go on, as would be the case for the classical material implication. An enriched representation of the conditional as a ternary connective shows more clearly what is at issue here: "if *turn switch* and *nothing funny is going on* then *light on*." If we turn the switch but find that the light is not on, we conclude that something is amiss and start looking for that something. But – and this is the important point – in the absence of positive information to the effect that something is amiss, we assume that there is nothing funny going on. This is the closed–world assumption for reasoning with abnormalities, CWA(ab).

   This phenomenon can be seen in a controlled setting in an experiment designed by Claire Hughes and James Russell ([131]), the "box task," which lends itself particularly well to a logical analysis using closed world reasoning. This task was designed for analyzing autistic behavior, to which we return in Chapter 9 below.

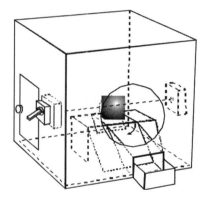

Figure 2.4   Hughes and Russell's box task. Reprinted from [236,p. 316] by permission of Dunitz.

   The task is to get the marble, which is lying on the platform, inside the box. However, when the subject puts her hand through the opening, a trapdoor in the platform opens and the marble drops out of reach. This is because there is an infrared light beam behind the opening, which, when interrupted, activates the trapdoor mechanism. The switch on the left side of the box deactivates the whole mechanism, so that to get the marble you have to flip the switch first. In the standard setup, the subject is shown how manipulating the switch allows one to retrieve the marble after she has first been tripped up by the trapdoor mechanism.

   A more formal analysis of the box task could go as follows. The main premise can be formulated as

(1)   If you reach for the marble through the opening *and there is nothing funny going on*, you can retrieve the marble.

where the italicized conjunct is the variable, assumed to be present always, for an unknown precondition. This conjunct occasions closed world reasoning of the form

(2)   I haven't *seen* anything funny.
           :: There *is* nothing funny going on.

Backward chaining then leads to the plan

(3)   To get the marble, put your hand through the opening.

Now a problem occurs: the marble drops out of reach before it can be retrieved. Premise (1) is not thereby declared to be false, but is now used to derive

(4)   Something funny is going on.

To determine what's so funny, the information about the switch is recruited, which can be formulated as a rule "repairing" (1) as in (5a) or (5b)

(5a)   If you reach for the marble, set the switch to the right position, *and there is nothing funny going on*, then you can retrieve the marble.
(5b)   If the switch is in the wrong position, there is something funny going on.

Closed–world reasoning with (5b) now yields

(6)   If the switch is in the wrong position, there is something funny going on, *but only then*.

Backward chaining then leads to a new plan

(7)   To get the marble, set the switch to the right position and put your hand through the opening.

One interesting feature of this analysis is thus that the new plan (7) is constructed from the old one by utilising the variable for the unknown precondition.

   This is not reasoning as it is usually studied in the psychology of reasoning, but it is reasoning nonetheless, with a discernible formal structure, and applicability across a wide range of domains. In fact CWA(ab) can be viewed as a definition of validity, as follows. Suppose we have an enriched conditional of the form $p \wedge \neg ab \to q$, where ab is a proposition letter indicating some abnormality. Suppose furthermore that we have as information about ab the following implications: $q_1 \to ab, \ldots, q_k \to ab$, and that this is *all* the available information about ab. Since the implication $\perp \rightarrow ab$ is always true,[15] we may include this (admittedly trivial) statement in the information available about ab.

We now want to say that, given $p, \neg q_1, \ldots, \neg q_n$, q may be concluded. This is tantamount to replacing the information about ab by the single premise

$$ab \leftrightarrow q_1 \vee \ldots \vee q_k \vee \perp,$$

and applying classical validity. Note that as a consequence of this definition, if there is no nontrivial information about ab, the right–hand side of the preceding bi-implication reduces to a falsehood (i.e., $\perp$), and the bi-implication itself to $ab \leftrightarrow \perp$, which is equivalent to $\neg ab$. In short, if there is no nontrivial information about ab, we may infer $\neg ab$. Note that although classical reasoning is used here in explaining the machinery, the closed-world inference itself is non-classical: in classical logic nothing can be concluded from the premises $p, \neg q_1, \ldots, \neg q_n$.

A famous observation can be illuminated from this point of view: Scribner's study of reasoning among the illiterate Kpelle tribe in Liberia (see [243]). Here is a sample argument given to her subjects

> All Kpelle men are rice farmers.
> Mr. Smith[16] is not a rice farmer.
> Is Mr. Smith a Kpelle man?

Subjects refused to answer the question definitively, instead giving evasive answers such as "If one knows a person, one can answer questions about him, but if one doesn't know that person, it is difficult." Scribner then went on to show that a few years of schooling in general led to the classical competence answer.

This result, like those of Luria in the 1930s (see [177]) has been taken as evidence that the illiterate subjects do not understand what is being asked of them: to answer the question solely on the basis of (an inference from) the premises given. Instead, so it is argued, they prefer to answer from personal experience, or to refrain from answering if they have no relevant experience. But this explanation presupposes that the Kpelle subject adopts the material implication as the logical form of the first premise. If, as is more plausible, he adopts a meaning of the conditional which allows exceptions (as we did in discussing the box task), he can only be charged with not applying closed–world reasoning to Mr. Smith. That is, if the Kpelle subject believes he has too little information to decide whether Mr. Smith is abnormal, he is justified in refusing to draw the modus tollens inference. On this account, what the couple of years elementary schooling teaches the child is a range of kinds of discourse in which exactly what to close the world on, and what to leave open, varies with some rather subtle contextual cues.

---

15. $\perp$ stands for an arbitrary contradiction, while $\top$ is a formula which is always true.
16. "Mr. Smith" is not a possible Kpelle name.

2.3.3   Causal and Counterfactual Reasoning

Counterfactual reasoning occurs when one starts from an assumption known to be false and tries to derive consequences. What would have happened if Hitler had invaded Britain? is a famous example. Such reasoning involves causal reasoning, because one needs to set up plausible chains of events. Counterfactual reasoning has been investigated in preschool children with the aim of establishing correlations with "theory of mind"

Riggs and Peterson [227] devised a "counterfactual" adaptation of the standard false belief task, in which a mother doll bakes a chocolate cake, in the process of which the chocolate moves from the fridge (its original location) to the cupboard. The question asked of the child is now

(*) Where *would* the chocolate *be* if mother hadn't baked a cake?

This question is about alternative courses of events and hence seems to use causal reasoning.

Pragmatically, the formulation of question (*) suggests it must have an answer. The answer cannot come from classical logic, starting from the description of the situation alone: classical logic compels one to ask What else could be the case? reflecting the obligation to consider all models of the data. In particular there would be models to consider in which mother eats all the chocolate, or in which the chocolate evaporates inside the fridge (an event of extremely small, but still nonzero, probability). Of course nothing of the sort happens in actual causal reasoning. There a "principle of inertia" applies, which roughly says: "things and properties remain as they are, unless there is explicit information to the contrary." This can be further spelled out as the closed–world assumption for reasoning about causality (CWA(c)):[17]

1. One assumes that only those events (affecting the entity of interest) occur which are forced to occur by the data – here the only such event is the chocolate's change of location from fridge to cupboard.

2. One also assumes that events only have those causal effects which are described by one's background theory – e.g., turning on the oven does not have a causal effect on the location of the chocolate.

3. No spontaneous changes occur, that is, every change of state or property can be attributed to the occurrence of an event with specified causal influence.

Together these principles suffice to derive an answer to (*). In fact this type of reasoning can be fully formalized in the "event calculus" originally developed in artificial intelligence (see [282] for extensive treatment and references).

---

17. A fully formal analysis will be given in chapter 9.

Its logical structure is similar to the one detailed in section 2.3.2 as regards properties (1) and (2), but property (3) brings in a new ingredient relating to development over time.

Formally, this can be viewed as yet another twist to the definition of validity: one now obtains a notion according to which the conclusion is evaluated at a later instant than the evaluation time of the premises. The classical definition of validity assumes that the conclusion of an argument is evaluated on models of the premises, thus validating a property like $p \models p$, that is, "on every model on which p is true, p is true." The definition of validity used in CWA(c) allows that models of the conclusion are temporal developments of models of the premises, and in this case we need no longer have $p \models p$. Suppose the models for the premises are evaluated at time t, and the models for the conclusion are temporal developments of these models considered at time $t' > t$. Clearly, even if p is true at time t, that same proposition p may be false at t'.

These considerations allow us to see the connection between closed world reasoning and planning. One feature distinguishing human planning from that of other species is the much increased capacity for offline planning. This involves mentally constructing a model, a structure representing the relevant part of the world, and computing the effect of actions in that model *over time*, taking into account likely events and the causal consequences of the actions performed. The various forms of closed–world reasoning introduced so far have to be combined here to enable the construction of the model and the computation of its development over time. What is interesting here for discussions of domain specificity is that the procedures used to construct models in offline planning can be used as well to construct models of linguistic discourse, for instance the structure of the events described by the discourse (see [282]). It is proposed in the reference cited that offline planning has been exapted[18] for the purposes of language comprehension, viewed as the ability to construct discourse models. If true, this would show an incursion of very general reasoning procedures into the purportedly domain–specific language module. Issues of modularity will crop up throughout.

2.3.4   Attribution of Beliefs and Intentions

An important step in cognitive development is the acquisition of a "theory of mind," the ability to understand that someone else may have beliefs different from one's own. A standard experimental paradigm to test theory of mind is the "false belief task," of which the following is an example (due to Wimmer and Perner [305])

> Children are first told the story:"Maxi and Mummy are in the kitchen. They put some
> chocolate in the fridge. Then Maxi goes away to play with his friend. Mummy decides to

---

18. See section 6.2.3 for a definition and discussion of the contrast between exaptation and adaptation.

bake a cake. She takes the chocolate from the fridge, makes the cake, and puts the rest of the chocolate in the cupboard. Maxi is returning now from visiting his friend and wants some chocolate." Children are then asked the test question: "Where does Maxi think the chocolate is?"

Normally developing children will be able to attribute a "false belief" to Maxi and answer "In the fridge" from around age 4 or so.

Another version[19] uses an episode from the Bob the Builder children's television series, in which Bob climbs a ladder to do some repair work on the roof of a house. While Bob is happily hammering, the series' resident gremlin Naughty Spud takes away the ladder to steal apples from a nearby apple tree. After Bob has finished his work on the roof, he makes preparations to climb down. At this point the video is stopped and the child who has been watching this episode is asked: "Where does Bob think that the ladder is?" Again, children below the cut-off age answer: "At the tree."

It is illuminating to view the reasoning leading up to these answers as an instance of closed–world reasoning. What is needed first of all is an awareness of the causal relation between perception and belief, which can be stated in the form: "if φ is true in scene S, and agent a sees S, then a comes to believe φ," where φ is a metavariable ranging over proposition letters $p, q, \ldots$. In other words, seeing is a cause of believing. Thus Maxi comes to believe that the chocolate is in the fridge. An application of the principle of inertia (cf. (3) above) yields that Maxi's belief concerning the location of the chocolate persists unless an event occurs which causes him to have a new belief, incompatible with the former. The story does not mention such an event, whence it is reasonable to assume – using 1 and 2 – that Maxi still believes that the chocolate is in the fridge when he returns from visiting his friend. Viewed in this way, attribution of belief is a special case of causal reasoning, and some correlation with performance on counterfactual reasoning tasks is to be expected. The tasks are not quite the same, however. The causal relation between perception and belief is an essential ingredient in the false belief task, absent in the counterfactual task. There are two sides to this: positively, that a belief may form after seeing something, and negatively, that there are only a few specified ways in which beliefs can form, e.g., by seeing, by being told, and by inference – this negative aspect is an application of closed–world reasoning. Children failing the false belief task could master causal reasoning generally, but fail on the aspects just mentioned. So, assimilating the reasoning involved in theory of mind tasks as a kind of defeasible reasoning potentially provides both a basis for continuity with earlier developmental or evolutionary precursors, and a basis for discontinuity – it is causal reasoning by closed–world assumptions, but causal reasoning by closed–world assumptions of a specific kind. Reasoning

---

19. Investigated experimentally by the van Lambalgen's students David Wood and Marian Counihan.

about minds is reasoning in a specific domain, but its characterization may be possible by a rather small extension of a logical framework for other domains.

We viewed classical logic as resulting from setting parameters for syntax, semantics, and the consequence relation. We have seen that these settings are appropriate for the domain of classical mathematics, but that they cannot claim universal validity. Other domains require different settings; e.g., closed–world reasoning about databases has only bivalence in common with classical logic. In fact, a wide range of everyday tasks involve closed–world reasoning: e.g., planning, and adapting to failures of plans during their execution, diagnosis of causes, causal reasoning itself, reasoning about mental behavior and states, interpreting speaker's intentions underlying discourse. Each of these domains leads to a logic especially suited to that domain. Reasoners have in general little trouble in selecting the logic appropriate to a domain, although, as we shall see in the course of this book, some psychiatric disorders are accompanied, and perhaps even caused, by inappropriately applied reasoning schemes.

In the following chapters, we will look at several experimental reasoning paradigms to discover evidence of parameter setting at work. It will turn out that for a subject, discovering the right parameters is often the hardest part of a laboratory reasoning task.

At this point, the psychologist reader, from our experience, is likely to be puzzled. "Subjects don't know these logics! These formalisms are just theorists' tools! All these squiggles don't happen in minds! Anyway, all you are doing is redescribing stuff which psychologists know about in terms of pragmatics!" are among typical objections, so we had perhaps better attempt to defuse them. Of course we agree that subjects don't "know these logics" just in the sense that they don't know the grammar of English, but they *do* know these logics just in the sense that they *do* know the grammar of English. Yes, they are also theorists' tools, but we take seriously the possibility that something computationally equivalent is implemented in the mind. In chapter 8 we will show that that implementation doesn't require squiggles. And yes, many of the phenomena we are describing as applying reasoning in non-standard logics have been given descriptions already by psychologists. Our claim is that those descriptions remain ad hoc until they are systematized as we are trying to do here. It is very important that the psychological reader takes us seriously when we claim that these logics are in the mind, but equally important that they realise that that claim does not bring all the baggage usually ascribed to it.

3 A Little Logic Goes a Long Way

The psychology of reasoning studies how subjects draw conclusions from premises – the process of derivation. But premises have to be interpreted before any conclusions can be drawn. Although premise interpretation has received recurrent attention (e.g., Henle [122], Gebauer and Laming [92], Newstead [201], Byrne [28]), the full range of dimensions of interpretation facing the subject has not been considered. Nor has interpretation been properly distinguished from derivation *from* an interpretation in a way that enables *interactions* between interpretation and derivation to be analysed. Our general thesis is that integrating accounts of interpretation with accounts of derivation can lead to deeper insight into cognitive theory generally, and human reasoning in particular. This chapter exemplifies this general claim in the domain of Wason's selection task [295], an important reference point for several prominent cognitive theories of reasoning. What is meant by interpretation in this context? Interpretation maps representation systems (linguistic, diagrammatic, etc.) onto the things in the world which are represented. Interpretation decides such matters as: which things in the world generally correspond to which words; which of these things are specifically in the domain of interpretation of the current discourse; which structural description should be assigned to an utterance; which propositions are assumed and which derived; which notions of validity of argument are intended; and so on. Natural languages such as English sometimes engender the illusion that such matters are settled by general knowledge of the language, but it is easy to see that this is not so. Each time a sentence such as "The presidents of France were bald" is uttered, its users must decide, for example, who is included, and how bald is bald, *for present purposes*. In the context of the selection task we shall see that there are quite a few such decisions which subjects have to make, each resolvable in a variety of ways, and each with implications for what response to make in the task.

Of course, interpretation, in this sense, is very widely studied in philosophy, logic and linguistics (and even psycholinguistics), as we document in our references throughout the chapter. Our thesis is that interchange between these studies and psychological studies of reasoning has been inadequate. Perhaps because the methods of the fields are so divergent, there has been a reluctance to take semantic analyses seriously as a guide to psychological processes, and many of the concepts of logic are loosely employed in psychology, at best. There are, of course, honorable exceptions which we will consider in our discussion.

In this chapter we take Wason's selection task and argue that the mental processes it evokes in subjects are, quite reasonably, dominated by interpretive processes. Wason's task is probably the most intensively studied task in the psychology of reasoning literature and has been the departure point, or point of passage, for several high–profile cognitive theories: mental models theory (Johnson-Laird and Byrne [144]), relevance theory (Sperber, Cara, and Girotto [252]), "evolutionary psychology" (Cosmides [47]), rational analysis (Oaksford and Chater [205]). We will argue and present empirical evidence that each of these theories misses critical contributions that logic and semantics can make to understanding the task. For various reasons the materials of the task exert contradictory pressures leading to conflicting interpretations, and we argue that what we observe are subjects' various, not always very successful, efforts to resolve these conflicts. The results of our experiments expose rich individual variation in reasoning and learning and so argue for novel standards of empirical analysis of the mental processes involved.

3.1   The Mother of All Reasoning Tasks

Wason's original task was presented by means of a form as depicted in figure 3.1. The reader, who has probably seen the task before, should realise that this is all the information provided to the subjects, in order to appreciate the tremendous difficulty posed by this task. We will later present a variant of the task (the "two rule task") which may recreate in the cognoscenti the feelings of perplexity experienced by the untutored subject.

> Below is depicted a set of four cards, of which you can see only the exposed face but not the hidden back. On each card, there is a number on one of its sides and a letter on the other.
>
> Also below there is a rule which applies only to the four cards. Your task is to decide which if any of these four cards you *must* turn in order to decide if the rule is true. Don't turn unnecessary cards. Tick the cards you want to turn.
>
> **Rule:** *If there is a vowel on one side, then there is an even number on the other side.*
>
> **Cards:** | A | | K | | 4 | | 7 |

Figure 3.1   Wason's selection task

This experiment has been replicated many times. If one formulates the rule

If there is a vowel on one side, then there is an even number on the other side.

as an implication $p \rightarrow q$, then the observed pattern of results is typically given as in table 3.1.

Thus, the modal response[1] (around half of the undergraduate subjects) is to turn A and 4. Very few subjects turn A and 7. Wason (and, until fairly recently, the great majority of researchers) assumed, without considering alternatives, that the correct performance is to turn the A and 7 cards only. Oaksford and Chater's inductive rational choice model [205] was the first to challenge this assumption, by rejecting deductive models entirely – more on this below. Wason adopted this criterion of good reasoning from a classical logical interpretation of the rule.

In a very real sense, however, Wason got his own task wrong in stipulating that there was a particular "obviously correct" answer. This holds on the assumption that the rule is interpreted using the material implication, but nothing in the experimental material itself forces this interpretation. Undergraduate subjects come to this task with their own interpretation of the conditional "if ... then," and more often than not this interpretation is as a defeasible rule robust to exceptions. In this case, the "competence" answer would be to respond that *no* combination of card choices can falsify the rule, because any possible counterexamples are indistinguishable from exceptions. And no finite combination of choices can prove the rule is true.[2] Alternatively, subjects with other plausible interpretations of the task and rule might reasonably want to respond that several alternative sets of cards would test the rule equally well, and this again is not an available response. There are of course many psychological reasons why we should not expect subjects to make these kinds of responses even if they were offered as possibilities. There are strong demand characteristics and authority relations in the experimental situation. Furthermore, subjects are not accustomed to reflecting on their language use and also lack a vocabulary for talking about and distinguishing the elementary semantic concepts which are required to express these issues. Taking interpretation seriously does not mean we thereby assume reasoning is perfect, nor that we reject classical logic as one (possibly educationally important) logical model. But the unargued adoption of classical logic as a criterion of correct performance is thoroughly antilogical. In our discussion we review some of the stances toward logic exhibited by the prominent cognitive theories that have made claims about the selection task, and appraise them from the viewpoint advocated here.

---

1. The mode of a data sample is the element that occurs most often in the sample.
2. It is true that Wason's instructions explicitly state that the rule applies only to the four cards, but, as we shall see below, this is not a reasonable restriction on one dominant interpretation, and is widely ignored.

Table 3.1 Typical proportions of choices in the selection task

p	p, q	$p, \neg q$	$p, q, \neg q$	misc.
35%	45%	5%	7%	8%

3.2   A Preliminary Logical Distinction

The program of empirical investigation that ensued from Wason's original experiment can be seen as a search for those contents of rules that make the task "easy" or "hard" according to the classical competence criterion. Differences in accuracy of reasoning are then explained by various classifications of content.

For example, when the original "abstract" (i.e., descriptive) form of the selection task proved so counterintuitively hard, attention rapidly turned to finding materials that made the task easy. Johnson-Laird, Legrenzi, and Legrenzi [142] showed that a version of the task using a UK postal regulation ("If a letter has a second class stamp, it is left unsealed") produced near-ceiling performance. They described the facilitation in terms of *familiarity* of the materials. Griggs and Cox [109] showed that reasoning about a drinking age law ("if you drink alcohol here, you have to be over 18") was easy. Wason and Green[296] similarly showed that a rule embedded in a "production-line inspection" scenario (e.g., "If the wool is blue, it must be 4 feet long") also produced good performance. Cosmides [47, 48] went on to illustrate a range of materials which produce "good" reasoning, adding the claim this facilitation only happened with social contract rules. Cosmides and her collaborators used the argument that only social contract material was easy, to claim that humans evolved innate modular "cheating detector algorithms" which underpin selection task performance on social contract rules. Note that nonsocial contract examples such as the "wool" example just quoted were prominent in the literature before Cosmides made these claims. Recent work has extended the evolutionary account by proposing a range of detectors beyond cheating detectors which are intended to underpin reasoning with, for example, precautionary conditionals (Fiddick, Cosmides, and Tooby [81]).[3] These observations of good reasoning were reported as effects of *content* on reasoning with rules of the same *logical form*. Cosmides and Tooby are explicit about logic being their target:

> On this view [the view Cosmides and Tooby attack], reasoning is viewed as the operation of content-independent procedures, such as formal logic, applied impartially and uniformly to every problem, regardless of the nature of the content involved. (Cosmides and Tooby [48,p. 166])

---

3. Cummins [53] has argued, against this proliferation, that the innate module concerned is more general and encompasses all of deontic reasoning.

Johnson-Laird equally claims that the effect of content on reasoning contradicts the formal-logical model of reasoning:

> [F]ew select the card bearing [7], even though if it had a vowel on its other side, it would falsify the rule. People are much less susceptible to this error of omission when the rules and materials have a sensible content, e.g., when they concern postal regulations ... Hence the content of a problem can affect reasoning, and this phenomenon is contrary to the notion of formal rules of inference (Johnson-Laird [146,p. 225])

Wason himself, discussing an example from [299] which used the rule: "If I go to Manchester I go by train," rejects the idea that there are structural differences between thematic and abstract tasks:

> The thematic problem proved much easier than a standard abstract version which was *structurally equivalent...* ([300,p. 643]; emphasis added)

We argue here that by far the most important determinant of ease of reasoning is whether interpretation of the rule assigns it descriptive or deontic *logical form*, and we explain the effect of this interpretive choice in terms of the many problems descriptive interpretation creates in this task setting, as contrasted with the ease of reasoning with deontic interpretations.

Descriptive conditionals describe states of affairs and are therefore true or false as those states of affairs correspond to the conditionals' content. Deontic conditionals, as described in the previous chapter, state how matters *should* be according to some (perhaps legal) law or regulation, or preference.[4] The semantic relation between sentence and case(s) for deontics is therefore quite different than for descriptives. With descriptives, *sets* of cases may make the conditional true, or make it false. With deontics, cases *individually* conform or not, but they do not affect the status of the law (or preference, or whatever). This is of course a crude specification of the distinction. We shall have some more specific proposals to make below. But it is important for the empirical investigation to focus on these blunt differences that all analyses of the distinction agree on.[5]

Returning to the examples given, we see that a rule like "if you drink alcohol here, you have to be over 18" is deontic, not descriptive. If everybody drinking whiskey in a particular pub is under 18, the rule may be massively violated, but it is still in force. We have a different situation if the rule is intended to be descriptive, an intention which can be suggested, but not fixed, by the formulation "if someone drinks alcohol here, he is over 18." In this case a primary school boy sipping his whiskey may be taken to falsify the rule. The other examples can be analysed similarly.

---

4. There are a great variety of specific deontic stances which all share the feature that they deal in what is ideal relative to some criterion.

5. This is an important invocation to be born in mind by the formalist concerned to contribute to experimental investigation: "Use the bluntest formal analysis which is sharp enough to make the necessary distinctions!"

In English, the semantic distinction between descriptives and deontics is not reflected simply on the surface of sentences. Deontics are often expressed using subjunctives or modals – *should, ought, must* – but are equally often expressed with descriptive verbs. It is impossible to tell without consultation of context, whether a sentence such as "In the UK, vehicles drive on the left" is to be interpreted descriptively or deontically – as a generalization or a legal prescription. Conversely, subjunctive verbs and modals are often interpreted descriptively. (e.g., in the sentence "If it is 10 am, that should (must) be John," said on hearing the doorbell, the modal expresses an inference about a description). This means that we as experimenters cannot determine this semantic feature of subjects' interpretation of conditionals simply by changing auxiliary verbs in rules. A combination of rule, content, and subjects' knowledge influences whether to assign a deontic or descriptive *form*.

Our proposal about the selection task at its simplest is that the semantic difference between descriptive and deontic conditionals leads to a processing difference when these conditionals are used in the selection task. In barest outline, the semantic difference is this. Deontic conditionals such as the drinking age law cannot be false, they can only be violated. Hence turning a card never affects the status of the rule. Now, whether a given customer violates the drinking age law is independent of whether another customer does so. This seems a trivial observation, but a comparison with the case of descriptive rules will show its importance.

A descriptive rule can be true or false, and here the purpose of turning cards is to determine which is the case; in this case, unlike the previous one, the result of turning a card can affect the status of the rule. A consequence of this is a form of dependence between card choices, in the following sense: turning A to find 7 already decides the status of the rule by showing it to be false; it does not seem necessary to turn the 7 card as well. On the other hand, if upon turning A one finds a 4, it is necessary to turn the 7 as well. We will see that this situation is confusing to subjects, who sometimes believe that the task is unsolvable because of this dependence. It is not, of course, once one realises that the cards are not real but depicted, and hence cannot be turned at all. These blunt semantic differences mean that the original descriptive (abstract) task poses many difficulties to naive reasoners not posed by the deontic task.[6] A formal analysis of the differences will be given below, but these indications should suffice for the present.

We will derive a variety of particular difficulties to be expected from the inter-

---

6. Previous work has pointed to the differences between the deontic and descriptive tasks (e.g., Manktelow and Over [180]; Oaksford and Chater [205]). Cheng and Holyoak [37] developed the theory that success on deontic selection tasks was based on *pragmatic reasoning schemata*. Although they present this theory as an alternative to logic-based theories, it arguably presents a fragmentary deontic logic with some added processing assumptions (theorem prover) about the "perspective" from which the rule is viewed. However, Cheng and Holyoak did not take the further step of analyzing abstractly the contrasting difficulties which descriptive conditionals pose in this task.

action of semantics and task, and the presentation of an experimental program to demonstrate that subjects really do experience these problems. Deriving a spectrum of superficially diverse problems from a single semantic distinction supports a powerful empirical generalization about reasoning in this task, and an explanation of why that generalization holds. It also strongly supports the view that subjects' problems are highly variable and in doing so reveals an important but much neglected level of empirical analysis.

It is important to distinguish coarser from finer levels of semantic analysis in understanding our predictions. At finer levels of analysis, we will display a multiplicity of interpretive choices and insist on evidence that subjects adopt a variety of them – both across subjects and within a single subject's episodes of reasoning. At this level we certainly do not predict any specific interpretation. At coarser levels of analysis such as between truth–functional and non-truth–functional conditionals, and between descriptive and deontic conditionals, it is possible to predict highly specific consequences of adopting one or the other kind of reading in different versions of the task, and to show that these consequences are evident in the data. If they do appear as predicted, then that provides strong evidence that interpretive processes are driving the data. In fact, many of these consequences have been observed before, but have remained unconnected with each other, and not appreciated for what they are – the various consequences of a homogeneous semantic distinction. The take-home message is: semantics supplies an essential theoretical base for understanding the psychology of reasoning.

The plan of the remainder of the chapter is as follows. We begin by presenting in the next section what we take to be essential about a modern logical approach to such cognitive processes as are invoked by the selection task. The following section then uses this apparatus to show how the logical differences between descriptive and deontic selection tasks can be used to make predictions about problems that subjects will have in the former but not the latter. The following section turns these predictions into several experimental conditions, and presents data compared to Wason's original task as baseline. Finally, we discuss the implications of these findings for theories of the selection task and of our interpretive perspective for cognitive theories more generally.

3.3 Logical Forms in Reasoning

The selection task is concerned with reasoning about the natural language conditional "if . . . then." The reasoning patterns that are valid for this expression can only be determined after a *logical form* is assigned to the sentence in which this expression occurs. The early interpretations of the selection task all assumed that the logical form assigned to "if . . . then" should be the connective $\rightarrow$ with the semantics given by classical propositional logic. We want to argue that this easy identification is not in accordance with the modern conception of logic outlined in chapter 2. By this, we do not just mean that modern logic has come up with other competence models besides classical logic. Rather, the easy identification downplays the complexity of the process of assigning logical form. In a nutshell, modern logic sees itself as concerned with the mathematics of reasoning systems. It is related to a concrete reasoning system such as classical propositional logic as geometry is related to light rays. It is impossible to say a priori what is the right geometry of the physical world; however, once some coordinating definitions (such as "a straight line is to be interpreted by a light ray") have been made, it is determined which geometry describes the behavior of these straight lines, and hypotheses about the correct geometry become falsifiable. Similarly, it does not make sense to determine a priori what is the right logic. This depends on one's notion of truth, semantic consequence, and more. But once these parameters have been fixed, logic, as the mathematics of reasoning systems, determines what is, and what is not, a valid consequence. In this view it is of prime importance to determine the type of parameter that goes into the definition of what a logical system is, and, of course, the psychological purposes that might lead subjects to choose one or another setting in their reasoning. This parameters setting generally involves as much reasoning as does the reasoning task assigned to the subject. We are thus led to the important distinction between reasoning *from* an interpretation and reasoning *to* an interpretation. The former is what is supposed to happen in a typical inference task: given premises, determine whether a given conclusion follows. But because the premises are formulated in natural language, there is room for different logical interpretations of the given material and intended task. Determining what the appropriate logical form is in a given context itself involves logical reasoning which is far from trivial in the case of the selection task.

We have seen in chapter 2 that the parameters characterizing logical form come in at least three flavors: pertaining to syntax, to semantics, and to the notion of logical consequence. In short, therefore, the interpretive problem facing a subject in a reasoning task is to provide settings for all these parameters – this is what is involved in assigning logical form. It has been the bane of the psychology of reasoning that it operates with an oversimplified notion of logical form. Typically, in the psychology of reasoning, assigning logical form is conceived of as translating a natural language sentence into a formal language whose semantics is supposed to be given, but this is really only the beginning: it fixes just one parameter. We do not claim that subjects know precisely what they are doing; that is, most likely subjects do not know in any detail what the mathematical consequences of their choices are. We do claim, however, that subjects worry about how to set the parameters, and below we offer data obtained from tutorial dialogues to corroborate this claim. This is not a descent into postmodern hermeneutics. This doomful view may be partly due to earlier

psychological invocations of interpretational defenses against accusations of irrationality in reasoning, perhaps the most cited being Henle [122]: "there exist
no errors of reasoning, only differences in interpretation." It *is* possible, however, to make errors in reasoning: the parameter settings may be inconsistent,
or a subject may draw inferences not consistent with the settings.

From the point of view of the experimenter, once all the parameters are fixed,
it is mathematically determined what the extension of the consequence relation
will be; and the hypotheses on specific parameter settings therefore become
falsifiable. In particular, the resulting mathematical theory will classify an infinite number of reasoning patterns as either valid or invalid. In principle there
is therefore ample room for testing whether a subject has set his parameters
as guessed in the theory: choose a reasoning pattern no instance of which is
included in the original set of reasoning tokens. In practice, there are limitations to this procedure because complex patterns may be hard to process. Be
that as it may, it remains imperative to obtain independent confirmation of the
parameter settings by looking at arguments very different from the original set
of tokens. This was, for instance, our motivation for obtaining data about the
meaning of negation in the context of the selection task (more on this below):
while not directly relevant to the logical connectives involved in the selection
task,[7] it provided valuable insight into the notions of truth and falsity.

Psychology is in some ways harder once one acknowledges interpretational
variety, but given the overwhelming evidence for that variety, responding by
eliminating it from psychological theory is truly the response of the drunk beneath the lamppost. In fact, in some counterbalancing ways, psychology gets a
lot easier because there are so many independent ways of getting information
about subjects' interpretations – such as tutorial dialogues. Given the existence
of interpretational variety, the right response is richer empirical methods aimed
at producing convergent evidence for deeper theories which are more indirectly
related to the stimuli observed. What the richness of interpretation does mean
is that the psychology of reasoning narrowly construed has less direct implications for the rationality of subjects' reasoning. What was right about the earlier
appeals to interpretational variation is that it indeed takes a lot of evidence to
confidently convict subjects of irrationality. It is necessary to go to great lengths
to make a charitable interpretation of what they are trying to do and how they
understand what they are supposed to do before one can be in a position to assert that they are irrational. Even when all this is done, the irrational element
can only be interpreted against a background of rational effort.

---

7. Though see [74] to see how negation is not far away.

3.4   Logical Forms in the Selection Task

We now apply the preceding considerations to the process of assigning a logical form to the standard selection task. An important component of this process is determining a meaning of the conditional, but this is not all there is to logical form in the selection task. To see this, it is useful to reformulate the task as an *information processing task* as intended by Marr [183].[8] Here we run into an immediate ambiguity: the information–processing task may be meant as the one intended by the experimenter, or as understood by the subject. In both cases the input consists of the form with instructions, but the output can be very different.

The intentions of the experimenter are clear: the output should consist of checks under the cards selected. The output in the subject's interpretation of the task can vary considerably. Some subjects think the output can be a plan for showing the rule to be true or false. Other subjects interpolate a process of information gathering and view the task as "what information do I require to decide the rule, and how do I obtain that information." This gets them in considerable trouble, since they tend to rephrase the minimality condition "do not turn unnecessary cards" as the condition "determine the minimum information necessary to decide the rule," which is importantly different. In this section we will describe several formal models corresponding to different understandings of the task.

Wason had in mind the interpretation of the conditional as a truth–functional implication, which together with bivalence yields the material implication. Truth–functional, because the four cards must decide the truth–value of the conditional; bivalent, because the task is to determine *truth or falsity* of the conditional, implying that there is no other option. All this is of course obvious from the experimenter's point of view, but the important question is whether this interpretation is accessible to the subject. Given the wide range of other meanings of the conditional, the subject must *infer* from the instructions, and possibly from contextual factors, what the intended meaning is. Reading very carefully, and bracketing her own most prominent meanings for the key terms involved, the subject may deduce that the conditional is to be interpreted truth–functionally, with a classical algebra of truth–values, hence with the material implication as resulting logical form. (Actually the situation is more complicated; see the next paragraph.) But this bracketing is what subjects with little logical training typically find hard to do.

The subject first has to come up with a formal language in which to translate the rule. It is usually assumed that the selection task is about propositional logic, but in the case of the "abstract" rule 1 actually needs predicate logic,

---

8. Marr's ideas will be explained in greater detail in chapter 5 in section 5.1.4 and in chapter 11.

mainly because of the occurrence of the expression "one side ... other side." One way (although not the only one) to formalise the rule in predicate logic uses the following predicates:

$V(x, y)$ "x is on the visible side of card y"
$I(x, y)$ "x is on the invisible side of card y"
$O(x)$ "x is a vowel"
$E(x)$ "x is an even number"
and the rule is then translated as the following pair:

$$\forall c(\exists x(V(x, c) \wedge O(x)) \rightarrow \exists y(I(y, c) \wedge E(y)))$$
$$\forall c(\exists x(I(x, c) \wedge O(x)) \rightarrow \exists y(V(y, c) \wedge E(y)))$$

This might seem pedantic were it not for the fact that some subjects go astray at this point, replacing the second statement by a biconditional

$$\forall c(\exists x(I(x, c) \wedge O(x)) \leftrightarrow \exists y(V(y, c) \wedge E(y))),$$

or even a reversed conditional

$$\forall c(\exists x(V(x, c) \wedge E(x)) \rightarrow \exists y(I(y, c) \wedge O(y))).$$

This very interesting phenomenon will be studied further in section 3.5.5.[9]

For simplicity's sake, in the following we will focus only on subjects' problems at the level of propositional logic.

3.4.1 The Big Divide: Descriptive and Deontic Conditionals

It was noticed early on that facilitation in task performance could be obtained by changing the abstract rule to a familiar rule such as

If you want to drink alcohol, you have to be over 18

though the deontic nature of the rule was not initially seen as important, in contrast to its familiarity. This observation was one reason why formal logic was considered to be a bad guide to actual human reasoning. Logic was not able to explain how statements supposedly of the same logical form lead to vastly different performance – or so the argument went. However, using the expanded notion of logical form given above one can see that the abstract rule and the deontic rule *are not of the same form.*

Descriptive Interpretation of the Task

We assume first that the subject views the task descriptively, as determining whether the rule is true or false of the four cards given, no exceptions allowed.[10]

---

9. The fact that Gebauer and Lamming [92] accept this reversed reading in this context provides a timely reminder that subjects and experimenters are sometimes equally prone to accept interpretations which would be held to be quite incongruous in a more neutral context.
10. Some subjects have a descriptive interpretation which does allow exceptions; see section 3.5.2.

We also assume that cards with false antecedent (i.e., a consonant) are viewed as complying with the rule[11] This dictates an interpretation of the descriptive conditional as material implication.

Wason viewed his task in terms of bivalent classical logic, but even in the descriptive case this holds only for an omniscient being, who can view both sides of the cards. The human subject who comes to this task is at first confronted with a lack of information, and may apply a logic which is appropriate to this situation: a semantics which is sensitive to the information available to the subject. It will turn out that there are two subtly different ways of taking into account the incomplete information, which will be seen to correspond to different behaviors of subjects. In the process of formalization, we will also have occasion to introduce two different notions of truth that persistently confuse subjects.

The first formalization of the selection task views it as an information–processing task whose output is the information the subject requires for deciding the rule. Suppose for simplicity that the letters on the cards can only be A, K, and the numbers only 4,7. Define a model, consisting of "information states" as follows. For brevity, we will sometimes call information states "states." There are four states corresponding to the visible sides of the cards; denote these by $A, K, 4, 7$. These correspond to incomplete information states. Then there are eight states corresponding to the possibilities for what is on the invisible side; denote these by $(A, 4)$, $(A, 7)$, $(K, 4)$, $(K, 7)$, $(4, A)$, $(4, K)$, $(7, A)$, and $(7, K)$. These correspond to complete information states (about a single card). This gives as domain W of the model twelve states in all, each pertaining to a single card. Starting from W one may define the set W_4 consisting of all consistent information states relating to the four cards simultaneously. W_4 contains sets such as $\{(A, 4), K, 4, 7\}$, $\{A, K, (4, A), (7, A)\}$, $\{(A, 4), K, (4, A), 7\}$, or $\{(A, 7), (K, 4), (4, K), (7, K)\}$. On W_4 one can define an ordering $\leqslant$ by $w \leqslant v$ if the information contained about a given card in v is an extension of, or equal to, the information about that card in w. So we have, e.g., $\{(A, 4), K, 4, 7\} \leqslant \{(A, 4), K, (4, A), 7\}$ and $\{A, K, 4, 7\} \leqslant \{(A, 7), (K, 4), (4, K), (7, K)\}$, but $\{(A, 4), (4, A), K, (7, A)\} \nleqslant \{A, (4, A), K, (7, A)\}$.

To represent the different relations of truth that cards and rule can bear toward each other, we introduce a support-relation $\Vdash$ and the standard "makes true" relation $\models$. The latter relation is in a sense symmetric: if for a model $\mathcal{A}$ and a formula φ one has $\mathcal{A} \models \varphi$ one may say equivalently that $\mathcal{A}$ makes φ true, or that φ is true of $\mathcal{A}$. This is different for the support-relation $\Vdash$, holding between a "piece of information" v and a formula φ: $v \Vdash \varphi$ must be read as the asymmetric relation "v contains evidence for φ." It is the interplay between the asymmetric and the symmetric relation that causes many subjects a headache.

---

11. It would not be appropriate to give the implication the truth–value "undecided" (as in Kleene's three–valued logic) in this case, since no amount of additional information can affect this truth–value.

The support-relation $w \Vdash \psi$ is defined between states in W_4 and formulas ψ as follows. Let p be the proposition "the card has a vowel," and q the proposition "the card has an even number." The referent of the expression "the card" is determined by the information state on which p, q are interpreted; we assume that in an expression $p \wedge (\neg)q$ the referent of "the card" in q is bound by that in p. Then we have

1. $A \Vdash p$, $K \Vdash \neg p$, p undecided on 4 and 7 (i.e., neither $4 \Vdash p$ nor $4 \Vdash \neg p$, and similarly for 7);

2. $4 \Vdash q$, $7 \Vdash \neg q$, q undecided on A and K;

3. $(A, 4) \Vdash p \wedge q$, $(A, 7) \Vdash p \wedge \neg q$, $\ldots (4, A) \Vdash p \wedge q$, $(4, K) \Vdash \neg p \wedge q$, etc.

For a state v in W_4, define $v \Vdash p \wedge \neg q$ as: "there is a card (x, y) in u such that $(x, y) \Vdash p \wedge \neg q$." We say that the rule is supported by a piece of information v, and write $v \Vdash p \rightarrow q$, if $v \not\Vdash p \wedge \neg q$. Lastly we say that v makes the rule true, and write $v \models p \rightarrow q$, if for all $u \geqslant v : u \Vdash p \rightarrow q$. Clearly $v \models p \rightarrow q$ implies $v \Vdash p \rightarrow q$, but the converse does not hold, and this is one source of confusion for subjects, as we will see in section 3.5.2. In this "information-seeking" version of the task the subject now must compute the information states that decide the rule. A combinatorial exercise involving the truth–table for $\rightarrow$ shows that these are: $\{(A, 7), K, 4, 7\}$, $\{A, K, 4, (7, A)\}$, $\{(A, 4), K, 4, (7, K)\}$ and their extensions. Suppose the subject now views the task as: "what information must I gather in order to decide the rule," and interprets the instruction not to turn unnecessary cards in this light, thus looking for minimal information states only. The subject must then perform an action, or actions, which bring her from $\{A, K, 4, 7\}$ to one of the desired minimal information states. The trouble is that sometimes turning a single card suffices to achieve a minimal information state, and that sometimes turning two cards is necessary, and it depends on the unknown hidden side of the cards which situation one is in. Subjects interpreting the task in this way therefore think that it is unsolvable. To make the task solvable, a different interpretation is needed, in which the subject does not think in terms of the information which must be *gathered*, but in terms of information which becomes *available*. The formalization appropriate to this interpretation involves a game in which the subject plays against an adversary who makes the information available; the subject's optimal choice corresponds to a winning strategy in this game. A formal characterization goes as follows.

The game is played between two players, I (the subject) and II (the experimenter). The game is played on sixteen boards simultaneously, corresponding to what can be on the back of the cards whose visible sides are $A, K, 4, 7$. Player I selects a set of cards which she claims will decide the rule on every board. Player II has two options:

(a) II picks a card outside I's selection and chooses a board;

(b) II picks a card in I's selection and chooses two boards.

In case (a), II's move is winning if I's selection makes the rule true, but II's card makes it false on the chosen board. In case (b), II's move is winning if II's selected card has different values on the two boards, but the rule is true on both. Player I wins if II does not win. Clearly a winning strategy for player I consists in the selection of A and 7. Less, and player II can win via a move of type (a); more, and II can win via a move of type (b). To compute the winning strategy is again a combinatorial exercise.

It is essential for this version of the task that the game is played on sixteen boards simultaneously. If the game were to be played on a single board about which player I knows nothing, the concept of strategy would not make sense, and we find subjects saying that it is only luck that a selection turns out be relevant; see for instance, subject 5 in section 3.5.3. Hence if the game corresponding to the selection task is formalized as being played on one board only, the subject must consider the task to be unsolvable.

There is thus much more to the descriptive selection task than a simple computation in propositional logic which subjects cannot do because they are partly irrational, or have no general logical competence. Indeed, that subjects find the purely propositional part easy is witnessed by the fact that they do not have trouble evaluating the impact of a card correctly (e.g., subject 3 in the introduction to section 3.5). It is the choosing that creates the difficulty, and here the instructions provide little guidance on how to construct the proper information–processing task, or they may even actively interfere with the construction.

Deontic Interpretation of the Task

The logic appropriate to a deontic interpretation of the task is very different. One difference is in the structure of the models associated with deontic statements.

As we have seen in chapter 2, a deontic model $\mathcal{A}$ is given by a set of "worlds" or "cases" W, together with a relation $R(w, v)$ on W intuitively meaning: "v is an ideal counterpart to w." That is, if $R(w, v)$, then the norms posited in w are never violated in v. The relation R is used to interpret the modal operator O ("it ought to be the case that"). On such a model, we may define a deontic conditional by writing $O(p \rightarrow q)$, but it is convenient to introduce a special notation for this conditional, namely $p \prec q$, and to define for any world $w \in W$

$$w \models p \prec q \text{ iff for all } v \text{ such that } R(w, v): \ v \models p \text{ implies } v \models q,$$

and

$$\mathcal{A} \models p \prec q \text{ iff for all } w \text{ in } W: w \models p \prec q.$$

The satisfaction relation for atomic propositions is the same as that in the descriptive case.

The definition thus introduces an additional parameter R. If W is the set of worlds defined above, define R on W by $R(A, (A, 4))$, $R(7, (7, K))$, $\neg R(A, (A, 7))$, $\neg R(7, (7, A))$, $R(K, (K, 4))$, $R(K, (K, 7))$, $R(4, (4, A))$, and $R(4, (4, K))$.[12] R encodes the evaluation of each card against the norm, and this is what subjects can easily do.

As the reader will have no trouble verifying, the deontic model $(W, R, \models)$ then satisfies $p \prec q$, i.e., for all w in W: $w \models p \prec q$. For example, to verify that $A \models p \prec q$, one notes that the only world v satisfying $R(A, v)$ is $(A, 4)$, which satisfies both p and q. That is, in contrast to the previous case the rule is true from the start, hence there is no need to gather evidence for or against the rule, and the conflicts between $\models$ and $\Vdash$, and between two views of information, cannot arise in this case. The information–processing task becomes rather different: the output is the set of cases which possibly violate the norm, and inspection of the definition of R shows that only A and 7 are candidates. Turning 7 to find A just means that $(7, A)$ is not an ideal counterpart to 7, in the sense that it does not satisfy the norms holding in 7. The computation is accordingly just a simple lookup. The set W_4 and the strategic choices it gives rise to do not enter into the picture.[13]

Deontic Connectives

This is actually a general phenomenon, which is not restricted to just conditionals. As we shall see, if one gives subjects the following variation on the selection task,

> There is a vowel on one side of the cards *and* there is an even number on the other side,[14]

they typically respond by turning the A and 4 cards, instead of just replying "this statement is false of these four cards" (see below, section 4.1.5). One reason for this behavior is given by subject 22 in section 3.5.6, who now sees the task as checking those cards which could still satisfy the conjunctive rule, namely A and 4, since K and 7 do not satisfy in any case. Such a response is only possible if one has helped oneself to a predicate such as R. Formally, one may define a deontic conjunction $p \sqcap q$ by putting, for all w in W,

$$w \models p \sqcap q \text{ iff for all } v \text{ such that } R(v, w): v \models p \wedge q.$$

---

12. We shall assume that if v is an ideal counterpart to w, then v is maximally ideal, that is, v is the ideal counterpart of itself. Thus we assume $\forall w \forall v (R(w, v) \rightarrow R(v, v))$.

13. In the psychological literature one may sometimes find a superficially similar distinction between descriptive and deontic conditionals. See, e.g., Oaksford and Chater [205], who conceive of a deontic conditional as material implication plus an added numerical utility function. The preceding proposal introduces a much more radical distinction in logical form.

14. Emphasis added.

In this case the worlds $(K, 4)$ and $(K, 7)$ are both non-ideal counterparts to the partial world K, and similarly for the partial world 7. In other words, no completion of K or 7 can be ideal, and therefore the subject has to turn only A and 4, to see whether perhaps *these* worlds are ideal.

Domains

Above we have seen that subjects may be in doubt about the structure of the relevant model: whether it consists of cards, or of cards plus a distinguished predicate. An orthogonal issue is, which set of cards should form the domain of the model. The experimenter intends the domain to be the set of four cards. The subjects may not grasp this; indeed there are good reasons why they shouldn't. Section 3.5.2 gives some reasons why natural language use suggests considering larger domains, of which the four cards shown are only a sample, and it presents a dialogue with a subject who has a probabilistic concept of truth that comes naturally with this interpretation of the domain.

Other Logical Forms

Some subjects believe a conditional allows exceptions, and cannot be falsified by a single counterexample (see section 3.5.2). These subjects' concept of conditional is more adequately captured by the following pair of statements

1. $p \wedge \neg e \rightarrow q$

2. $p' \wedge \neg q' \rightarrow e$

Here e is a proposition letter standing for "exception," whose defining clause is (2). (In the second rule, we use p', q' rather than p, q to indicate that perhaps only some, but not all, cards which satisfy p but not q qualify as bona fide exceptions.) Condition (1) then says that the rule applies only to nonexceptional cards. There are no clear falsifying conditions for conditionals allowing exceptions, so (1) and (2) are best viewed as premises. This of course changes the task, which is now seen as identifying the exceptions. These robust default conditionals were mentioned above in chapter 2, section 2.3 and will be used below in chapter 7 to model discourse interpretation in the suppression task.

This concludes our survey of what is involved in assigning logical form in this task. We now turn to the demonstrations that subjects are indeed troubled by the different ways in which they can set the parameters, and that clearer task instructions can lead to fewer possibilities for the settings.

3.5   Giving Subjects a Voice

A standard selection task experiment consists in giving subjects a form which contains the instructions and shows four cards; the subjects then have to mark the cards they want to select. The type of data obtainable in this way is highly abstracted from the reasoning process. The subjects' approach to the task may be superficial in the sense of not engaging any reasoning or comprehension process which would be engaged in plausible real-world communication with the relevant conditionals.   One loses information about subjects' vacillations (which can be very marked) and thus one has little idea at what moment of their deliberations subjects make a choice. It is also possible that the same answer may be given for very different reasons. Furthermore, the design implies that the number of acceptable answers is restricted; for instance, some subjects are inclined to give an answer such as "A or 4," or "any card," or "can't say, because it depends on the outcomes," and clearly the standard design leaves no room for such answers. Early on, Wason and Johnson-Laird [297] investigated the relationship between insight and reasoning by also using dialogue protocols. They distinguished two kinds of feedback: (1) feedback from hypothetical turnings –"suppose there is an A on the back of the 7, what would you then conclude about the rule?"; (2) actual feedback in which the subject turns the 7 card and finds the A – "are you happy that you did/didn't select the 7 card?." It seems to us that this type of design is much more conducive to obtaining information about the whys and wherefores of subjects' answers.

We report here excerpts from Socratic tutorial dialogues with subjects engaged in the task, to illustrate the kinds of problems subjects experience.[15] Observational studies of externalized reasoning can provide prima facie evidence that these problems actually are real problems for subjects, although there is, of course, the possibility that externalizing changes the task. Only a controlled experiment can provide evidence that the predicted mental processes actually do take place when subjects reason in the original noninteractive task. A controlled experiment whose hypotheses derive from a combination of the present material with a logical analysis will be reported in the next chapter.

We present these observations of dialogues in the spirit of providing plausibility for our semantically based predictions. We assure the reader that they are representative of episodes in the dialogues – not one-offs. But rather than turn these observations into a quantitative study of the dialogues which would still only bear on this externalized task, we prefer to use them to illustrate and motivate our subsequent experimental manipulations which do bear directly on the original task. We acknowledge that we cannot be certain that our interpretations of the dialogues are correct representations of mental processes – the

---

15. Some of these excerpts were reported in [264] and [265]. Others come from a tutorial experiment performed by the our student Marian Counihan.

reader will often have alternative suggestions. Nevertheless, we feel that the combination of rich naturalistic, albeit selective observations with controlled experimental data is more powerful than either would be on its own. At the very least, the dialogues strongly suggest that there are multiple possible confusions, and often multiple reasons for making the very same response, and so counsel against homogeneous explanations.

As an appetiser we present two examples of dialogues, both of kinds observed by Wason. The first example would be considered a case of "irrationality" by Wason (but not by us), the second shows a possibly related and initially perplexing dissociation between logical evaluation and selection of cards which Wason also found striking.

The first example shows that subjects may fail to understand the implication of the 7/A combination. Here, as in the sequel, we denote by "7/A" the card which has 7 on the visible face and A on the invisible back.

> *Subject* 14
> S. I would just be interested in As and 4s, couldn't be more than that.
> E. So now let's turn the cards, starting from right to left. [Subject turns 7 to find A.]
> E. Your comments?
> S. It could be an A, but it could be something else. E. So what does this tell you about the rule?
> S. About the rule . . . that if there is an A then maybe there is a 7 on the other side.
> E. So there was a 7.
> S. But it doesn't affect the rule.

The second example shows that a subject sometimes hypothesises (or discovers) an A on the back of the 7, and notes that this would mean the rule was false of the card, but then declines to choose the card (or revise an earlier failure to choose it).

> *Subject* 3
> E. OK. Lastly the 7.
> S. Well I wouldn't pick it.
> E. But what would it mean if you did?
> S. Well, if there is an A then that would make the rule false, and if there was a K, it wouldn't make any difference to the rule.

Following the theory outlined in chapter 2 and section 3.3, we view these confusions as a consequence of subjects' trying to fix one of the many parameters involved in deciding upon a logical form. Here is a list of the interpretational problems faced by subjects, as witnessed by the experimental protocols. Illustrations will be provided below.

What is truth?
 What is falsity?
 Pragmatics: the authority of the source of the rule
 Rules and exceptions

Reasoning and planning
Interaction between interpretation and reasoning
Truth of the rule vs. "truth" for a case
Cards as viewed as a sample from a larger domain
 Obtaining evidence for the rule vs. evaluation of the cards
Existential import of the conditional
Subjects' understanding of propositional connectives generally

Interestingly, most of these problems simply cannot occur on a deontic interpretation of the task, and we take this to be the reason why performance on this task is so much 'better' than on the descriptive task.

3.5.1 The Design of the Tutorial Experiment: High-Energy Phenomenology[16]

The experiment to be reported in the next section[17] consisted of two parts. First we gave subjects a booklet with the standard Wason task and the two–rule task (for which see below), which also contained a so–called *paraphrase* task, in which the subjects were asked to judge entailment relations between sentences involving propositional connectives and quantifiers. This task continues the classical work of Fillenbaum [82] on subjects' understandings of natural language connectives. For example, the subject could be given the sentence "if a card has a vowel on one side, it has an even number on the other side," and then be asked to judge whether "every card which has a vowel on one side, has an even number on the other side" follows from the given sentence. This example is relatively innocuous,[18] but we will see below that these judgments can be logically startling. The results of this task gave us some information about subjects' understanding of logical connectives, which could then be related to their performance in the selection task.

The second part of the experiment consisted of a series of dialogues with the subject while she or he was engaged in solving the Wason task or one of its variants. The dialogues were recorded on video and transcribed. In the case of the standard task, the setup was as follows. The subject received a form giving the same instructions as we saw in figure 3.1, except that the pictures of the card were replaced by real cards, again showing A,K, 4, and 7. We first asked the subjects to select cards. We then asked them to reflect on what might be on the other side, given the instructions, and to evaluate the imagined outcomes with respect to the truth–value of the rule. Subjects were then allowed to revise

---

16. We first came across this phrase in an ad for a physics job, but it seemed to capture the feeling of Wason's materials scattering into a thousand interpretations when they impinged on the subjects' expectations, as well as the amount of effort expended by both E and S in struggling to understand events.
17. The experiment was performed in 1999 in Edinburgh by us together with Magda Osman.
18. Although not quite, as it brings to the fore issues about the existential import of the conditional, to which we will return in section 3.5.6.

their initial selection. Lastly, we asked them to turn each card and to explain to us what the result implies for the truth–value of the rule. We also followed this procedure for variants of the standard task, such as the one explained next.

A Two–Rule Task

This task, whose standard form is given as figure 3.2, is the first in a series of manipulations which try to alleviate some of the difficulties subjects have in interpreting the task. The classical logical competence model specifies that cor-

> Below is depicted a set of four cards, of which you can see only the exposed face but not the hidden back. On each card, there is an 8 or a 3 on one of its sides and a U or I on the other.
>
> Also below there are two rules which apply only to the four cards. It is given that exactly one rule is true. Your task is to decide which if any of these four cards you *must* turn in order to decide which rule is true. Don't turn unnecessary cards. Tick the cards you want to turn.
>
> 1. *If there is a U on one side, then there is an 8 on the other side.*
>
> 2. *If there is an I on one side, then there is an 8 on the other side.*

Cards:

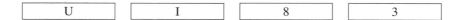

| U | I | 8 | 3 |

Figure 3.2   Two–rule task.

rect performance is to turn just the 3 card. We conjectured that explicitly telling the subject that one rule is true and one false, should background a number of issues concerned with the notion of truth, such as the possibility of the rule withstanding exceptions. The experimental manipulation turned out to be un-expectedly fruitful; while struggling through the task, subjects made comments very suggestive of where their difficulties lay. Below we give excerpts from the tutorial dialogues which highlight these difficulties. In the tutorial version of this experiment, subjects were presented with real cards lying in front of them on the table. The cards shown were U, I, 8 and 3. In this case, both U and I carried an 8, 8 carried an I, and 3 a U.

The task is pragmatically somewhat peculiar in that the two rules different in the antecedent, not the consequent, and are still said to be mutually exclusive. Naturally occurring mutually exclusive rules seem to have the same antecedent but different consequents. The antecedent of a conditional often acts as a topic (in the linguistic sense), and the two conditionals then say something different of this topic. It is much less common to have two topics, each corresponding to an antecedent. Occasionally one therefore observes pragmatic normalization in the dialogues, which inverts the conditionals to "if 8 then U" and "if 8 then I."

We are now in a position to present subjects' musings, insights and perplexities while working through the various tasks.

3.5.2 Subjects' Understanding of Truth and Falsity

'Truth' and 'falsity' are among the most important parameters to be set, and the reader should recall from chapter 2 that they can be set independently: only classical logic forces "not true" to be the same as "false." This stipulation corresponds to a definition of semantics, in which one defines only "true on a model" ($\models$), not "false on model" ($\not\models$). It is, however, equally possible to give a recursive definition of semantics in which $\models$ and $\not\models$ are defined by simultaneous recursion. We therefore give 'true' and 'false' separate headings.

The Logic of 'True'

On a classical understanding of the two–rule task, the competence answer is to turn the 3; this would show which one of the rules is false, hence classically also which one is true. This classical understanding should be enforced by explicitly instructing the subjects that one rule is true and the other one false. Semantically this means, for a given model $\mathcal{A}$ that if not $\mathcal{A} \not\models p \rightarrow q$, then $\mathcal{A} \models p \rightarrow q$. Interestingly, some subjects refuse to be moved by the explicit instruction, insisting that "not-false" is not the same as "true." These subjects are thus guided by some nonclassical logic.

> *Subject* 17.
> *S.* [Writes miniature truth–tables under the cards.]
> *E.* OK. so if you found an I under the 3, you put a question mark for rule 1, and rule 2 is false; if you turned the 3 and found a U, then rule 1 is false and rule 2 is a question mark. So you want to turn 3 or not?
> *S.* No.
> *E.* Let's actually try doing it. [First] turn over the U ... you find a 3, which rule is true and which rule is false?
> *S.* (Long pause)
> *E.* Are we none the wiser?
> *S.* No, there's a question mark.
> *E.* It could have helped us, but it didn't help us?
> *S.* Yes.
> ⋮
> *E.* OK, and the 3.
> *S.* Well if there is a U then that one is disproved [pointing to the first rule] and if there is an I then that one is disproved [pointing to the second rule]. But neither rule can be proved by 3.
> ⋮

E. Turn over the last card [3] and see what's on the back of it... so it's a U. What does that tell us about the rule?
S. That rule 1 is false and it doesn't tell us anything about rule 2?
E. Can't you tell anything about rule 2?
S. No.

The subject thinks falsifying rule 1 does not suffice and now looks for additional evidence to support rule 2. In the end she chooses the 8 card for this purpose, which is of course not the competence answer even when "not-false" is not equated with "true" (this answer may reflect the pragmatic normalization of the two conditionals referred to above). Here are two more examples of the same phenomenon.

> *Subject 8.*
> *S.* I wouldn't look at this one [3] because it wouldn't give me appropriate information about the rules; it would only tell me if those rules are wrong, and I am being asked which of those rules is the correct one. Does that make sense?

> *Subject 5.*
> *E.* What about if there was a 3?
> *S.* A 3 on the other side of that one [U]. Then this [rule 1] isn't true.
> *E.* It doesn't say...?
> *S.* It doesn't say anything about this one [rule 2].
> *E.* And the I?
> *S.* If there is a 3, then this one [rule 2] isn't true, and it doesn't say anything about that one [rule 1].

The same problem is of course present in the standard Wason task as well, albeit in a less explicit form. If the cards are A, K, 4, and 7, then turning A and 7 suffices to verify that the rule is not false; but the subject may wonder whether it is therefore true. For instance, if the concept of truth of a conditional involves attributing a law-like character to the conditional, then the absence of counterexamples does not suffice to establish truth; a further causal connection between antecedent and consequent is necessary.[19] Since the truth of $p \rightarrow q$ cannot be established on the model w in W_4, the semantics implicitly adopted by these subjects for $p \rightarrow q$ is a form of intensional semantics, following the terminology introduced in chapter 2. That is, to determine $w \models p \rightarrow q$ one has to refer to information extraneous to w, for example a much larger population of cards. A subject faced with this difficulty will be unable to solve the task as given, because of lacking information.

Let us note here that this difficulty is absent in the case of deontic rules such as

If you drink alcohol in this bar, you have to be over 18.

---

19. Such a causal connection is present in the "production line scenarios" which ask the subject to imagine that there is a machine producing cards which on one side ..., etc.

Such a rule cannot, and in fact need not, be shown to be true by examining cases; its truth is given, and the subjects need only establish that it is not violated. So in the deontic case, subjects have no worries about the meaning of "truth."

Another twist to the concept of truth was given by those subjects, who, when reading the rule(s) aloud, actually inserted a modality in the conditional:

> *Subject* 13. [Standard Wason task]
> *S.* ...if there is an A, then there is a 4, necessarily the 4...[somewhat later]...if there is an A on one side, necessarily a 4 on the other side....

If truth involves necessity, then the absence of counterexamples is not sufficient for truth. Again this leads to an intensional semantics for $p \rightarrow q$.

The Logic of 'False'

Interesting things happen when one asks subjects to meditate on what it could mean for a conditional to be false. As indicated above, the logic of "true" need not determine the logic of "false" completely; it is possible to give a separate definition of $w \not\models p \rightarrow q$.

The paraphrase task alluded to above showed that a conditional $p \rightarrow q$ being false is often ($> 50\%$) interpreted as $p \rightarrow \neg q$! (We will refer to this property as *strong falsity*.) This observation is not ours alone: Fillenbaum [82] observed that in 60% of the cases the negation of a causal temporal conditional $p \rightarrow q$ ("if he goes to Amsterdam, he will get stoned") is taken to be $p \rightarrow \neg q$; for contingent universals (conditionals, such as the rule in the selection task, where there is no salient connection between antecedent and consequent) the proportion is 30%. In our experiment the latter proportion is even higher. Here is an example of a subject using strong falsity when asked to imagine what could be on the other side of a card.

> *Subject* 26 [Standard Wason task; subject has chosen strong falsity in paraphrase task]
> *E.* So you're saying that if the statement is true, then the number [on the back of A] will be 4. ...What would happen if the statement were false?
> *S.* Then it would be a number other than 4.

Note that strong falsity encapsulates a concept of necessary connection between antecedent and consequent in the sense that even counterexamples are no mere accidents, but are governed by a rule. If a subject believes that true and false in this situation are exhaustive (i.e., that the logic is bivalent), this could reflect a conviction that the cards have been laid out according to *some* rule, instead of randomly. It is interesting to see what this interpretation means for card choices in the selection tasks. If a subject has strong falsity and applies the (classical) tautology $(p \rightarrow q) \vee (p \rightarrow \neg q)$, then (in the standard Wason task) *either* of the cards $A, 4$ can show that $p \rightarrow q$ is not-false, hence true. Unfortunately, in the standard setup 'either of A, 4' is not a possible response offered.

In the tutorial experiment involving the two–rule task subjects were at liberty to make such choices. In this case strong falsity has the effect of turning each of the two rules into a biconditional, "U if and only if 8" and "I if and only if 8" respectively. *Any* card now distinguishes between the two rules, and we do indeed find subjects emphatically making this choice:

> *Subject* 10
> *E.* OK, so you want to revise your choice or do you want to stick with the 8?
> *S.* No no . . . I might turn all of them.
> *E.* You want to turn all of them?
> *S.* No no no just one of them, any of them.

Perhaps the customary choice of p, q in the standard task is the projection of "either of p, q" onto the given possibilities. These considerations just serve to highlight the possibility that a given choice of cards is made for very different reasons by different subjects, so that by itself statistical information on the different card choices in the standard task must be interpreted with care.

Truth and Satisfaction

Subjects are persistently confused about several notions of truth that could possibly be involved. The intended interpretation is that the domain of discourse consists of the four cards shown, and that the truth–value of the rule is to be determined with respect to that domain. This interpretation is, however, remarkably difficult to get at. An alternative interpretation is that the domain is some indefinitely large population of cards, of which the four cards shown are just a sample; this is the intuition that lies behind Oaksford and Chater's Bayesian approach [205]. We will return to this interpretation in section 3.5.2 below. The other extreme is that each card defines a domain of its own: each card is to be evaluated against the rule independently.

This interpretation is the one suited to deontic conditionals, though it is also possible with descriptive interpretations and is sometimes encouraged by "seek violations" instructions (see [308]). What is perhaps most tantalizing reading the early literature on the task is how little the experimenters themselves noticed that deontic interpretation was critical. There was a good deal of attention to the effects of "seek violators" instructions, but these were interpreted against the background of Wason's focus on falsification, not on their effect of making the cards independent of each other, or of removing the ambiguity between judging the cases and judging the truth of the rule.

An intermediate position is that there are cards which by themselves suffice to determine the truth–value of the rule; we saw an instance of this while discussing examples of "strong falsity," where the A and 4 cards are each decisive. The phenomenon may be more general, however, a failure to appreciate the relativity of the relation "the rule is true of the card." That is, even if a card satisfies the rule (what we called 'support' in section 3.4.1), it need not make it true.

> *Subject* 10.
> *E.* If you found an 8 on this card [I], what would it say?
> *S.* It would say that rule 2 is true, and if the two cannot be true then rule 1 is wrong....(Subject turns 8.)
> *E.* OK. so it's got an I on the back, what does that mean?
> *S.* It means that rule 2 is true.
> *E.* Are you sure?
> *S.* I'm just thinking whether they are exclusive, yes because if there is an I then there is an 8. Yes, yes, it must be that.

One experimental manipulation in the tutorial dialogue for the two–rule task addressed this problem by making subjects first turn U and I, to find 8 on the back of both. This caused great confusion, because the subjects' logic (equating truth with satisfaction) led them to conclude that therefore both rules must be true, contradicting the instruction.

> *Subject* 18 [Initial choice was 8].
> *E.* Start with the U, turn that over.
> *S.* U goes with 8.
> *E.* OK. now turn the I over.
> *S.* Oh God, I shouldn't have taken that card, the first ...
> *E.* You turned it over and there was an 8.
> *S.* There was an 8 on the other side, U and 8. If there is an I there is an 8, so they are both true. [Makes a gesture that the whole thing should be dismissed.]

> *Subject* 28.
> *E.* OK, turn them.
> *S.* [turns U, finds 8] So rule 1 is true.
> *E.* OK, for completeness' sake let's turn the other cards as well.
> *S.* OK. so in this instance if I had turned that one [I] first then rule 2 would be true and rule 1 would be disproved. Either of these is different. [U or I]
> *E.* What does that actually mean, because we said that only one of the rules could be true? Exactly one is true.
> *S.* These cards are not consistent with these statements here.

On the other hand, subjects who ultimately got the two–rule task right also appeared to have an insight into the intended relation between rule and cards.

> *Subject* 6.
> *E.* So say there were a U on the back of the 8, then what would this tell you?
> *S.* I'm not sure where the 8 comes in because I don't know if that would make the U one right, because it is the opposite way around. If I turned that one [pointing to the U] just to see if there was an 8, if there was an 8 it doesn't mean that rule 2 is not true.

We claim that part of the difficulty of the standard task involving a descriptive rule is the possibility of confusing the two relations between rule and cards.

Transferring the "truth of the card" to the "truth of the rule" may be related to what Wason called "verification bias," but it seems to cut deeper. One way to transfer the perplexity unveiled in the above excerpts to the standard task would be to do a tutorial experiment where the A has a 4 on the back, and the 7 an A. If a subject suffering from a confusion about the relation between cards and rule turns the A and finds 4, he should conclude that the rule is true, only to be rudely disabused upon turning 7.

It is clear that for a deontic rule no such confusion can arise, because the truth–value of the rule is not an issue.

Exceptions and Brittleness

The concept of truth Wason intended is that of "true without exceptions," what we call a brittle interpretation of the conditional. It goes without saying that this is not how a conditional is generally interpreted in real life. And we do find subjects who struggle with the required transition from a notion of truth which is compatible with exceptions, to exceptionless truth.

In terms of logical form, this is the issue of the formal expression into which the natural language conditional is translated. As we observed in section 3.4, the proper formal correlate is a formula $p \wedge \neg e \rightarrow q$, where e is a proposition letter denoting an exceptional state of affairs, which can be given further content by a clause of the form "$\ldots \rightarrow e$."

> *Subject* 18.
> *S*. [Turns 3 and finds U] OK.. well no...well that could be an exception you see.
> *E*. The U?
> *S*. The U could be an exception to the other rule.
> *E*. To the first rule?
> *S*. Yes, it could be an exception.
> *E*. So could you say anything about the rule based on this? Say, on just having turned the U and found a 3?
> *S*. Well yes, it could be a little exception, but it does disprove the rule so you'd have to...
> *E*. You'd have to look at the other ones?
> *S*. Yes.

Similarly in the standard Wason task:

> *Subject* 18.
> *S*. If I just looked at that one on its own [7/A] I would say that it didn't fit the rule, and that I'd have to turn that one [A] over, and if that was different [i.e., if there wasn't an even number] then I would say the rule didn't hold.
> *E*. So say you looked at the 7 and you turned it over and you found an A, then?
> *S*. I would have to turn the other cards over ...well it could be just an exception to the rule so I would have to turn over the A.

Clearly, if a counterexample is not sufficient evidence that the rule is false, then it is dubious whether card turnings can prove the rule to be true or false at all. Subjects may accordingly be confused about how to interpret the instructions of the experiment. In our data, the term "(possible) exception" was reserved for the $\neg q$ card; the p card qualified as a potential falsifier. We have no explanation for this phenomenon, but if it is pervasive, it would give yet another reason why subjects don't bother to look at the $\neg q$ card, even when they are clear about its logical meaning.

The Cards as Sample

Above we noted that there are problems concerning the domain of interpretation of the conditional rule. The intended interpretation is that the rule applies only to the four cards shown. However, the semantics of conditionals is such that they tend to apply to an open-ended domain of cases. This can best be seen in contrasting universal quantification with the natural language conditional. Universal quantification is equally naturally used in framing contingent contextually determined statements as open-ended generalizations. So, to develop Goodman's example [102], "All the coins in my pocket this morning are copper" is a natural way to phrase a local generalization with a fixed enumerable domain of interpretation. However, "If a coin is in my pocket this morning, it's copper" is a distinctly unnatural way of phrasing the same claim. The latter even invites the fantastical interpretation that if a silver coin were put in my pocket this morning it would become copper – that is an interpretation in which a larger open-ended domain of objects is in play.

Similarly in the case of the four–card task, the clause that "the rule applies only to the four cards" has to be explicitly included. One may question whether subjects take this clause on board, since this interpretation is an unnatural one for the conditional. It is further unnatural to call the sentence a *rule* if its application is so local. Formally, this means that the set W of possible worlds introduced in section 3.4.1 must be replaced by a much richer structure.

A much more natural interpretation is that the four cards are a sample from a larger population. Indeed this is the point of purchase of Oaksford and Chater's proposals [205] that performance is driven by subjects' assumptions about the larger domain of interpretation. Some subjects raise this issue explicitly.

> *Subject* 3.[20] [in standard Wason task; has chosen A, 4.]
> *S.* Well in that case you would have to turn all the cards, if you couldn't work with just a start point. Because then if you turned.... take a random set of cards, imagine a random set of cards. If you had three A faces, and five 7 faces, but you couldn't have any assumption that that was a starting point, you would have to turn all the cards, because then you might get a 60%, 40% divide, and you would have to take an average, and say the rule isn't right, but the majority of cards suggest that if there's an A on one side then there's a 4. A likelihood, in that case.

---

20. In Marian Counihan's experiment.

E. But if there was a likelihood, what would that mean?

S. It wouldn't be a rule, it would be invalidated.

Here is another subject who thinks that truth or falsity can only be established by (crude) probabilistic considerations.

> *Subject* 26.
>
> *S.* [has turned U,I, found an 8 on the back of both] I can't tell which one is true.
>
> *E.* OK, let's continue turning.
>
> *S.* [turns 3] OK, that would verify rule 2. [...] Well, there are two cards that verify rule 2, and only one card so far that verifies rule 1. Because if this [3] were verifying rule 1, it should be an I on the other side.
>
> *E.* Let's turn [the 8].
>
> *S.* OK, so that says that rule 2 is true as well, three of the cards verify rule 2 and only one verifies rule 1.
>
> *E.* So you decide by majority.
>
> *S.* Yes, the majority suggests rule 2.

It is interesting that 3/U is described as *verifying* rule 2, rather than *falsifying* rule 1; U→8 is never ruled out:

> *S.* It's not completely false, because there is one card that verifies rule 1.

Asked to describe her thought processes, the subject later comments

> *S.* Well, when there's two rules then you can't say that they should both be true because they are mutually exclusive ... so depending on which way the cards are there is basically a 50 per cent probability that either one is going to be true. ... With one rule I think it will be true or if it wouldn't be true, then it seems more likely that it would be true.

3.5.3   Dependencies between Card Choices

The tutorial dialogues suggest that part of the difficulty of the selection task consists in having to choose a card *without being able to inspect what is on the other side of the card*. This difficulty can only be made visible in the dialogues because there the subject is confronted with real cards, which she is not allowed to turn at first. It then becomes apparent that some subjects would prefer to solve the problem by "reactive planning," i.e., by first choosing a card, turning it, and deciding what to do based on what is on the other side. This source of difficulty is obscured by the standard format of the experiment. The form invites the subjects to think of the cards depicted as real cards, but at the same time the answer should be given on the basis of the representation of the cards on the form, i.e., with inherently unknowable backs. The instruction "Tick the cards you want to turn ..." clearly does not allow the subject to return a reactive plan.

The tutorials amply show that dependencies are a source of difficulty. Here is an excerpt from a tutorial dialogue in the two–rule condition.

Subject 1.
E. Same for the I, what if there is an 8 on the back?
S. If there is an 8 on the back, then it means that rule 2 is right and rule one is wrong.
E. So do we turn over the I or not?
S. Yes. Unless I've turned the U already.

And in a standard Wason task:

Subject 10.
S. OK, so if there is a vowel on this side then there is an even number, so I can turn A to find out whether there is an even number on the other side or I can turn the 4 to see if there is a vowel on the other side.
E. So would you turn over the other cards? Do you need to turn over the other cards?
S. I think it just depends on what you find on the other side of the card. No I wouldn't turn them.
$\vdots$

E. If you found a K on the back of the 4?
S. Then it would be false.
$\vdots$

S. But if that doesn't disclude [*sic*] then I have to turn another one.
E. So you are inclined to turn this over [the A] because you wanted to check?
S. Yes, to see if there is an even number.
E. And you want to turn this over [the 4]?
S. Yes, to check if there is a vowel, but if I found an odd number [on the back of the A], then I don't need to turn this [the 4].
E. So you don't want to turn . . .
S. Well, I'm confused again because I don't know what's on the back, I don't know if this one . . .
E. We're only working hypothetically now.
S. Oh well, then only one of course, because if the rule applies to the whole thing then one would test it.
$\vdots$

E. What about the 7?
S. Yes, the 7 could have a vowel, then that would prove the whole thing wrong. So that's what I mean, do you turn one at a time or do you . . . ?
$\vdots$

E. Well if you needed to know beforehand, without having turned these over, so you think to yourself I need to check whether the rule holds, so what cards do I need to turn over? You said you would turn over the A and the 4.
S. Yes, but if these are right, say if this [the A] has an even number and this has a vowel [the 4], then I might be wrong in saying "Oh it's fine," so this could have an odd number [the K] and this a vowel [the 7] so in that case I need to turn them all.
E. You'd turn all of them over? Just to be sure?
S. Yes.

Once one has understood Wason's intention in specifying the task, it is easy to assume that it is obvious that the experimenter intends subjects to decide what cards to turn *before* any information is gained from any turnings. Alternatively, and equivalently, the instructions can be interpreted to be to assume the minimal possible information gain from turnings. However, the obviousness of these interpretations is possibly greater in hindsight, and so we set out to test whether they are a source of difficulty in the task. Note that no contingencies of choice can arise if the relation between rule and cards is interpreted deontically. Whether one case obeys the law is unconnected to whether any other case does. Hence the planning problem indicated above cannot arise for a deontic rule, which might be one explanation for the good performance in that case.

In this connection it may be of interest to consider the so-called *reduced array selection task*, or RAST for short, due to Wason and Green [296] and discussed extensively by Margolis [182]. In its barest outline[21] the idea of the RAST is to remove the p and $\neg p$ cards from the array of cards shown to the subject, thus leaving only q and $\neg q$. The p and $\neg p$ cards cause no trouble in the standard task in the sense that p is chosen almost always, and $\neg p$ almost never, so one would expect that their deletion would cause little change in the response frequencies for the remaining cards. Surprisingly, howevers, the frequency of the $\neg q$ response increases dramatically. From our point of view, this result is less surprising, because without the possibility to choose p, dependencies between card choices can no longer arise. This is not to say that this is the only difficulty the RAST removes.

Getting Evidence for the Rule vs. Evaluation of the Cards

A related planning problem, which can, however, occur only on a nonstandard logical understanding of the problem, is the following. Some subjects interpret the instruction not to choose unnecessary cards as the injunction not to choose a card whose turning may yield a nondecisive outcome.

In a few early tutorial dialogues involving the two–rule experiment, the background rule incorrectly failed to specify that the cards have one side either U or I and on the other side either 3 or 8, owing to an error in the instructions. In this case the competence response is not to turn 3 only, but to turn U, I, and 3. But several subjects did not want to choose the 3 for the following reason.

> *Subject* 7.
> *S.* Then I was wondering whether to choose the numbers. Well, I don't think so because there might be other letters [than U,I] on the other side. There could be totally different letters.
> *E.* You can't be sure?
> *S.* I can't be sure. I can only be sure if there is a U or an I on the other side. So this is not very efficient and this [3] does not give me any information. But I could turn the U or the I.

---

21. The actual experimental setup is much more complicated and not quite comparable to the experiments reported here.

Apparently the subject thinks that he can choose between various sets of cards, each sufficient, and the choice should be as parsimonious as possible in the sense that every outcome of a turning must be relevant. To show that this is not an isolated phenomenon, here is a subject engaged in a standard Wason task:

Subject 5.
E So you would pick the A and you would pick the 4. And lastly the 7?
S. That's irrelevant.
E. So why do you think it's irrelevant?
S. Let me see again. Oh wait, so that could be an A or a K again [writing the options for the back of 7 down], so if the 7 would have an A then that would prove me wrong. But if it would have a K then that wouldn't tell me anything.
E. So?
S. So these two [pointing to A and 4] give me more information, I think.
E. . . . You can turn over those two [A and 4].
S. [turns over the A]
E. So what does that say?
S. That it's wrong.
E. And that one [4]?
S. That it's wrong.
E. Now turn over those two [K and 7].
S. [Turning over the K] It's a K and 4. Doesn't say anything about this [pointing to the rule]. [After turning over the 7] Aha.
E. So that says the rule is . . . ?
S. That the rule is wrong. But I still wouldn't turn this over, still because I wouldn't know if it would give an A, it could give me an a K and that wouldn't tell me anything.
E. But even though it could potentially give you an A on the back of it like this one has.
S. Yes, but that's just luck. I would have more chance with these two [referring to the A and the 4].

These subjects have no difficulty evaluating the meaning of the possible outcomes of turning 3 (in the two–rule task), or 7 (in the standard Wason task), but their choice is also informed by other considerations, in particular a perceived tradeoff between the 'information value' of a card and the penalty incurred by choosing it. Here is a subject very explicit about the trade-off.

Subject 3. [Standard Wason task; he realises the meaning of the 7 card, but that doesn't change his choice of only A]
S.... if there's an A on this side (pointing to the underside of the 7), it would invalidate the rule.
E. OK. So would that mean that you should turn the 7, or not?
S. Well you could turn the 7, but it says don't turn any cards you don't have to, and you only have to turn the A.
E. OK. So the 7 could have an A on it, which would invalidate the rule, but..
S. [interrupting] It could have, but it could also have a K on it, so if you turned that [the 7]) and it had a K, it would make no difference to the rule, and you would have turned a card that was unnecessary, which it says not to do.
E. But what if it had an A on it?
S. But what if it had a K on it?

Of course this does not yet explain the observed evaluation of the 4/K card as showing that the rule is wrong, and simultaneously taking the K/4 card to be irrelevant. The combined evaluations seem to rule out a straightforward biconditional interpretation of the conditional, and also the explanation of the choice of 4 as motivated by a search for confirmatory evidence for the rule, as Wason would have it. This pattern of evaluations is not an isolated phenomenon, so an explanation would be most welcome. Even without such an explanation it is clear that the problem indicated, how to maximise information gain from turnings, cannot play a role in the case of deontic conditionals, since the status of the rule is not an issue.

3.5.4   The Pragmatics of the Descriptive Selection Task.

The descriptive task demands that subjects seek evidence for the truth of a statement which comes from the experimenter. The experimenter can safely be assumed to know what is on the back of the cards. If the rule is false its appearance on the task sheet amounts to the utterance, by the experimenter, of a knowing falsehood, possibly with intention to deceive. It is an active possibility that doubting the experimenter's veracity is a socially uncomfortable thing to do.

Quite apart from the possible sociopsychological effects of discomfort, the communication situation in this task is bizarre. The subject is first given one rule to the effect that the cards have letters on one side and numbers on the other. This rule they are supposed to take on trust. Then they are given another rule by the same information source and they are supposed *not* to trust it but seek evidence for its falsity. If they do not continue to trust the first rule, then their card selections should diverge from Wason's expectations. If they simply forget about the background rule, the proper card choice would be A,K, and 7; and if they want to test the background rule as well as the foreground rule, they would have to turn *all* cards. Notice that with the deontic interpretation, this split communication situation does not arise. The law stands and the task is to decide whether some people other than the source obey it. Here is an example of a subject who takes both rules on trust:

> *Subject* 3. [Standard Wason task; has chosen A and 4]
> *E.* Why pick those cards and not the other cards?
> *S.* Because they are mentioned in the rule and I am assuming that the rule is true.

Another subject was rather bewildered when upon turning A he found a 7:

> *Subject* 8.
> *S.* Well there is something in the syntax with which I am not clear because it does not say that there is an exclusion of one thing, it says "if there is an A on one side there is a 4 on the other side." So the rule is wrong.
> *E.* This [pointing to A] shows that the rule is wrong.
> *S.* Oh, so the rule is wrong, it's not something I am missing.

Although this may sound similar to Wason's "verification bias," it is actually very different. Wason assumed that subjects would be in genuine doubt about the truth–value of the rule, but would then proceed in an "irrational," verificationist manner to resolve the issue. What transpires here is that subjects take it on the authority of the experimenter that the rule is true, and then interpret the instructions as indicating those cards which are evidence of this.

> *Subject* 22.
> S. Well, my immediate [inaudible] first time was to assume that this is a true statement, therefore you only want to turn over the card that you think will satisfy the statement.

The communicative situation of the two–rule task is already much less bizarre, since there is no longer any reason to doubt the veracity of the experimenter. The excerpts also suggest that a modified standard task in which the rule is attributed not to the experimenter but to an unreliable source might increase the number of competence responses. It hardly needs emphasising anymore that these problems cannot arise in the case of a deontic rule.

3.5.5 Interaction between Interpretation and Reasoning

The tutorial dialogues reveal another important source of confusion, namely the interpretation of the anaphoric expression "one side ... other side" and its interaction with the direction of the conditional. The trouble with "one side ... other side" is that in order to determine the referent of "other side," one must have kept in memory the referent of "one side." That may seem harmless enough, but in combination with the various other problems identified here, it may prove too much. Even apart from limitations of working memory, subjects may have a nonintended interpretation of "one side ... other side," wherein "one side" is interpreted as "*visible* side" (the front, or face of the card) and "other side" is interpreted as "*invisible* side" (the back of the card). The expression "one side ... other side" is then interpreted as deictic, not as anaphoric. That is, both "one side" and "other side" can be identified by direct pointing, whereas in the case of an anaphoric relationship the referent of "other side" depends on that of "one side." This possibility was investigated by Gebauer and Laming [92], who argue that deictic interpretation of "one side ... other side" and a biconditional interpretation of the conditional, both singly and in combination, are prevalent, persistently held, and consistently reasoned with. Gebauer and Laming present the four cards of the standard task six times to each subject, pausing to actually turn cards which the subject selects, and to consider their reaction to what is found on the back. Their results show few explicitly acknowledged changes of choice, and few selections which reflect implicit changes. Subjects choose the same cards from the sixth set as they do from the first. Gebauer and Laming argue that the vast majority of the choices accord with normative reasoning from one of the four combinations of interpretation achieved by permuting the conditional/biconditional with the deictic/anaphoric interpretations.[22]

We tried to find further evidence for Gebauer and Laming's view, and presented subjects with rules in which the various possible interpretations of 'one side ... other side' were spelled out explicitly; e.g., one rule was

(1)   If there is a vowel on the face of the card, then there is an even number on the back.

To our surprise, subjects seemed completely insensitive to the wording of the rule and chose according to the standard pattern whatever the formulation; for discussion see Stenning and van Lambalgen [264]. This result made us curious to see what would happen in tutorial dialogues when subjects are presented with a rule like (1), and indeed the slightly pathological (2)

(2)   If there is a vowel on the back of the card, there is an even number on the face of the card.

After having presented the subjects with these two rules, we told them that the *intended* interpretation of "one side ... other side" is that "one side" can refer to the visible face or to the invisible back. Accordingly, they now had to choose cards corresponding to

(3)   If there is a vowel on one side (face or back), then there is an even number on the other side (face or back).

We now provide a number of examples, culled from the tutorial dialogues, which demonstrate the interplay between the interpretations chosen for the anaphora and the conditional. The first example shows us a subject who explicitly changes the direction of the implication when considering the back/face anaphora, even though she is at first very well aware that the rule is not biconditional.

> *Subject* 12. [experiments (1), (2), (3)]
> *E.* The first rule says that if there is a vowel on the face of the card, so what we mean by face is the bit you can see, then there is an even number on the back of the card, so that's the bit you can't see. So which cards would you turn over to check the rule?
> *S.* Well, I just thought 4, but then it doesn't necessarily say that if there is a 4 that there is a vowel underneath. So the A.
> *E.* For this one it's the reverse, so it says if there is a vowel on the back, so the bit you can't see, there is an even number on the face; so in this sense which ones would you pick?
> *S.* [Subject ticks 4] This one.
> *E.* So why wouldn't you pick any of the other cards?

---

22. Four combinations, because the deictic back/face reading of "one side ... other side" appeared to be too implausible to be considered. But see below.

S. Because it says that if there is an even number on the face, then there is a vowel, so it would have to be one of those [referring to the numbers].

$\vdots$ [Now in the standard Wason task]

E. [This rule] says that if there is a vowel on one side of the card, either face or back, then there is an even number on the other side, either face or back.

S. I would pick that one [the A] and that one [the 4].

E. So why?

S. Because it would show me that if I turned that [pointing to the 4] over and there was an A then the 4 is true, so I would turn it over. Oh, I don't know. This is confusing me now because I know it goes only one way.

$\vdots$

S. No, I got it wrong didn't I? It is one way, so it's not necessarily that if there is an even number then there is a vowel.

The second example is of a subject who gives the normative response in experiment (3), but nonetheless goes astray when forced to consider the back/face interpretation.

Subject 4. [experiments (1), (2), (3)]

E. OK. This says that if there is a vowel on the face [pointing to the face] of the card, then there is an even number on the back of the card. How is that different to ...

S. Yes, it's different because the sides are unidirectional.

E. So would you pick different cards?

S. If there is a vowel on the face ... I think I would pick the A.

E. And for this one? [referring to the second statement] This is different again because it says if there is a vowel on the back ...

S. [completes sentence] then there is an even number on the face. I think I need to turn over the 4 and the 7. Just to see if it [the 4] has an A on the back.

E. OK. Why wouldn't you pick the rest of the cards?

S. I'm not sure, I haven't made up my mind yet. This one [the A] I don't have to turn over because it's not a vowel on the back, and the K is going to have a number on the back so that's irrelevant. This one [the 4] has to have a vowel on the back otherwise the rule is untrue. I still haven't made up my mind about this one [the 7]. Yes, I do have to turn it over because if it has a vowel on the back then it would make the rule untrue. So I think I will turn it over. I could be wrong.

[When presented with the rule where the anaphor has the intended interpretation]

S. I would turn over this one [the A] to see if there is an even number on the back and this one [the 7] to see if there was a vowel on the back.

Our third example is of a subject who explicitly states that the meaning of the implication must change when considering the back/face anaphora.

Subject 16. [experiments (1), (2), (3); subject has correctly chosen A in condition (1)]

E. The next one says that if there is a vowel on the back of the card, so that's the bit you can't see, then there is an even number on the face of the card, so that's the bit you can see; so that again is slightly different, the reverse, so what would you do?

S. Again I'd turn the 4 so that would be proof but not ultimate proof but some proof ...

E. With a similar reasoning as before?
S. Yes, I'm pretty sure what you are after . . . I think it is a bit more complicated this time, with the vowel on the back of the card and the even number, that suggests that if and only if there is an even number there can be a vowel, I think I'd turn others just to see if there was a vowel, so I think I'd turn the 7 as well.
[In condition (3) chooses A and 4]

And here is the most striking example, in which the interaction can clearly be seen to go both ways.

Subject 23. [Standard Wason task]
S. Then for this card [4/K] the statement is not true.
E. Could you give a reason why it is not?
S. Well, I guess this also assumes that the statement is reversible, and if it becomes the reverse, then instead of saying if there is an A on one side, there is a 4 on the other side, it's like saying if there was a 4 on one side, then there is an A on the other.

$$\vdots$$

E. Now we'll discuss the issue of symmetry, you said you took this to be symmetrical.
S. Well, actually it's effectively symmetrical because you've got this either exposed or hidden clause, for each part of the statement. So it's basically symmetrical.
E. But there are two levels of symmetry involved here. One level is the symmetry between visible face and invisible back, and the other aspect of symmetry is involved with the direction of the statement "if . . . then."
S. Right, OK. so I guess in terms of the "if . . . then" it is not symmetrical . . . In that case you do not need that one [4], you just need [A]. . . . [while attempting the two-rule task he makes some notes which indicate that he is still aware of the symmetry of the cards]
S. For U, if there is an 8 on the other side, then rule 1 is true, and you'd assume that rule 2 is false. And with I, if you have an 8, then rule 1 is false and rule 2 is true. . . . [the subject has turned the U and I cards, which both carry 8 on the back, and proceeds to turn the 3 and 8 cards]
S. Now the 3, it's a U and it's irrelevant because there is no reverse of the rules. And the 8, it's an I and again it's irrelevant because there is no reverse of the rules. . . . Well, my conclusion is that the framework is wrong. I suppose rules one and two really hold for the cards.
E. We are definitely convinced only one rule is true . . .
S. Well . . . say you again apply the rules, yes you could apply the rules again in a second stab for these cards [3 and 8] here.
E. What do you mean by "in a second stab?"
S. Well I was kind of assuming before you could only look at the cards once based on what side was currently shown to you. . . . This one here [8] in the previous stab was irrelevant, because it would be equivalent to the reverse side when applied to this rule, I guess now we can actually turn it over and find the 8 leads to I, and you can go to this card again [3], now we turn it over and we apply this rule again and the U does not lead to an 8 here. So if you can repeat turns rule 2 is true for all the cards.
E. You first thought this card [3] irrelevant.
S. Well it's irrelevant if you can give only one turn of the card.

What's interesting in this exchange is that in the first experiment the variable, "symmetric" reading of the anaphora seems to trigger a symmetric reading of the implication, whereas in the second experiment asymmetric readings of the anaphora and the implications are conjoined, even though he was at first aware that the intended reading of the anaphora is symmetric. (The fact that the subject wants to turn the cards twice is evidence for the constant (asymmetric) reading of the anaphora.)

We thus see that, in these subjects, the direction of the conditional is related to the particular kind of deixis assumed for "one side … other side." This shows that the process of natural language interpretation in this task need not be compositional, and that, contrary to Gebauer and Laming's claim, subjects need not have a persistent interpretation of the conditional, at least when asked to justify themselves. Two questions immediately arise:

1. Why would there be this particular interaction?

2. What does the observed interaction tell us about performance in the standard Wason task?

Question (2) can easily be answered. *If* subjects were to decompose the anaphoric expression "one side… other side" into two deictic expressions "face/back" and "back/face" and were then to proceed to reverse the direction of the implication in the latter case, they should choose the p and q cards. Also, since the expression "one side … other side" does not appear in a deontic rule such as "if you want to drink alcohol, you have to be over 18," subjects will not be distracted by this particular difficulty.

Question (1) is not answered as easily. There may be something pragmatically peculiar about a conditional of which the consequent, but not the antecedent, is known. These are often used for diagnostic purposes (also called *abduction*): if we have a rule which says "if switch 1 is down, the light is on," and we observe that the light is on, we are tempted to conclude that switch 1 must be down. This, however, is making an inference, not stating a conditional; but then subjects are perhaps not aware of the logical distinction between the two.

It is of interest that the difficulty discussed here was already identified by Wason and Green [296] albeit in slightly different terms: their focus is on the distinction between a *unified* and a *disjoint* representation of the stimulus (i.e., a card). A unified stimulus is one in which the terms referred to in the conditional cohere in some way (say as properties of the same object, or as figure and ground), whereas in a disjoint stimulus the terms may be properties of different objects, spatially separated.

Wason and Green conjectured that it is disjoint representation which accounts for the difficulty in the selection task. To test the conjecture they conducted three experiments, varying the type of unified representation. Although they use a reduced array selection task (RAST), in which one chooses only between q and $\neg q$, relative performance across their conditions can still be compared.

Their contrasting sentence rule pairs are of great interest, partly because they happen to contain comparisons of rules with and without anaphora. There are three relevant experiments numbered 2 to 4. Experiment 2 contrasts unified and disjoint representations without anaphora in either, and finds that unified rules are easier. Experiment 3 contrasts unified and disjoint representations with the disjoint rule having anaphora. Experiment 4 contrasts unified and disjoint representations but removes the anaphora from the disjoint rule while adding another source of linguistic complexity (an extra tensed verb plus pronominal anaphora) to the unified one. For a full discussion of their experiments we refer the reader to Stenning and van Lambalgen [264]; here we discuss only their experiment 2.

In experiment 2, cards show shapes (triangles, circles) and colors (black, white), and the two sentences considered are

(4)   Whenever they are triangles, they are on black cards.

(5)   Whenever there are triangles below the line, there is black above the line.

That is, in (4) the stimulus is taken to be unified because it is an instance of figure/ground, whereas in (5) the stimulus consists of two parts and hence is disjoint. Performance for sentence (5) was worse than for sentence (4) (for details, see Wason and Green [296,pp. 604-607]).

We would describe the situation slightly differently, in terms of the contrast between deixis and anaphora. Indeed, the experimental setup is such that for sentence (5), the lower half of the cards is hidden by a bar, making it analogous to condition (2), where the object mentioned in the antecedent is hidden. We have seen above that some subjects have difficulties with the intended direction of the conditional in experiment (2). Sentence (5) would be the "difficult half" of the anaphora-containing sentence "Whenever there are triangles on one side of the line, there is black on the other side of the line." Sentence (4) does not contain any such anaphora. With Wason and Green we would therefore predict that subjects find (5) more difficult.

3.5.6   Subjects' Understanding of Propositional Connectives

We have discussed some aspects of the interpretation of the conditional above, in particular those which are connected with the interpretation of the task, such as the distinction between descriptive and deontic conditionals. This section is devoted to some of the wilder shores of the semantics of conditionals: the existential import of the conditional, and the related interpretation of the conditional as a conjunction.

Existential Import of the Conditional

In a second set of tutorial experiments[23] all the interpretational difficulties reviewed above were apparent. This is encouraging, because it points to the stability of the factors identified. Interestingly, a new difficulty surfaced while subjects went through condition (2), which involves the rule "if there is a vowel on the back of the card, there is an even number on the face of the card." To understand what is going on here, it is important to make the quantification over cards in the rule explicit: "for all cards, if there is a vowel on one side of the card, there is an even number on the other side of the card." A well-known issue in the semantics of the universal quantifier, first raised by Aristotle, is whether this quantifier has "existential import": if "all A are B" is true, does this entail that there *are* As which are Bs? Aristotle thought so, and he makes his point by means of two examples: of the two statements, "Some man is white" and "Some man is not white" one or the other must be true; and "Every pleasure is good" implies "Some pleasure is good." The examples show that Aristotle takes subjects and predicates to denote nonempty sets. This is precisely what our subjects appear to be doing, in requiring that, in order for the conditional to be true, there must be at least one card which satisfies both antecedent and consequent. They consider the rule to be undecided if there is no such instance, even in the absence of counterexamples.[24]

> *Subject* 1. [in experiment (2)].
> *S.* In this case I think you would need to turn the 7. And... that would be the only one you need to turn. ... 'Cause, these two [A and K] have to have numbers on the back, so they don't apply ... Which leaves these two [4 and 7]. Erm. And if there's an A on the back then it fits the rule [pointing to the 4] and if there is a K on the back then it doesn't apply to the rule, so it doesn't matter, which leaves this one [pointing to the 7], 'cause if there's an A on the back of here, and it's a 7, then you've disproved the rule.
> *E.* OK, and if there is not an A on the back of that [the 7]?
> *S.* If there's not an A on the back. [thinks] then ... maybe you do need to turn that one [pointing to the 4]. If there's not an A on the back [of the 7], then it doesn't disprove the rule and it doesn't prove it. So you'd have to turn the 4 I think.
> *E.* And what if the 4 also didn't have an A on the back - what would that mean for the rule?
> *S.* Well then ... for this set of cards, the rule... it would disprove the rule I suppose. Cause if there is not an A on the back of this card [pointing to the 4], [pause] then... there isn't a 4 on the face of it. OK, if there's not an A on the back, then none of these cards have an A on the back, and a 4 on the face, which is what the rule states. So for this set of cards it's disproved, it's not true.

It is abundantly clear that the subject considers existential import to be a necessary requirement for the truth of the conditional. The next subject expresses this insight by means of the modal "could" :

---

23. Performed in Edinburgh in 2003 by the our student Marian Counihan. The design was the same as that of the first experiment.
24. We will have more to say on this phenomenon in section 3.5.6 below.

Subject 7. [in experiment (2)].

S. If there's a A on the back of this card [the 7] then it's finished, you basically don't care anymore. Whereas if there's a K, all it seems to prove really is that this [the rule] could be true. ... I suppose we do... need to turn this card [the 4], just to affirm the rule.

The next subject has a slightly different interpretation, and says that if there is no card instantiating the rule (and no falsifying card), the rule is still undecided. This probably reflects a different understanding of what the domain of the rule is: the cards on the table, or a wider set of cards.

Subject 2. [in experiment (2): has stated he wants to turn 4 and 7]

E. OK, now say you turned both of those [pointing to 4 and 7] and you found an A on both.

S. Then the rule would be ... wrong. Because if there's an A on the back of both of them, then the rule says that there would be a 4 on the front of both of them, but, there's not, so, I mean there's a 4 on one of them, but then there is also a 7 on one of them, so, the rule's wrong, I mean, it doesn't always follow, so it's wrong. [Pause] Although it doesn't say always, there [pointing at the rule], but I am presuming it means always. I don't know [laughs].

E. Yes, it is meant to apply to any of them.

S. Yeah, OK, so the rule would be wrong if there's an A on both [4 and 7].

$\vdots$

S. ... hang on, with an A and 7 there [on the 7 card], and an A and a 4 there [pointing to the 4] it would be wrong, still ... because of the A and 7, yeah, the A and the 4's correct, but because that [pointing to the 7 card] is incorrect, that's, the whole rule would be incorrect.

E. So, in either case, if there was an A on this side [pointing to the overturned 7 card], this other side of the 7, it would make the rule incorrect?

S. Yeah.

E. And despite what was on the [pointing to the 4]?

S. Oh, yeah, yeah. No OK, so you only need to turn that one [the 7]. Do you? [looks at rule] No you don't. No, sorry, no [indicates 4 and 7 cards again] you do need to turn them both, because if that is a K [turning over the 7], then you need to turn that one to check that one [the 4] to check that that is not a K as well.

E. And if that was a K as well?

S. Then the rule ... [pause] then you wouldn't know ... because ... there's nothing saying you can't have a K and a 4, but all it is saying is whether or not there's an A on the back, if there's a K on the back of both of these [the 4 and the 7] then you don't know, the rule might be right, or might be wrong.

These observations have some relevance to performance in the standard task. Suppose again, as we did in section 3.5.5, that subjects split the rule into the components (1) and (2). The first component yields the answer A; this card simultaneously establishes existential import. Interestingly, existential import as applied to the second condition yields the answers 4,7, so that we have found yet another way to justify the mysterious $p, q, \neg q$ response in the original task.

Interpreting the Conditional as a Conjunction

We now return to the possible interpretations of conditionals and their relevance to subjects' understanding of the task. In the literature on Wason's task only two types are distinguished: the unidirectional material implication, and the biconditional. When one turns to the linguistics literature, the picture is dramatically different. An interesting source here is Comrie's paper Conditionals: A Typology [44], where conditionals are distinguished according to the degree of hypotheticality of the antecedent. In principle this is a continuous scale. Viewed cross-linguistically, the degree of hypotheticality ranges from certain, a case where English uses *when* ("when he comes, we'll go out for dinner," [25] via neutral ("if a triangle is right-angled, it satisfies Pythagoras' theorem") to highly unlikely ("if we were to finish this paper on time, we could submit it to the proceedings") and even false, the counterfactual ("if we had finished this paper on time, we would have won the best paper prize"). If conditionals come with expectations concerning the degree of hypotheticality of the antecedent, this might affect the truth condition for the conditional that the subject implicitly applies. For example, we have seen in section 3.5.6 that some subjects claim the conditional has existential import; this may be viewed as the implicature that the antecedent of the conditional is highly likely.

Indeed we claim that, in order to understand performance in Wason's task, it is imperative to look into the possible understandings of the conditional that a subject might have, and for this, language typology appears to be indispensable. An interesting outcome of typological research is that the conditional ostensibly investigated in Wason's task, the hypothetical conditional, where one does not want to assert the truth of the antecedent, may not even be the most prevalent type of conditional. We include a brief discussion of the paper Typology of *if*-Clauses by Athanasiadou and Dirven [4] (cf. also [5]) to corroborate this point; afterward we will connect their analysis to our observations.

In a study of 300 instances of conditionals in the COBUILD corpus [42], the authors observed that there occurred two main types of conditionals, *course of event* conditionals, and *hypothetical* conditionals. The hypothetical conditionals are roughly the ones familiar from logic; an example is

If there is no water in your radiator, your engine will overheat immediately. [42,17]

A characteristic feature of hypothetical conditionals is the events referred to in antecedent and consequent are seen as hypothetical, and the speaker can make use of a whole scale of marked and unmarked attitudes to distance herself from claims concerning likelihood of occurrence. The presence of "your" is what makes the interpretation more likely to be hypothetical: the antecedent need not ever be true for "your" car. Furthermore, in paradigmatic cases (temporal

---

25. Dutch, however, can also use the conditionals marker "als" here.

and causal conditionals) antecedent and consequent are seen as consecutive. By contrast in course–of– event conditionals such as

> If students come on Fridays, they get oral practice in Quechua (from [44])

or

> If there is a drought at this time, as so often happens in central Australia, the fertilised egg in the uterus still remains dormant [42,43]

the events referred to in antecedent and consequent are considered to be generally or occasionally recurring, and they may be simultaneous. Generic expressions such as "on Fridays" or "as so often happens ..." tend to force this reading of the conditional. e.g., the first example invokes a scenario in which some students do come on Fridays and some don't, but the ones who do get oral practice in Quechua. The generic expression "on Fridays," together with implicit assumptions about student timetables and syllabuses, causes the sentence to have the habitual "whenever" reading. It is also entailed that some students do come on Fridays, generally. These examples also indicate that course–of–event conditionals refer to events situated in real time, unlike hypothetical conditionals. It should now be apparent that the logical properties of course–of–event conditionals are very different from their hypothetical relatives. For example, what is immediately relevant to our concerns is that course–of–event conditionals refer to a population of cases, whereas hypothetical conditionals may refer to a single case; this *is* relevant, because it has frequently been claimed that subjects interpret the task so that the rule refers to a population of which the four cards shown are only a sample (cf. section 3.5.2). Interestingly, Athanasiadou and Dirven estimated that about 44% of conditionals in COBUILD are of the course–of–events variety, as opposed to 37% of the hypothetical variety. Needless to say, these figures should be interpreted with caution, but they lend some plausibility to the claim that subjects may come to the task with a nonintended, yet perfectly viable, understanding of the conditional. We will now discuss the repercussions of this understanding for subjects' card selections.

One of the questions in the paraphrase task asked subjects to determine which of four statements follow from the rule "Every card which has a vowel on one side has an even number on the other side." More than half of our subjects chose the possibility "It is the case that there is a vowel on one side and an even number on the other side." Fillenbaum [82] already observed that there are high frequencies for conjunctive paraphrases for positive conditional threats ("if you do this I'll break your arm" becomes "do this and I'll break your arm") (35%), positive conditional promises ("if you do this you'll get a chocolate" becomes "do this and I'll get you a chocolate") (40%) and negative conditional promises ("if you don't cry I'll get you an ice cream" becomes "don't cry and I'll get you an ice cream") (50%). However, he did not observe conjunctive paraphrases for contingent universals (where there is no intrinsic connection between antecedent and consequent) or even law-like universals. Clearly, the statements we provided are contingent universals, so Filenbaum's observations on promises and threats are of no direct relevance. However, if the course–of–event conditional is a possible reading of the conditional, the inference to a conjunction observed in many of our subjects makes much more sense. Clearly the truth–conditions for conditionals of this type differ from the intended interpretation; to mention but one difficult case, when is a generic false? Thus, a generic interpretation may lead to different evaluations and selections. Here is an example of what a conjunctive reading means in practice.

> *Subject* 22. [subject has chosen the conjunctive reading in the paraphrase task]
> E. [Asks subject to turn the 7]
> S. That one ... that isn't true. There isn't an A on the front and a 4 on the back. ... you turn over those two [A and 4] to see if they satisfy it, because you already know that those two [K and 7] don't satisfy the statement.
> E. [baffled] Sorry, which two don't satisfy the rule?
> S. These two don't [K and 7], because on one side there is K and that should have been A, and that [7] wouldn't have a 4, and that wouldn't satisfy the statement.
> E. Yes, so what does that mean ... you didn't turn it because you thought that it will not satisfy?
> S. Yes.

Clearly, on a conjunctive reading, the rule is already falsified by the cards as exhibited (since the K and 7 cards falsify); no turning is necessary. The subject might, however, feel forced by the experimental situation to select some cards, and accordingly reinterprets the task as *checking* whether a given card satisfies the rule. This brings us to an important consideration: how much of the problem is actually caused by the conditional, and how much is caused by the task setting, no matter what binary logical connective is used?

The literature on the selection task, with very few exceptions, has assumed that the problem is a problem specific to conditional rules. Indeed, it would be easy to infer also from the foregoing discussion of descriptive conditional semantics that the conditional (and its various expressions) is unique in causing subjects so much difficulty in the selection task, and that our only point is that a sufficiently rich range of interpretations for the conditional must be used to frame psychological theories of the selection task.

However, the issues already discussed – the nature of truth, response to exceptions, contingency, pragmatics – are all rather general in their implications for the task of seeking evidence for truth. One can distinguish the assessment of truth of a sentence from truthfulness of an utterer for sentences of any form. The robustness or brittleness of statements to counterexamples is an issue which arises for any generalization. The sociopsychological effects of the experimenter's authority, and the communicative complexities introduced by having to take a cooperative stance toward some utterances and an adversarial one toward others is also a general problem of pragmatics that can affect statements of any logical form. Contingencies between feedback from early evidence on choice of subsequent optimal evidence seeking are general to any form of sentence for which more than one case is relevant. What would happen, for example, if the rule were stated using the putatively least problematical connective, conjunction? Chapter 4 gives the answer.

3.6   Matching Bias: the "No-Processing" Explanation

We have paid scant attention to more traditional interpretations of the selection task, focusing instead on the logical difficulties experienced by subjects in the descriptive task. This is not to imply that the traditional explanations are completely without foundation. We provide one example here: Evans's "matching strategy." This was proposed as a shallow processing strategy, operating automatically. We will have more to say on the distinction between shallow and deep processing in chapter 7 on the suppression task; but for now we give some examples showing that this type of response also occurs when subjects fully engage with the task.

Evans (see, for example, the review in Evans, Newstead, and Byrne [76]) defines the "matching strategy" as the choice of cards which match the atomic parts of the content of a clause in a rule. So for the rule *If p then q*, *p* and *q* cards match: for the rule *If p then not q* still *p* and *q* cards match: and the same for *If not p then q*. Here is a particularly striking example.

> *Subject* 9. [experiment (1)]
> *E.* [This rule] says that if there is a vowel on the face, then there is an even number on the back. So what we mean by face is the bit you can see, and by back the bit you can't see. Which cards would you need to turn over to check if the rule holds?
> *S.* This one [ticks A] and this one [ticks 7]
> *E.* So why would you pick those two?
> *S.* One has a vowel on the face and the other one an even number. If you turn it, if it's true, then it should have an even number [pointing to the A] and this should have a vowel [pointing to the 7].
> *E.* [baffled] So you picked, Oh you were saying if there was a vowel underneath [pointing to the 7]
> *S.* That's because I'm stupid. Even number is 1,3,5, . . .
> *E.* No, 2,4,6, . . .
> *S.* [Corrects 7 to 4, so her final choice was A and 4] OK. So these.

The next example is straightforward:

> *Subject* 3. [Standard Wason task; has chosen A and 4]
> *E.* Why pick those cards and not the other cards?
> *S.* Because they are mentioned in the rule and I am assuming that the rule is true.

Evans conceptualises the use of this strategy as a "superficial" response to both rule and task which subjects adopt prior to processing the information to the level of a coherent interpretation of the whole sentence. As such, the strategy may be applied prior to or alongside other processing strategies. It is taken to explain the modal response of turning the p and q cards in the abstract task. It must assume that something else is going on (perhaps superimposed on matching) when subjects adopt other responses. Thematic effects have to be explained in terms of contentful processes engaging other processes at deeper levels than matching.[26]

3.7 The Subject's Predicament

So what is the upshot of this extended semantic analysis of the range of subjects' interpretations and factors influencing them which were revealed by these Socratic dialogues? We feel the need to provide some more synoptic integration of this mass of rich observations, though what we offer here should be understood as a very partial view.

Some effects are global. For example, content may strongly shift subjects toward a deontic interpretation, and then few interpretational problems arise. The two cards Wason expected to be turned are the only possible violators of the "law." To produce an integrated sketch of some of these global effects, table 3.2 presents some of the global parameters an interpretation must fix, and hints at their relations. Under descriptive interpretations, robust ones (tolerating exceptions) lead immediately to conflict with finite sets of cases determining truth–value, and problems of distinguishing exceptions from counterexamples, which in turn may lead to the "cards as sampled from a population" interpretation. Brittle interpretation allays these problems but raises the issue of contingencies between card choices. Both robust and brittle interpretations are susceptible to both kinds of reversibility – of physical cards, and of logical rule. Deontic interpretations suffer from none of these problems: cards are independent of each other, only cases are judged (not rule), the veracity of the experimenter is not at stake. The content triggering a deontic reading generally makes for logical irreversibility, and there are no anaphors to interact with card reversibility issues.

But many of the factors affecting interpretation are local and interact with other parameters in determining the interpretive outcome, defying tabulation. A useful supplementary way to draw together the complex threads is to tabulate some ranges of interpretations which can lead to each of the four dominant choice combinations in table 3.1, which jointly account for 92% of the subjects. Table 3.3 lays out some of the parameters leading to these common choice combinations.

---

26. Oaksford and Stenning [204] by investigating a full range of clause negations in both selection and evaluation tasks, showed that matching is not a particularly good explanation of performance with the full range of negated conditionals. They argue that a better summary of the data is in terms of the degree to which the material and instructions allow negative clauses to be processed as corresponding positive characterizations.

Table 3.2 Global parameters as they contrast between descriptive and deontic interpretation

descriptive		deontic
robust	brittle	
conflict with task "population" reading	dependencies between cards	independent cards judging cases–not rule
reversibility		no reversibility
of cards	of rule	
discomfort with challenging E		no calling E a liar

Table 3.3   Some interpretation features and the main choice-combinations to which they may lead in the descriptive selection task: some choices on other tasks are mentioned with their interpretational feature.

Main card choice combinations				Interpretational Feature
p	p, q	$p, \neg q$	$p, q, \neg q$	(in italics)
x	x			*strong negation*: choose either (both) letter(s), or $\neg q$ in two–rule task
			x	*not-false doesn't mean true*: ruling out counterexamples, but also seeking positive case
		x		*truth vs. satisfaction ambiguity*: if resolved, removes contingency issues if unresolved in two-rule task, reject materials
	x			*robustness*: immediate conflict with task, may invoke sample reading
x				*choice contingencies*: choose true antecedent first RAST and two-rule tend to remove problem
	x			*can't call E a liar!*: assume rule true, seek cases that make rule true
	x			*in conjunction task*: test cards of unknown truth–value
			x	*existential import of universal* rule out counterexamples but positive instance required too
x	x			*assume cards irreversible*: maintain logical irreversibility, or convert and conjoin conditional
	x			*superficial mention in rule* determines relevance "matching"
			x	*deontic conjunctive interpretation* or *one-card-at-a-time* *descriptive interpretation*

3.8   Conclusion

The explorations by dialogue reported here have cast their net somewhat wider than is customary, to obtain information about subjects' processing and semantic understanding of the task. The picture that emerges is complex. The differences between subjects, even when they make the same selection, are huge and defy any single explanation. All choice combinations reflect more than one interpretation and some combinations we are still struggling to explain. For example, there appears to be no explanation for a very common pattern of evaluation and selection: p, q is selected, $q/\neg p$ is evaluated as falsifying, and $\neg p/q$ is evaluated as irrelevant, although we ventured a hypothesis in section 3.5.5. It does not seem very helpful to dismiss such behavior as "irrational." It is more interesting to relate this and other behavior to subjects' understanding of the task, but much richer data are required than the four "bits" received from each subject in the classical task. We have seen that understanding interpretation sometimes leads to clarification of what subjects are trying to do, and that often turns out to be quite different than the experimenter assumes.

The granularity of these data is very much finer than experimental psychologists have deemed necessary for the analysis of this task (though this fine granularity is rather ordinary in lots of areas of psychology such as visual perception). A common reaction is that this interpretational variety is all very well for linguistics, but surely it is obvious that this is not what is going on in the few seconds that subjects think about what cards to turn over in the original task, and besides, if this is what is going on, it's far too hard to study. This attitude was crystallized for KS by a remark made after he had given a talk on the material (ironically in Wason's old department). "You have given a very interesting analysis of the task from a semantic point of view," the questioner commented, "but what we need is a psychological explanation." The questioner seemed to assume that when linguists and logicians substantiate an analysis, that they are claiming "ordinary speakers" have conscious access to the analysis within its own terminology. Equally, they assume that even demonstrating the formal semantics is correct doesn't have the implication that ordinary speakers actually mean by the expression, what the analysis says they mean.

We would be the first to acknowledge that our analysis isn't more than a beginning, but what is striking here is the idea that it is not a "psychological" analysis. Cognitive psychology is founded on the idea that people interpret their fresh experience in the light of their long–term knowledge and that the resulting rich structures furnish them the wherewithal to reason to their decisions. If we don't know how subjects interpret a task, or its materials, then how are we to start understanding what they do? And if they do lots of different things which are each comprehensible on the basis of their different interpretations, then hadn't we better have different explanations for their different acts? In some subfields of psychology, the questioner's comment might have been taken to mean that what is needed is a *mental process* model and that that is what sets semantics off from psychology. We have some sympathy since we agree that process models would be really nice to have, and we certainly don't have one, although the logical models in section 3.4 are an essential prerequisite for a process model. None of the theories of this task are any more process theories than the approach offered here – most of them less so. And if reasoning to an interpretation among a rich set of possibilities is the mental process going on, then how can we get a process model without any account of the range of interpretations in play? In the next chapter we will bring evidence that the gap between the interpretational problems appearing in these dialogues and what goes on in the traditional controlled experiments is not so great as it might at first appear.

These dialogues may also provide challenges to natural language semantics. While it is of course possible to attribute the vacillations in interpretation (of conditionals and anaphora, for example) to performance factors, it seems more interesting to look into the structure of the linguistic competence model to see how the observed interferences may arise. It seems to us that dialogues such as these provide a rich source of data for semantics and pragmatics, which promises to yield deeper insight into interpretation and processing of natural language.

What we hope to have demonstrated in this chapter is that the data do not warrant abandoning the search for formal models to provide bases for explaining subjects' reasoning behavior. Instead, formal models embodying insights from neighboring fields are useful guides for a richer program of empirical exploration and testing. There is a danger that deceptively simple models obscure the phenomena in need of explanation, and in so doing likewise obscure the educational relevance of the logical competence models and their highly objectified stance toward language. Stanovich [254] shows how closely related this stance is to other educational achievements. The tutorial dialogues presented here provide some insight into the variety of students' problems which may be of some help to those involved in teaching reasoning skills.

4 From Logic via Exploration to Controlled Experiment

In chapter 2 we presented logical analysis suggesting a wide range of possibilities for interpreting conditionals, and in chapter 3 this was followed by prima facie evidence that subjects experience severe interpretational problems in the original descriptive selection task and that they respond to these problems in many different ways. The analysis uncovered a range of difficulties with abstract descriptive conditionals that do not arise if deontic interpretation is strongly suggested by familiar content. But the fact that these problems surface in Socratic dialogues does not mean that they occurred in the original experiments. This chapter examines how to get from the evidence of exploration to evidence of controlled experiment. We present experimental evidence, but we are just as much concerned with the process of design of such experiments. In accordance with our comments in chapter 1 about the need for exploration, and the establishment and bridging of substantial gaps between theory and data, the issues that go into designing experiments to interact with formal theories are more important than this particular task.

The backbone of this chapter is an experiment reported in [265], augmented with some material from subsequent experiments. The results of several experimental manipulations are compared with baseline performance on the classical descriptive task. Each manipulation is designed to assess contributions of different interpretational problems proposed by semantic analysis, and found in the subjects' dialogues, to Wason's original results. So the logic of the research plan is rather simple. We proposed that Wason did not understand the conflicts that his subjects experienced between their initial interpretations of instructions and materials, and that these interpretational conflicts can explain why their behavior does not conform to the classical logical model which Wason unquestioningly assumed to be the relevant competence model for performance.

So our research plan will be to design manipulations which alleviate several interpretational conflicts and show that each alleviation produces more of the responding which Wason expected. Our second important claim is that the chief factor determining whether subjects conform to Wason's expectations is whether they adopt a descriptive or a deontic interpretation – we claim that the "easy tasks" are easy because they invoke deontic interpretation. This claim presents our first design choice: we elect to study how to make Wason's original descriptive task "easy" i.e., to get a descriptive task to invoke the classical interpretation he assumed. We could instead have chosen to systematically make the deontic tasks "hard" by introducing the factors which produce problems of interpretation. Why do we choose the first fork? There are important issues about deontic reasoning, so the second path is not without interest.[1] But the overwhelmingly most important factor in our choice is that we want to study descriptive conditionals, and in particular robust non-truth-functional descriptive conditionals, because we claim they are crucial for understanding a wide range of other tasks in the psychology of reasoning. So we will present in chapter 7 a range of logical models of these robust conditionals applied to understanding human interpretation. In chapter 9 we study the very distinct attitudes of autistic people toward descriptive rules, and these rules will be central again in chapter 11 when we return to the relation between interpretation and derivation.

If this is the long-term strategy, what are the tactics? We have to design manipulations to alleviate each of several interpretational problems. We cannot do them all. Why choose the ones we choose? This is a partly pragmatic question. One may have a feeling for which are the most important problems – important theoretically, and important in terms of what difficulty of problem they present to what proportion of subjects. One's wish list of manipulations may be ordered but still one needs inspiration as to how to test. However elegant one's description of an interpretational problem, there is no guarantee that there is a simple way of testing whether subjects actually experience the problem. One can but try to design such manipulations. Good experimentalists are, among other things, good at designing workable tests. Even having designed what looks like the perfect test, there is no guarantee that it will produce a result either way. It may not engage subjects in a way that impinges on their responses, and of course it may be hard to tell from a negative result that subjects don't experience the problem the manipulation was designed to exhibit. Negative evidence is weak evidence, and means hard work ruling out the alternatives.

Of course our design problems are not finished once we have found workable manipulations which produce the predicted effects. Having insisted on the need for abstract theory and its distance from the data, we need bridging theory to get from observation to theoretical conclusion. Our manipulations may have

---

1. We have pilot data which bear on this issue. We tried to make a version of the deontic task (the drinking age rule) harder by introducing some of the difficulties found in the descriptive task. For instance, the instruction "Your task is to decide which if any of these four cards you must turn in order to decide *if a customer violates the law*" was replaced by "Your task is to decide which if any of these four cards you must turn in order to decide *whether the rule is violated*." The idea was that in the second formulation the attention is directed away from the customers (i.e., the cards) and toward the rule; a single card would now suffice to show that the rule is violated. This manipulation could therefore reintroduce the problems with dependencies that are usually absent in the deontic task. Indeed, we found a decrease in correct answers to 50%. Since the design contained some flaws, these results are at most suggestive.

the predicted effect, but for some reason other than the one intended.

All this laboratory wisdom is very obvious, but for logic students unused to experimentation, it is easy to forget, and they will not be reminded by what appears in psychological journals since most of this process of discovery and design is concealed, along with practically all negative results. The problems of bridging will be discussed with our results.

4.1 Designing Experiments Following Observations

This section describes the experiment reported in [265], with particular attention to the why and wherefore of the design. In what follows we describe each manipulation we settled on as a condition in the experiment, and then present the results together. In each case we try to motivate the design choices.

4.1.1 Conditions: Classical "Abstract" Task

To provide a baseline of performance on the selection task with descriptive conditionals, the first condition repeats Wason's classical study [295] with the following instructions and materials (see instructions in section 3.1). The other conditions are described through their departures from this baseline condition. This is obviously important to get an exact baseline for behavior in the original task *in this population of subjects*. For example, it is not unusual for absolute frequencies of Wason's "correct" response to vary between 4% and 10% in different undergraduate populations.

4.1.2 Conditions: Two–Rule Task

The motivation for introducing this manipulation was twofold. First, we saw robustness of natural language conditionals as central to the problems subjects have in descriptive tasks. Presenting the task as a comparison of two rules, and explicitly telling the subjects that one rule is true and one false should background a number of issues concerned with the notion of truth, such as the possibility of the rule withstanding exceptions. If we are right that robustness is a problem, and in these assumptions about the effects of the manipulation, then this should move performance toward Wason's classical logical competence model where the conditionals are treated as truth–functional.

Second, we wanted to estimate the contribution of a Bayesian information–gain explanation to subjects' behavior, an explanation introduced in section 3.5.2. This second purpose does not seek to remove an obstacle to classical logical interpretation, but rather to explore the power of an alternative explanation of subjects' behavior based on a different competence model than Wason's. The information-gain model postulates that in solving the standard Wason task, subjects always compare the rule given to the unstated null hypothesis that its antecedent's and consequent's truth–values are statistically independent in a population of cards. We were thus interested in seeing what would happen if subjects were presented with explicit alternative non-null hypotheses. Information gain must make different predictions in this case. Although elaborations of the information-gain theory might make prediction complicated, it seems that in its simple application, it must predict that the $\neg q$ card offers the most information, and that subjects will therefore pick this as the competence response on this theory.

After repeating the preliminary instructions for the classical task, the instructions continued as follows:

> Also below there appear two rules. One rule is true of all the cards, the other isn't. Your task is to decide which cards (if any) you *must* turn in order to decide which rule holds. Don't turn unnecessary cards. Tick the cards you want to turn.
> **Rule 1:** *If there is a vowel on one side, then there is an even number on the other side.*
> **Rule 2:** *If there is a consonant on one side, then there is an even number on the other side.*

Normative performance in this task, according to the classical logical competence model, is to turn only the not-Q card. The rules are chosen so that the correct response is to turn exactly the card that the vast majority of subjects fail to turn in the classical task. This has the added bonus that it is no longer correct to turn the P card which provides an interesting comparison with the original task. This is the only descriptive task we know of for which choosing the true-antecedent case is an error.

By any obvious measure of task complexity, this task is more complicated than the classical task. It demands that two conditionals are processed and that the implications of each case is considered with respect to both rules and with respect to a distribution of truth–values. Nevertheless, our prediction was that performance should be substantially nearer the logically normative model for the reasons described above.

4.1.3 Conditions: Contingency Instructions

The "contingency instructions," designed to remove any difficulties in understanding that choices have to be made ignoring possible interim feedback, after an identical preamble, read as follows, where the newly italicized portion is the change from the classical instructions:

> Also below there appears a rule. Your task is to decide which of these

four cards you *must* turn (if any) in order to decide if the rule is true. *Assume that you have to decide whether to turn each card before you get any information from any of the turns you choose to make.* Don't turn unnecessary cards. Tick the cards you want to turn.

If the contingencies introduced by the descriptive semantics are a source of difficulty for subjects, this additional instruction should make the task easier. In particular, since there is a tendency to choose the P card first, there should be an increase in not-Q responding.

After conducting this experiment we found a reference in Wason [300] to the use of essentially similar instructions in his contribution to the Science Museum exhibition of 1977, and there are mentions in other early papers. Clearly he had thought about assumed contingencies between card choices as a possible confusion. Wason reports no enhancement in his subjects' reasoning, but he does not report whether any systematic comparison between these and standard instructions was made, or quite what the population of subjects was. He certainly did not observe that this problem for subjects doesn't arise under deontic interpretations.

4.1.4 Conditions: Judging Truthfulness of an Independent Source

We chose to investigate the possible contribution of problems arising from the authoritative position of the experimenter and the balance of cooperative and adversarial stances required toward different parts of the task materials through instructions to assess truthfulness of the source instead of truth of the rule, and we separated the source of the rule from the source of the instructions (the experimenter). The instructions read as follows:

Also below there appears a rule *put forward by an unreliable source*. Your task is to decide which cards (if any) you *must* turn in order to decide *if the unreliable source is lying*. Don't turn unnecessary cards. Tick the cards you want to turn.

With these instructions there should be no discomfort about seeking to falsify the rule. Nor should any falsity of the rule throw any doubt on the truthfulness of the rest of the instructions, since the information sources are independent.

These "truthfulness" instructions are quite closely related to several other manipulations that have been tried in past experiments. In the early days of experimentation on this task, when it was assumed that a failure to try and falsify explained the correct response, various ways of emphasizing falsification were explored. Wason [295] instructed subjects to pick cards which could break the rule and Hughes [132] asked them whether the rule was a lie. Neither instruction had much effect. However, these instructions fail to separate the source of the rule from the experimenter (as the utterer of the rule) and may fail for that reason.

Kirby [158] used a related manipulation in which the utterer of the rule was a machine said to have broken down, needing to be tested to see if it was working properly again after repair. These instructions did produce significant improvement. Here the focus of the instruction is to tell whether the machine is "broken," not simply whether the utterance of the rule is a falsehood. This might be expected to invoke a deontic interpretation involving comparisons of the actual world with an ideal world in which the machine works correctly (Kirby's condition is akin to the "production line inspection scenarios" mentioned before), and so it might be that the improvement observed is for this reason.

Platt and Griggs [217] explored a sequence of instructional manipulations in what they describe as abstract tasks which culminate in 81% correct responding. One of the changes they make is to use instructions to "seek violations" of the rule, which is relevant here for its relation to instructions to test the truth of an unreliable source. Their experiments provide some insight into the conditions under which these instructions do and don't facilitate performance. Platt and Griggs study the effect of "explications" of the rule and in the most effective manipulations actually replace the conditional rule by explications such as: "A card with a vowel on it can only have an even number, but a card with a consonant on it can have either an even or an odd number." Note that this explication removes the problematic anaphora (see above, section 3.5.5), explicitly contradicts a biconditional reading, and removes the conditional, with its tendency to robust interpretation. But more significantly still, the facilitation of turning not-Q is almost entirely effected by the addition of seek violations instructions, and these instructions probably switch the task from a descriptive to a deontic task.

In reviewing earlier uses of the 'seek violations' instructions, Platt and Griggs note that facilitation occurs with abstract permission and obligation rules but not with the standard abstract task. So, merely instructing to seek violations doesn't invoke a deontic reading when the rule is still indicative, and the content provides no support for a deontic reading – "violations" presumably might make the rule false. But combined with an "explication" about what cards *can* have on them (or with a permission or obligation schema) they appear to invoke a deontic reading. As we shall see, 80% seems to be about the standard rate of correct responding in deontically interpreted tasks regardless of whether they contain material invoking social contracts.

So the present manipulation does not appear to have been explored before. We predicted that separating the source of the rule from the experimenter while maintaining a descriptive reading of the rule should increase normative responding.

4.1.5   Conditions: Exploring Other Kinds of Rules than Conditionals

This condition of the experiment was designed to explore the malleability of subjects' interpretations of rules other than conditionals. In particular we chose a conjunctive rule as arguably the simplest connective to understand. As such this condition has a rather different status from the others in that it is not designed to remove a difficulty from a logically similar task but to explore a logical change. Since it was an exploration we additionally asked for subjects' justification of their choices afterward.

A conjunctive rule was combined with the same instructions as are used in the classical abstract task.

> **Rule**: *There is a vowel on one side, and there is an even number on the other side.*

The classical logical competence model demands that subjects should turn no cards with such a conjunctive rule – the rule interpreted in the same logic as Wason's interpretation of his conditional rule can already be seen to be false of the not-P and not-Q cards. Therefore, under this interpretation the rule is already known to be false and no cards should be turned.

We predicted that many subjects would not make this interpretation of this response. An alternative, perfectly rational, interpretation of the experimenter's intentions is to construe the rule as having deontic force (every card *should* have a vowel on one side and an even number on the other) and to seek cards which might flout this rule other than ones that obviously can already be seen to flout it. One factor making this interpretation more salient may be that in a card-turning experiment, there is what psychologists call a "demand characteristic" to turn something. If this interpretation were adopted, then the P and Q cards would be chosen. Note that this interpretation is deontic even though the rule is syntactically indicative.

4.1.6   Subjects

Subjects were 377 first–year Edinburgh undergraduates, from a wide range of subject backgrounds.

4.1.7   Method

All tasks were administered to subjects in classroom settings in two large lectures. Subjects were randomly assigned to the different conditions, with the size of sample in each condition being estimated from piloting on effect sizes. Adjacent subjects did different conditions. The materials described above were preceded by the following general instruction:

The following experiment is part of a program of research into how people reason. Please read the instructions carefully. We are grateful for your
help.

4.1.8 Results

Those subjects (twelve across all conditions) who claimed to have done similar
tasks before or to have received any instruction in logic were excluded from
the analysis. Table 4.1 presents the data from all of the conditions. Subjects
were scored as making a completely correct response, or as making at least
some mistake, according to the classical logical competence model. For all the
conditions except the two–rule task and the conjunction condition, this 'competence model' performance is choice of P and not-Q cards. For the two–rule
task the correct response is not-Q. For the conjunction condition it is to turn no
cards.

Table 4.1 Frequencies of card choice combinations by conditions: classical logical competence
responses are marked *. Any response made by at least three subjects in at least one condition is
categorized: everything else is miscellaneous.

Condition	P Q	Q	P	P ¬Q	¬Q	¬P,Q	P,Q, ¬Q	¬P,¬Q	all	None	Misc.	Total
Classical	56	7	8	4*	3	7	1	2	9	8	5	108
Two-rule	8	8	2	1	9*	2	1	0	0	2	4	37
Contingency	15	0	3	8*	1	6	4	8	3	0	3	51
Truthfulness	39	6	9	14*	0	7	3	6	8	15	5	112
Conjunction	31	2	9	7	2	0	0	1	0	9*	8	69

Table 4.2 presents the tests of significance of the percentages of correct/incorrect
responses as compared to the baseline classical condition. Of subjects in the
baseline condition 3.7% made the correct choice of cards.

  The percentages completely correct in the other conditions were two-rule
condition, 24%; "truthfulness" condition, 13%; in the "contingency" condition,
18%; and in the conjunction condition, 13%. The significance levels of these
proportions by Fisher's exact test appear in table 4.2.

The two–rule task elicits substantially more competence model selections than
the baseline task. In fact the completely correct response is the modal response.
More than six times as many subjects get it completely correct even though superficially it appears to be a more complicated task. The next most common
responses are to turn P with Q, and to turn just Q. The former is the modal
response in the classical task. The latter appears to show that even with unsuccessful subjects, this task shifts attention to the consequent cards – turnings of
P are substantially suppressed: 32% as compared to 80% in the baseline task.

Table 4.2 Proportions of subjects completely correct and significances of differences from baseline of each of the four manipulations

Condition	Wrong	Right	p	Percent Correct
Classical baseline	104	4		3.7
Two-Rule	28	9	.004	24
Contingency	37	8	.005	18
Truthfulness	98	14	.033	13
Conjunction	60	9	.022	13

Contingency instructions also substantially increase completely correct responding, and do so primarily at the expense of the modal P–with–Q response. In particular they increase the not-Q choice to 50%.

Instructions to test the truthfulness of an unreliable source have a smaller effect which takes a larger sample to demonstrate, but nevertheless 13% of subjects get it completely correct, nearly four times as many as the baseline task. The main change is again a reduction of P–with–Q responses, but there is also an increase in the response of turning nothing.

Completely correct performance with a conjunctive rule was 13% – not as different from the conditions with conditional rules as one might expect if conditionals are the main source of difficulty. The modal response is to turn the P and Q cards – just as in the original task. Anecdotally, debriefing subjects after the experiment reveals that a substantial number of these modal responses are explained by the subjects in terms construable as a deontic interpretation of the rule, roughly paraphrased as "The cards should have a vowel on one side and an even number on the other." The P-with-Q response is correct for this interpretation.

4.2 Discussion of Results

Each of the manipulations designed to facilitate reasoning in the classical descriptive task makes it substantially easier as predicted by the semantic/pragmatic theories that the manipulations were derived from. The fact that subjects' reasoning is improved by each of these manipulations provides strong evidence that subjects' mental processes are operating with related categories in the standard laboratory task. Approaches like those of Sperber's relevance theory and Evans's matching theory propose that the subjects solve the task "without thinking." The fact that these instructional manipulations have an impact on subjects' responses strongly suggests that the processes they impact on are of a kind to interact with the content of the manipulations. This still leaves the question, at what level of awareness? But even here, the tutorial dialogues suggest that the level is not so far below the surface as to prevent these processes being quite easily brought to some level of awareness.

It is important to resist the idea that if subjects were aware of these problems, that itself would lead to their resolution, and the conclusion that therefore subjects can't be suffering these problems. Extensive tutoring in the standard task which is sufficient to lead subjects to make their problems quite explicit generally does *not* lead, at least immediately, to stable insight. This is as we should expect. If, for example, subjects become aware that robustness to counterexamples makes the task instructions uninterpretable, that itself does not solve their problem of how to respond. Or, for another example, if subjects become aware of being unable to take account of contingencies between choices in their responses, that does not solve the problem of what response to make. General questions of what concepts subjects have for expressing their difficulties and in what ways they are aware of them are important questions, especially for teaching. These questions invite further research through tutoring experiments, but they should not be allowed to lead to misinterpretation of the implications of the present results. We take each condition in turn

4.2.1 The Two–Rule Task

There are other possible explanations as to how the novel task functions to facilitate competence model responding. If subjects tend to confuse the two situations, "this rule is true of this card" and "this card makes this rule true" then it may help them that the two–rule task is calculated to lead them early to a conflict that a single card (e.g., the true consequent card) "makes both rules true" even as the instructions insist that one rule is true and one false. Although some subjects may infer that there must therefore be something wrong with the instructions, others progress from this impasse to appreciate that cases can comply with a rule without making it true – the semantic relations are asymmetric even though the same word "true" can, on occasion, be used for both directions. This confusion between semantic relations is evidently closely related to what Wason early on called a "verification" strategy (searching for compliant examples) in that it may lead to the same selections, but it is not the strategy as understood by Wason. This confusion between semantic relations is in abundant evidence in the dialogues.

The two–rule task makes an interesting comparison with at least three other findings in the literature. First, the task was designed partly to make explicit the choice of hypotheses which subjects entertain for the kind of Bayesian information–gain modeling proposed by Oaksford and Chater. Providing two explicit rules (rather than a single rule to be compared with an assumed null hypothesis of independence) makes the false-consequent card unambiguously the most informative card and therefore the one which these models should predict will be most frequently chosen. In our data for this task, the false-consequent card comes in third, substantially behind the true–antecedent and true–consequent cards.

For a second comparison, Gigerenzer and Hug [96] studied a manipulation which is of interest because it involves both a change from deontic to descriptive interpretation and from a single to a two–rule task. One example scenario had a single rule that hikers who stayed overnight in a hut had to bring their own firewood. Cards represented hikers or guides and bringers or nonbringers of wood. As a single-rule deontic task with instructions to see whether people obeyed the rule, this produced 90% correct responding, a typical result. But when the instructions asked the subject to turn cards in order to decide whether this rule was in force, or whether it was the guides who had to bring the wood, then performance dropped to 55% as conventionally scored. Gigerenzer and Hug explain this manipulation in terms of "perspective change," but this is both a shift from a deontic task to a descriptive one (in the authors' own words "to judge whether the rule is *descriptively* wrong" (our emphasis), and from a single–rule to a two–rule task, albeit that the second rule is mentioned but not printed alongside its alternative. Gigerenzer and Hug's data appear to show a level of performance higher than single rule abstract tasks but lower than deontic tasks, just as we observe. Direct comparison of the two subject populations is difficult, however, as Gigerenzer and Hug's subjects score considerably higher on all the reported tasks than ours, and no baseline single-rule descriptive task is included.

The third comparison of the two–rule task is with work on "reasoning illusions" by Johnson-Laird and colleagues mentioned above (Johnson-Laird and Savary [147]; Johnson-Laird, Legrenzi, Girotto and Legrenzi [149]; Johnson-Laird and Byrne [143]. Johnson-Laird and Savary [147,p. 213] presented exactly comparable premises to those we used in our two–rule task but asked their subjects to choose a conclusion, rather than to seek evidence about which rule was true and which false. Their interest in these problems is that mental models theory[2] assumes that subjects "only represent explicitly what is true," and that this gives rise to "illusory inferences." The following material was presented with the preface that both statements are about a hand of cards, and one is true and one is false:

1. If there is a king in the hand, then there is an ace.
2. If there is *not* a king in the hand, then there is an ace.

Select one of these conclusions:

i. There is an ace in the hand.

ii. There is not an ace in the hand.

iii. There may or may not be an ace in the hand.

---

2. At this stage it is not necessary to know the ins and outs of this theory. Details will be supplied in chapter 5, section 5.1.2 and and chapter 10, section 10.6.

Johnson-Laird and Savary [147] report that fifteen out of twenty subjects concluded that that there *is* an ace in the hand, and the other five concluded that there might or might not be an ace in the hand. They claim that the fifteen subjects are mistaken in their inference.

> Hence, apart from one caveat to which we will return, there is no reasonable interpretation of either the disjunction or the conditionals that yields a valid inference that there is an ace [147,p. 204].

The caveat appears to be that there are interpretations on which the premises are inconsistent and therefore *anything* (classically) logically follows, including this conclusion [147,p. 220].

What struck us initially is that our subjects show some facility with reasoning about assumptions of the same form even when our task also requires added elements of selection rather than merely inference. Selection tasks are generally "harder" on classical notions of what is correct. Specifically, our two–rule task introduces the circumstance which Johnson-Laird and Savary claim mental models predicts to introduce fundamental difficulty, i.e., reasoning from knowledge that some as yet unidentifiable proposition is false. This introduction makes the selection task much *easier* for subjects than its standard form in our experiment.

On a little further consideration, there is at least one highly plausible interpretation which makes the "illusory" conclusion valid and is an interpretation which appears in our dialogues from the two–rule task. Subjects think in terms of one of the rules *applying* and the other not, and they confuse (not surprisingly) the semantics of applicability with the semantics of truth. This is exactly the semantics familiar from the *IF ... THEN ... ELSE* construct of imperative computer languages. If one clause applies and the other doesn't, then it follows that there is an ace. Whether the alternativeness of the rules is expressed metalinguistically by saying one is false and one true) or object-linguistically (with an exclusive disjunction), and whether the rules are expressed as implications or as exclusive disjunctions, thinking in terms of applicability rather than truth is a great deal more natural and has the consequence observed. Johnson-Laird (personal communication) objects that this interpretation just is equivalent to the mental models theory one. But surely this is a crisp illustration of a difference between the theories. If an interpretation in terms of applicability is taken seriously, subjects *should* draw this conclusion, and should stick to it when challenged (as many do). In fact, failure to draw the inference is an error under this interpretation. Only mental models theory's restriction to a range of classical logical interpretations makes it define the inference as an error. We put our money on the subjects having the more plausible interpretation of the conditionals here and the experimenters suffering an illusion of an illusion.

4.2.2   Contingency Instructions

As mentioned above, investigations of this manipulation have been reported by Wason in early studies, but his theory of the task did not assign it any great importance, or lead him to systematically isolate the effect, or allow him to see the connection between descriptive interpretation and this instruction. In the context of our hypothesis that it is descriptive vs. deontic interpretation which is the main factor controlling difficulty of the task through interactions between semantics and instructions, this observation that contingency has systematic and predicted effects provides an explanation for substantial differences between the abstract task and content facilitations which invoke deontic interpretations. None of the other extant theories assign any significant role to this observation.

The effectiveness of contingency instructions presents particular difficulties for current "rational analysis" models (the approach using Bayesian information gain [205]; see section 3.5.2), since the choice of false-consequent cards rises so dramatically with an instruction which should have no effect on the expected information gain. Indeed, the rational analysis approach assumes that subjects adopt a "sampling one card at a time from a population" interpretation and it is hard to see why contingencies between responses should arise as a problem on such interpretations.

Going further: Engaging Interactive Planning

To illustrate how any of the conditions of this experiment could give rise to further investigations, we here briefly present, with his kind permission, an experiment designed by our student Misha van Denderen, who used the resources of the web to investigate the role of "reactive planning" as a source of difficulty in the standard selection task ([280]; more on this experiment in section 4.2.5). Going beyond a simple instructional change, this experiment investigates what happens if subjects are actually allowed to really engage in reactive planning i.e., by first choosing a card, turning it, and deciding what to do based on what is on the other side. It is interesting to investigate whether more subjects end up giving the classical answer if they are given the opportunity to actually turn the cards and see what is on the other side. The question is therefore: if subjects get the opportunity to solve the task by reactive planning, will they continue to turn until they find a falsifying card?

The experiment presents the task in a graphical software interface, using graphical tokens of the kind that people have become familiar with. The four cards are presented with a check box beneath each and an OK button to submit the answers. Subjects can actually turn each card and are invited to do so until they think they can decide whether the rule is true or false. Here it is clear to subjects that they can only tick and see one card at a time. They can click the check boxes on and off as they please. Only when they press the OK button and confirm that they are sure are the answers recorded.

Apart from the clarification of the classical task, it is interesting to observe the behavior of subjects if they can actually turn the cards. Will subjects continue turning cards until they find a falsifying card? If, for example, subjects decide to turn the A/4 card and therefore show that the case fits the rule, will they continue to turn the 7 card in search of possible falsification? And will subjects draw the conclusion that the rule is false if they did find a falsifying card on the first turn? Or true if they found a case that fit?

To maximize the information, a tweak must be included in the software to ensure that falsification of the rule is never immediate after the first card turned. The experiment is therefore set up as follows. Each card can be clicked. When a subject clicks a card, he is asked: "You want to see the $< 1st, 2nd, 3rd, 4th >$ card to judge whether the claim is true or false. Correct? [Y/N]." If the subject answers N, the invisible side is not revealed. If he answers Y, the invisible side is revealed and the number or the letter is shown. If the subject clicks the 7 before the A, the 7/K-card is shown. If he clicks the A before the 7, the A/4 card is shown. Only if the subject clicks the 7 after the A or the A after the 7, is the A/7-card shown. If the user clicks the K, the K/7-card is shown and if he clicks the 4, the 4/K card is shown.

This online experiment drew 103 subjects. The population is likely to be different from the standard undergraduate population, since these subjects were recruited through a marketing agency. The results given in table 4.3 therefore may not be quite comparable, but they replicate even in the substantial subsample who are students. The results are striking: Wason's "competence" choice combination is now the modal response. There is a very marked decrease in "just p" and "p and q" answers, accompanied by an equally marked increase in "p and not-q" answers, together with a spreading out of the miscellaneous category. The results seem to suggest that in the standard task, the desire to do the task by reactive planning is indeed a considerable issue. As always, this variation changes the task in several ways. For example, it decreases working memory load. Perhaps this is why subjects reason "better". This is possible, but the experiment has most direct force for two points. The first is Wason's "verificationalist" explanation in terms of subjects' failure to seek falsification. Given the a clearly understood opportunity, subjects do seek falsification. The second is that the experiment illustrates vividly how the descriptive task differs from the deontic one in which no contingencies of response arise. We return to this experiment below in section 4.2.5 when we consider the joint impact of the subjsects' several problems.

Table 4.3   Scores in the web-based selection task with reactive planning

p	p, q	$p, \neg q$	$p, q, \neg q$	misc.
7%	23%	26%	10%	34%

4.2.3   Truthfulness Instructions

As described above, the truthfulness condition differs from past attempts to cue subjects to seek counterexamples. Its success in bringing about a significant if small improvement may have resulted from effects of the manipulation other than the sociopsychological effects or the more general pragmatic effects of the balance of cooperative and adversarial stances described above. For example it may well be that at least some subjects are more adept at thinking about the truthfulness of speakers than the truth–values of their utterances abstracted from such issues as ignorance or intent to deceive. We return to this issue when we consider experiments on illiterate subjects in chapter 5.

4.2.4   The Conjunctive Rule

The purpose behind the conjunctive version of the task was rather different from the other manipulations, namely to show that many features of the task militate against the adoption of Wason's intended interpretation of his instructions quite apart from difficulties specific to conditionals. The interpretation of sentence semantics is highly malleable under the forces of task pragmatics. The results show that a conjunctive rule is treated very like (even if significantly differently from) the *if . . . then* rule. A higher proportion of subjects make the 'classically correct' response than in the baseline task (13% as compared to 3.7%) but the modal response is the same (P and Q) and is made by similar proportions of subjects (45% conjunctive as compared to 52% baseline). One possibility is that a substantial number of subjects adopt a deontic interpretation of the rule and are checking for the cards that might be violators but are not yet known to be.

It is also possible that these results have more specific consequences for interpretation of the standard descriptive task. We know from Fillenbaum [82] and from our own paraphrase tasks [264] that about a half of subjects most readily entertain a conjunctive reading of *if . . . then* sentences. The developmental literature reviewed in Evans, Newstead, and Byrne [76] reveals this interpretation to be even commoner among young children. It is most implausible that this interpretation is due merely to some polysemy of the connective "if . . . then." Much more plausible is that the conjunctive reading is the result of assuming the truth of the antecedent suppositionally, and then answering subsequent questions from within this suppositional context.

Be that as it may, if subjects' selections in the conditional rule tasks correspond to the selections they would make given an explicit conjunction in the conjunction condition, and we are right that these selections are driven in this condition by an implicitly deontic interpretation of the conjunction, then this suggests a quite novel explanation of at least some "matching" responses in the original conditional task. Perhaps the similar rate of choice of P and Q in the conjunction and "if ... then" conditions points to a substantial number of subjects applying a deontic conjunctive interpretation in the standard task.

This hypothesis in turn raises the question how such a reading would interact with negations in the "negations" paradigm which is the source of the evidence for Evans's ' 'matching" theory [73] (see also section 3.6) and therefore the source of one leg of the "dual process" theory (Evans and Over [75], Evans [72]; see section 5.3). If interpretations stemming from deontic readings tend strongly toward wide scope for negation, then one would predict that the rule with negated antecedent ("not P and Q") would be read as "It's not the case that there is a vowel on one side and an even number on the other" which would lead to the same choices of A and 4, though for opposite reasons. That is, K and 7 are now seen as already compliant, and the A and the 4 have to be tested to make sure they *don't* have an even number or a vowel respectively. Pursuing this line of thought further suggests that negations in the second clause may not be interpretable in this framework because of their interactions with the anaphors ("if there is a vowel on one side then there is not an even number on the other side" gets interpreted as "if it's not the case that there is a vowel on one side, then there is an even number on the other") and subjects might be forced to interpret them with the same wide scope, again leading to the same card choices, and potentially explaining why "matching" appears to be unaffected by negation. Providing a semantic explanation, of course, leaves open the questions about what processes operate. Evidently, further research will be required to explore these possibilities. The semantic analyses may seem complex but they make some rather strong predictions about how subjects should react to card turnings. This is an interesting line for future research holding out the possibility of a semantic basis for matching behavior.

One objection to these various interpretations of the conjunction condition results might be that there are other interpretations of the rule used. Subjects might, for example, have interpreted the rule existentially, as claiming that at least one card had a vowel on one side and an even number on the other. This would lead normatively to the same A and 4 selections. Accordingly, in a follow-up experiment, we revised the conjunctive rule to

> **Rule**: *There are vowels on one side of the cards and even numbers on the other.*

4.2 Discussion of Results

It is implausible that this rule might be interpreted existentially. We ran this rule in another condition with its own baseline condition to ensure comparability of the new population. Table 4.4 shows the results of this experiment, with the earlier results repeated for convenient comparison. The result was slightly more extreme with this version of the conjunctive rule: 70% of subjects (rather than 45%) chose the P and Q cards. The proportion of classical logical competence model responses was identical to that for the baseline conditional task, and the baseline condition showed the population was comparable. The rewording raised the proportion of subjects giving the modal P and Q response. This rewording of the conjunctive rule appeared to make the universal deontic reading even less ambiguously the dominant reading.

Table 4.4 Frequencies of card choice combinations by conditions: the modified conjunction task and its new baseline condition are below the earlier results which are repeated here for convenience. Classical logical competence responses are marked *. Any response made by at least three subjects in at least one condition is categorized: everything else is miscellaneous

Condition	P Q	Q	P	P ¬Q	¬Q	¬P,Q	P,Q, ¬Q	¬P,¬Q	all	None	Misc.	Tot
Classical	56	7	8	4*	3	7	1	2	9	8	5	108
2-rule	8	8	2	1	9*	2	1	0	0	2	4	37
Contingency	15	0	3	8*	1	6	4	8	3	0	3	51
Truthfulness	39	6	9	14*	0	7	3	6	8	15	5	112
Conjunction	31	2	9	7	2	0	0	1	0	9*	8	69
Baseline 2	10	2	10	1*	1	0	0	0	0	1	3	30
Conjunction 2	21	1	3	1	0	0	0	0	0	1*	2	30
Subjunctive	13	2	8	3*	0	1	2	1	1	0	0	31

The results on the conjunctive rule illustrate several general issues: how easy it is to invoke a deontic reading of indicative wording; how unnatural it is for naive subjects to adopt an "is this sentence literally true?" perspective rather than a "what are the experimenter's intentions?" perspective; that the difficulty of classical interpretation can be as great with conjunction as with implication. Although the difficulties may be different difficulties, there is a real possibility that they are closely related through conjunctive suppositional interpretations of the conditional.

Finally, we explored one other obvious manipulation designed to follow up the malleability of subjects' interpretations exposed by the conjunctive rule. This is worth discussing as a "failed" negative result as much as for its own interest. If subjects' difficulties in the original descriptive task follow from the complexities of descriptive semantics, is it possible to restore deontic levels of performance in the abstract task merely by simply formulating the rule in the subjunctive mood? We ran a further condition in which the rule used was

If a card has a vowel on one side, then it *should* have an even number on the other.

and the instruction was to choose which of the four cards you *must* turn in order
to decide if the card complies with the rule.

The results of this condition are shown in table 4.4 in the "Subjunctive" row.
Three of thirty-one subjects turned P and not-Q, as compared to one of thirty in
the baseline. If this is a facilitation it is a small one (the probability of getting
this facilitation by chance is 0.32, i.e., statistically insignificant). Merely using
subjunctive wording may be insufficient to invoke a deontic reading. This is
not so surprising since there is an alternative "epistemic" interpretation of the
subjunctive modal here which might still be used with a descriptive semantics
for the underlying rule. Imagine that the rule is clearly a robust descriptive
scientific law (perhaps "All ravens are black"), then one might easily state in
this context, that a card with "raven" on one side *should* have "black" on the
other, implying something about what the cards have to be like to comply with
the scientific law (still with a descriptive semantics underlying), rather than
what the birds have to do to comply with a legal regulation. This possibility
of interpretation may make it hard to invoke a deontic interpretation without
further contentful support. Contentful support is, of course, what the various
"quality inspector" scenarios provide (e.g., [252]). Contentful support is also
what permission and obligation schemas, and the "seek violations" instructions
in combination with modal explications of the rule provide, as reported by Platt
and Griggs [217].

This failure of what is about the simplest direct manipulation that could test
the theory (that it is deontic interpretation which achieves most of the facilitations reported in the literature) is a very common kind of failure. Our interpretation is that the manipulation unfortunately fails to achieve its goal. An
opponent of our theory might claim it as evidence the theory is wrong. To settle this dispute one would need to get further evidence that the manipulation
doesn't succeed in invoking a deontic reading. Trying such direct tests is important – if they work they provide dramatic evidence. Generally when they
fail they are not reported. The problem is a problem of constructing a bridge
from a theory of interpretation to the effects of manipulations, and bridging is
unavoidable if theory is to be brought to bear on data.

4.2.5   Putting It All Together?

In summary of all the conditions, these results corroborate the findings of the
tutoring experiments, also reported in [264], that our manipulations alleviate
real sources of difficulty with interpretation for subjects in the original descriptive task – sources of difficulty which do not apply in the deontic task. This
evidence suggests that far from failing to think at all, subjects are sensitive to
several important semantic issues posed by the descriptive task. Since our manipulations only help to alleviate problems piecemeal in some subjects, they

cannot be expected to install a classical logical interpretation of the task and materials in all subjects, nor to produce performance levels comparable with the deontic tasks. It is difficult to assess what proportion of problems have been dealt with here. Several that we discussed in chapter 3 have not been treated (anaphora, card reversibility). It is an even harder methodological problem to find a way of estimating how much of the difficulties these problems jointly account for, because simply applying all the manipulations concurrently produces complicated instructions which themselves introduce their own problems.

Rather than presenting a complete model of what subjects are doing in this task, the experiment provides strong evidence that several of the major sources of interpretation problems identified by semantic analysis do contribute to subjects' difficulties in the original task. This is sufficient to make it very hard to defend any theory which assumes both that the correct interpretation is classical logic, and that it is the interpretation that subjects adopt. This includes all theories except the information-gain theory. As discussed above, both the two-rule and contingency conditions provide considerable evidence that the information–gain theory has its own problems.

The ingenious experiment by van Denderen [280], part of which was discussed in section 4.2.2, was actually aimed at the difficult task of assessing how many of these problems can be simultaneously alleviated. How many subjects can be induced to adopt the material implication interpretation Wason's criterion of correct reasoning requires, by simply simultaneously removing problems Wason strews in the subjects' path? And how many subjects then reason as their chosen interpretation requires? Platt and Griggs [217] induced very high selections of A and 7 cards in the descriptive task by focusing subjects on possibly noncompliant cases. But van Denderen's aim was to see what could be achieved without this focusing. The manipulations he used are as follows: (1) the task was run interactively on the web so that subjects could actually turn cards and alleviate the problems of wanting to make responses contingent on the feedback of early turns (this manipulation was discussed in section 4.2.2 above); (2) the conditional is not described as a *rule* (with the result of engendering a defeasible interpretation of the relevance of a larger population of cards) but rather as a simple expression of an observer's belief about four cards; (3) the conditionality (as opposed to biconditionality) of the rule is emphasized by inclusion of a clause explicitly disavowing the biconditional reading; (4) the source of the conditional was separated from the experimenter to avoid issues of the need to accuse an authority figure of lying; and (5) subjects are required to confirm their understanding of the instructions by answering some simple questions about the task before proceeding to the experiment.

The design of the experiment divided subjects into a group with a simple conditional (original conditional), and a group with the clause rejecting the biconditional added (extended rule). All subjects did two versions of the task:

one including all the enhancements just listed except for the possibility of inter-acting with the cards (noninteractive), and the other with this interaction (inter-active) , in that order. After these two selection tasks, subjects did an 'evalua-tion task' [297] where they judged each of the four card types as complying, not complying, or irrelevant to the conditional, in order to gather data on their inter-pretation. Armed with these data about individual interpretation, it is possible to assess not only whether subjects adopt Wason's intended interpretation of the conditional but also whether they reason correctly from it, or from whatever other interpretation they do adopt.

The results show a huge convergence on Wason's desired interpretation of the conditionals. Whereas with the original conditional, only a fifth of subjects chose the material implication interpretation (even with all the clarifications), with the extended rule this rose to 80%. There was a similarly large increase of A and 7 selections, from around 5% making this choice in Wason's original experiment, to 32% of subjects in the extended rule interactive task who chose just A and 7, and a further 16% chose A, 7, and 4. All told, 60% turned the 7 card compared to about 9% in Wason's original task. About 55% of subjects made all the card choices in the complex interactive task which normatively corresponded with their chosen interpretation, although more than half of these chose one or more cards they strictly need not have turned.

These results are a strong vindication of the theory we have proposed here. There is much interpretive variability, but a large majority of subjects can be induced to adopt the interpretation Wason intended, and when they do, a large proportion of them reason adequately from that interpretation. Reasoning is by no means perfect, but the hard part is getting to the interpretation which Wason hid. This experiment is rather revealing of the forest of problems the subject encounters, and therefore suggestive of why the ability to find Wason's inter-pretation and turn the A and 7 cards should be predictive of academic success, as Stanovich showed.

4.3   What Does This Say about Reasoning More Generally?

What implications do these results have for theories of reasoning, and for the place of interpretation in cognitive theory more generally? What do they tell us about the way the field has viewed the relation between logical and psycho-logical analyses of reasoning, and how that relation might be construed more productively? Each theory is a somewhat different case.

These results remove the founding evidence for "evolutionary" theories which propose that the difference in performance on "social contract" conditionals and descriptive conditionals needs to be explained by innate cheating detec-tion modules evolved in the Pleistocene. This topic will be discussed at greater length in chapter 6. As we will see, this reappraisal of the selection task provides a good example of how arguments for "massive modularity" in cognition should be treated with some skepticism (for further arguments, see [268]). The original experiments found variation in performance as a function of difference in materials. Sweeping generalizations were then made from the laboratory task without any consideration of the relation between that task and subjects' other communication and reasoning abilities. Just as our analysis directs attention to the differences between variations on the selection task and the continuities between natural language communication inside and outside the selection task, so our proposals return attention to the issue of how humans' generalized communication capacities arose in evolution. The interactions between logic's dual apparatus of interpretation and of derivation constitute an exquisitely context–sensitive conceptual framework for the study of human reasoning and communication, whether in evolution, development, or education. Chapter 5 takes up these themes.

The nonevolutionary theories of human reasoning are most generally affected by the present results through their implications for the relation between logic and psychology. We focus here particularly on relevance theory, mental models theory, and rational analysis models.[3]

Relevance Theory   Inasmuch as relevance theory [251, 99, 252] assumes that human reasoning and communication abilities are general abilities which interact with the specifics of the context, our general drift is sympathetic to relevance theory's conclusions. We agree with relevance theory, that the goal must be to make sense of what subjects are doing in the very strange situation of laboratory reasoning tasks – in a memorable phrase, to see subjects as "pragmatic virtuosos" (Girotto et al. [99]) – rather than to see them as logical defectives. Our divergences from relevance theory are about the granularity of interaction between semantic and pragmatic processes in subjects' reasoning; in the range of behavior we believe to be of theoretical concern; and in the program of research.

Relevance theory explains pragmatic effects in terms of very general factors – relevance to the task at hand and cost of inference to reveal that relevance. These factors must always operate with regard to some semantic characterization of the language processed. Condensing analysis into these two pragmatic factors, however, seems, in this case at least, to have led to relevance theorists missing the critical *semantic* differences which drive the psychological processes in this task – the differences between deontics and descriptives and their consequences for interpretation in this task's setting. Relevance theory's conclusion has been that not much reasoning goes on when undergraduate subjects get the abstract task "wrong." Our combination of tutoring observations and

---

3. The remainder of this section is therefore most useful to readers familiar with these theories. Other readers may skip ahead to the paragraph entitled "General Implications."

experiment strongly suggests that a great deal goes on, however speedily the "precomputed" attitudes are brought to bear in the actual task, and that the exact nature of the processes is highly variable from subject to subject. Taking logic more seriously leads us to seek more detailed accounts of mental processes.

Mental Models Theory   The current results have rather wide-ranging implications for mental models theory [144, 143]. Some implications specific to the theory's application to the selection task have already been discussed. Others are more general, about mental models theory's relation to logic and semantics. Since Johnson-Laird's early work with Wason on the selection task [297, 148, 298] mental models theory has been elaborated by a complex theory of the meanings of conditionals and the overlay of semantics by "pragmatic modulation," and the theory has been much exercised by the issue whether subjects' interpretations of the rule in the selection task is truth–functional or not [143]. However, this consideration of semantic possibilities has been divorced from any consideration of their implications for the subjects' interpretation of the *task*. If subjects' reading of the rule is non-truth–functional (by whatever semantic or pragmatic route), then the subjects should experience a *conflict* between their interpretation and the task instructions. This conflict has never been acknowledged by mental models theorists. What justification can there then be for applying the classical logical competence model as a criterion of correct performance while simultaneously rejecting it as an account of how subjects interpret the conditional? We shall return to some of the general logical issues raised by mental models in chapter 5, insection 5.1.4 and chapter 10, section 10.6.

Bayesian Models   Finally, where do our findings leave the Bayesian information–gain models of selection task behavior as optimal experiment (Oaksford and Chater [205, 206])? We applaud these authors' challenge to the uniqueness of the classical logical model of the task, and also their insistence that the deontic and descriptive versions of the task require distinct accounts. Their theory is clearly more sophisticated about the relations between formal models and cognitive processes than the theories it challenges. However, our proposals are quite divergent in their cognitive consequences. The rational analysis models reject any role for logic, claiming that the task is an inductive one. But this move smuggles logic in the backdoor. Applying optimal experiment theory requires assigning probabilities to propositions, and propositions are specified in some underlying language. The logic underlying the rational analysis model is the same old classical propositional calculus with all its attendant divergences from subjects' interpretations of the task materials. This has direct psychological consequences. The rational analysis models treat subjects' performances as being equally correct as measured by the two distinct competence models for descriptive and deontic tasks. Our analysis predicts that the descriptive task will be highly problematical and the deontic task rather straightforward. The tutorial evidence on the descriptive task and its experimental corroboration support our prediction about the descriptive task. Approaching through interpretation predicts and observes considerable variety in the problems different subjects exhibit in the descriptive task, and even variety within the same subject at different times. We can agree that some subjects may adopt something like the rational analysis model of the task, but disagree about the uniformity of this or any other interpretation. Most of all we do not accept that everyone is doing the same thing at the relevant level of detail.

General Implications   This situates our approach with regard to some prominent psychological theories of reasoning, and illustrates similarities and differences with extant approaches in the context of this one particular task. But our proposals also have general implications for how cognitive theories of reasoning relate to logical and linguistic theories of language and communication more generally. If we are anything like right about the selection task, it is both possible and necessary to bring the details of formal accounts of natural languages (semantics of deontics and descriptives, variable and constant anaphora, tense, definiteness, domain of interpretation, scope of negation) to bear in explaining the details of performance in laboratory reasoning tasks. This is necessary because subjects' behavior in these tasks is continuous with generalized human capacities for communication, and possible because although strange in many ways, laboratory tasks have to be construed by subjects using their customary communicative skills.

In fact laboratory tasks have much in common with the curious communicative situation that is formal education, and another benefit of the current approach is that it stands to reconnect the psychology of reasoning with educational investigations. With very few exceptions (e.g., Stanovich and West [253]), psychologists of reasoning have not asked what educational significance their results have. They regard their theories as investigating "the fundamental human reasoning mechanism" which is independent of education. On our account, the descriptive selection task is interesting precisely because it forces subjects to reason in vacuo and this process is closely related to extremely salient educational processes which are aimed exactly at equipping students with generalizable skills for reasoning in novel contexts more effectively. For example, the balance of required cooperative assumption of the background rule and adversarial test of the foreground rule in the descriptive selection task is absolutely typical of the difficulties posed in the strange communications involved in examination questions (cf. the quote from Ryle on p. 23). Many cross–cultural observations of reasoning can be understood in terms of the kinds of discourse different cultures invoke in various circumstances (see chapter 5). The discourses established by formal education are indeed a very distinctive characteristic of our culture (see, e.g., [20], [124]).

5 From the Laboratory to the Wild and Back Again

Instead of patiently explaining the state of the art in the psychology of reasoning, this book has started in medias res by taking one well-known experimental paradigm – the selection task – and showing both how traditional psychology of reasoning has treated it and what a cognitive science of reasoning might aspire to. It is now time to step back and introduce the most important concerns of the psychology of reasoning as it has been practiced. It has been argued by many outside the field that the kind of reasoning studied in this branch of psychology is totally irrelevant to real life, and this brings us to the question whether logical reasoning occurs in the wild, and more generally, whether it is a trick acquired by schooling or, on the contrary, a natural endowment.

5.1 The Laboratory

The psychology of reasoning is concerned with the experimental study of reasoning patterns also of interest to logicians, and in the literature we find experimental research on, for example,

- reasoning with syllogisms in adults,

- reasoning with propositional connectives in adults,

- acquisition of connectives and quantifiers in children,

- reasoning in subjects with various psychiatric or cognitive impairments,

- brain correlates of reasoning,

- reasoning in "primitive" societies.

As an example of the second area, an adult subject may be presented with the premises

If Julie has an essay, she studies late in the library.
Julie does not study late in the library.

and is then asked: what, if anything, follows? In this case (modus tollens) it may happen that half of the subjects reply that nothing can be concluded. In contrast, the analogous experiment for modus ponens, with the minor premise

> Julie has an essay.

typically yields "success" scores of around 95% drawing the conclusion. The psychologist is then interested in explaining the difference in performance, and believes that differences such as this actually provide a window on the cognitive processes underlying logical reasoning.[1] What is distinctive about the psychology of reasoning is that it views its task as uncovering *the mechanism* of logical reasoning: what goes on in the brain (and where) when it makes an inference? This issue can be framed in terms of what psychologists call the *representations* employed by reasoning, although we prefer the term *implementation* here. This level is concerned with how the abstract structures of informational analysis – discourses, sentences, models, proofs – are implemented, both in the world and in the mind. Is there something like a diagram or like a text implemented in the mind? Or perhaps on the paper the subject is using? Here one is concerned with memory, both long-term and working memory, with modalities (visuospatial, phonetic, orthographic), with the environment (as it functions representationally), and eventually with the brain – all the paraphernalia of psychological analysis. Here differences may certainly be expected between how the information specified in sentences and the information specified in models gets implemented. But remarkably little study has been aimed at this level until very recently, and much of what has been aimed at it has been based on dubious informational-level analyses. We will return to this issue after introducing three well-known "schools" in the psychology of reasoning, each identified by what it takes to be the mechanism underlying reasoning.

5.1.1 Mental Logic

This school, also known as the "mental rules" school [228], maintains that logical reasoning is the application of formal rules, which are more or less similar to natural deduction rules. Here is an example (from [229]): the theory tries to explain why humans tend to have difficulty with modus tollens, by assuming that this is not a primitive rule, unlike modus ponens; modus tollens has to be derived each time it is used; therefore it leads to longer processing time. Reasoning is thus assumed to be implemented as a syntactic process transforming sentences into other sentences via rewrite rules. Since on this view reasoning is similar to language processing, it has sometimes been maintained that it should be subserved by the same brain circuits:

---

1. We will in fact have something to say about this particular phenomenon in chapter 7.

> [Mental logic claims] that deductive reasoning is a rule governed syntactic process where internal representations preserve structural properties of linguistic strings in which the premises are stated. This linguistic hypothesis predicts that the neuro-anatomical mechanisms of language (syntactic) processing underwrite human reasoning processes . . . (Goel et al.[101,p. 504])

This would allow us to distinguish between "mental logic" and its foremost competitor, discussed next.

5.1.2   Mental Models

The founding father of the "mental models" school is Johnson-Laird [145]; applications of "mental models" to logic can be found in Johnson-Laird and Byrne [144]. The main claim of this school is that reasoners do not apply content-independent formal rules (such as, for example, modus ponens), but construct models for sentences and read off conclusions from these, which are then subject to a process of validation by looking for alternative models. Errors in reasoning are typically explained by assuming that subjects read off a conclusion from the initial model which turns out not to be true in all models of the premises. The "mental models" school arose as a reaction against "mental logic" because it was felt that formal, contentless rules would be unable to explain the so-called "content effects" in reasoning, such as were believed to occur in the selection task. It was also influenced by simultaneous developments in formal semantics, namely Kamp's discourse representation theory [152], which emphasized the need for the construction of "discourse models" as an intermediary between language and world.

On the representational side, "mental models" seems to point to spatial processing as the underlying mechanism.

> [Mental models claims] that deductive reasoning is a process requiring spatial manipulation and search. Mental model theory is often referred to as a spatial hypothesis and predicts that the neural structures for visuo-spatial processing contribute the basic representational building blocks used for logical reasoning. (Goel et al.[101,p. 504])

It then seems possible to set up an experiment to distinguish between the two theories, by using experimental evidence that language processing is localized in the left hemisphere, and spatial processing in the parietal cortex (chiefly on the right). If a subject shows no activation in the parietal cortex while reasoning, this is taken to be evidence against the involvement of spatial processing, and hence ultimately against mental models. A result of this kind was indeed obtained by Goel and colleagues [100]. Another example is Canessa et al. [30] which claims to identify the locations of social contract reasoning, and of abstract logical reasoning, in the brain on the basis of a scanning experiment of descriptive and deontic selection tasks. We will return to such arguments later, showing that the route from hypothesized mechanism to brain area is considerably less direct than claimed by Goel and other neuroscientists.

5.1.3   Darwinian Algorithms

Evolutionary psychology has also tried to shed its light on logical reasoning, beginning with the famous (or notorious) paper "The Logic of Social Exchange: Has Natural Selection Shaped how Humans Reason? Studies with the Wason Selection Task" by Leda Cosmides [47]. Here the main claim is that there is no role for (formal, domain–independent) logic in cognition; whenever we appear to reason logically, this is because we have evolved strategies ("Darwinian algorithms") to solve a problem in a particular domain. The first application is also the most vivid: the difference between bad performance on the abstract selection task and good performance on the drinking age rule is hypothesized to be due to the fact that the latter is a "social contract," and that we have evolved a mechanism for policing social contracts, the so-called cheater detector. This is just a very special instance of evolutionary psychology's general claim that the mind must be viewed as a collection of dedicated mechanisms (called "modules") each engineered by natural selection. We will discuss evolutionary psychology much more extensively in chapter 6, section 6.3; for the moment these brief indications suffice.

On the representational side, the picture is again a bit different. The hypothesis implies that there is a very specific brain area, located in the limbic system, dedicated to the vigorous pursuit of cheaters, and it has indeed been claimed by Cosmides and colleagues that this area can be identified from neuropsychological studies of selective impairments to the limbic system [272] (see also [30]).

5.1.4   Cold Water

There are more "schools" than have been mentioned here. But for now the most important point is that talk about *the* mechanism is apt to be highly misleading, because it does not take into account that any cognitive phenomenon can be studied at various levels. The classical discussion of this issue is David Marr's [183], where he points out that cognitive science should distinguish at least the following three levels of inquiry

1. identification of the information–processing task as an input–output function,

2. specification of an algorithm which computes that function,

3. neural implementation of the algorithm specified.

These distinctions between levels are of course familiar from computer science, as is the observation that there is no reason to stick to three levels only, since a program written in one language (say Prolog) may be implemented in another language (say C), and so on all the way down to an assembly language, machine code, and the several levels of analysis of hardware. What is important about Marr's three levels is that for any phenomenon analysed as an information system, three levels related in this way will figure. Furthermore, it is tempting to think that the neural implementation provides some kind of rock bottom, the most fundamental level of inquiry; but of course the neural implementation uses a *model* of what actual neurons do, and not the real things themselves. Neuroscience provides several further levels below the neuron.

The upshot of this discussion is that it makes no sense to ask for *the* mechanism underlying reasoning without first specifying a level at which one intends to study this question. As a consequence, a superficially sensible distinction such as that between mental logic and mental models may turn out to be empirically meaningless, at least in the form it is usually stated. The fact that the argument patterns studied by psychologists typically come from logics with a completeness theorem should already give one pause: at the input–output level manipulations with rules and manipulations with models cannot be distinguished in such systems. One can look at subtler measures such as error rates or reaction times; e.g., mental modelers like to point to a correlation between the difficulty of a syllogistic figure (as measured by error rate), and the number of models that the premises of the figure allow, but proof-theoretic rule systems often consider a series of "cases" which mimic these models, and so cast doubt on any empirical separation between rules and models at this level (see Stenning [258, 269] for discussions of this type of argumentation).

5.2   A View with No Room

Should the psychology of deduction be about these few well-known laboratory tasks in which subjects are presented with logical puzzles and asked to solve them: the selection task, syllogisms, the suppression task, conditional reasoning? And if our capacity of deduction is not just for performing these tasks, what is it for? What everyday functions does it serve? How are theoretical analyses of deductive performance in these laboratory tasks related to analyses of other cognitive functions?

As we remarked in the introduction, reasoning fell from the position of being absolutely central in the cognitive revolution, which was founded on conceptions of reasoning, computation, and the analysis of language, to become the deadbeat of cognitive psychology, pursued in a ghetto, surrounded by widespread skepticism as to whether human reasoning really happens outside the academy. Within the ghetto, the issue with the highest visibility has been about the nature of the mental representations underlying deduction – is it "rules" or is it "models"? There has been almost universal acceptance that the goal of the field is the characterization of "the fundamental human (deductive) reasoning mechanism," and that it must work on one or the other of these two kinds of representation. Along with confidence that there is a single fundamental human reasoning mechanism goes confidence that classical logic is the unchallenged arbiter of correct reasoning, although classical logic is often simultaneously rejected as a useful guide to mental representation or process. It is assumed that the classical logical form of the materials used in the experiments lies very near to their surface without any substantial interpretive process. This idea of interpretation as the superficial translation of natural language into logical form carries over into neglect of the processes whereby artificial logical languages are interpreted – assigned a mapping onto the world. Natural languages do not come with this mapping in anything like the detail required for discourse interpretation – artificial languages still less so (consider the introduction of our notion of interpretation in p. 21).

As we saw earlier in this chapter, there have been rejections of the appropriateness of logical deductive models of reasoning in favour of inductive information–gain models which turn reasoning into decision. But even those who have departed from accepting classical logic as the relevant competence model [205] have continued to accept that it makes sense to treat all subjects as "trying to do the same thing" and so the goal might be described as changing to that of characterizing the "fundamental human information–gain mechanism." But as both chapter 7 and the beginning of this chapter argue, even this apparently radical move to a completely different competence model still smuggles classical logic in at the backdoor.

The dissatisfactions of the ghetto have led even some prominent community members to depart entirely, claiming that once the ecological context of real life is considered seriously, what we find are decision processes, not reasoning processes, and that fast and frugal heuristics without any reference to competence models can replace logic, probability, and all other cumbersome systems of reasoning [95]. Reasoning is the idle pastime of the academy, but not the bread and butter of the real world. In fact several of the prominent researchers who earlier made much of their analyses of the selection task now claim the task is uninteresting.

As the last chapter suggested, the route out of this ghetto lies in taking interpretation seriously. In fact we believe that the mental processes mainly evoked by the laboratory tasks mentioned are interpretive processes – the processes of reasoning *to* interpretations. Modern logic provides a rich landscape of possibilities and we believe the empirical evidence is that subjects are engaged in setting a series of parameters in this space in order to formalise their understanding of what it is they are being asked to do. The evidence is that in these abstracted and unnatural settings student subjects are error-prone – so rich interpretation does not mean infallible reasoning. However, recasting the phenomena as interpretive provides a bridge between the laboratory and the wild.

Laboratory tasks force interpretation in a vacuum, and the scattering that results can tell us much about what happens at more normal pressures. Furthermore, the wild, at least in "developed" societies with extended formal schooling, is full of tasks which are abstracted in ways rather closely related to the laboratory tasks, which were, after all, originally collected or adapted from various teaching sources. The nature of this bridge is then a good guide to the tasks in the wild which most bring reasoning into play.

An immediate corollary of the formal stance of taking the multiplicity of interpretations seriously is the empirical consequence of needing to take individual differences seriously. Subjects do different things in the experiments, and this has so far been treated as simply stringing them out along a dimension of intelligence. They are all deemed to be trying to do the same thing, but succeeding or failing in different degrees. If there are many interpretations and each poses a qualitatively different task, then subjects are not even trying to do the same thing (at least at any finer grain than understanding what the hell they are being asked to do), and suddenly the data and the theoretical demands become far richer. And most important of all, the working relation between formalization and experiment changes entirely. Taking interpretation seriously and separating semantic from representational issues offers a room with a view quite panoramic enough to serve as foundations for human cognition.

The gulf of incomprehension between the logical and psychological communities is a source of great personal sadness. We must get away from the idea that these two disciplines are in competition and realise that logic is a theory at a much more abstract level than psychologists suppose, but nevertheless one that is indispensable for formulating empirical psychology. Trying to do without it is comparable to trying to study visual perception without geometry (only worse because of the variety of logics that are plainly required), and this analogy should make it clear that once one has done all one's geometry, visual perception still remains to be done. Logic is not about to replace psychology. Logic is about the specification of abstract systems, and is an indispensable guide to how those systems might or might not be implemented, at a number of different levels, in the mind. Of course, inappropriate logical analyses lead to bad psychological explanations (cf. the last chapter), but if logic analysis and psychological work are reasonably coupled, then that should become evident rather quickly, and a better logical analysis found. One moral of the last 35 years of the psychology of reasoning has been that the penalty of divorcing logic has been the reinvention of several pale imitations which have served only to confuse.

5.3   The Literate Wild

Psychology devised laboratory paradigms for reasoning, presumably on the assumption that reasoning is in some sense a natural cognitive capability, and therefore worth studying. Since there is room for doubt whether these experiments test what they were designed to test, it is useful to briefly adopt a more phenomenological approach and ask ourselves what can plausibly be classified as reasoning in natural environments. Here it is useful to introduce (and eventually adapt) the distinction between "system 1" and "system 2" processes discussed in dual process theories of reasoning [72]:

> system 1 is . . . a form of universal cognition shared between animals and humans. It is actually not a single system but a set of subsystems that operate with some autonomy. System 1 includes instinctive behaviors that would include any input modules of the kind proposed by Fodor . . . The System 1 processes that are most often described, however, are those that are formed by associative learning of the kind produced by neural networks. . . . System 1 processes are rapid, parallel and automatic in nature; only their final product is posted in consciousness [72,p. 454].

In these theories, logical reasoning is considered to belong to "system 2" which is

> slow and sequential in nature and makes use of the central working memory system. . . . [72,p. 454]

It is also sometimes said that system 1 and system 2 processes invoke different concepts of rationality [254]. This view of reasoning grew out of, and fed into, the standard experimental paradigms where subjects are given premises with the instruction to reason to a conclusion starting from the given premises only.

We believe that it is a mistake to maintain that fast and automatic processes are thereby not logical processes, as is implicit in the above quotation. On our view, the prime counterexample is discourse interpretation, which is by and large automatic *and* proceeds according to logical laws (albeit nonclassical), *and* involves the construction of representations in central working memory. Chapter 7 will treat this topic in detail; here we discuss what the wild looks like from the perspective of a different conceptualization of the boundary between system 1 and system 2 processes. In a nutshell, different goals require different assessments of what constitutes rational action, and accordingly determine an appropriate logic. *The formal properties of this logic then determine what kind of implementations are possible, and whether they can process quickly and automatically or only slowly and laboriously.* We conceptualise the part that logic plays in system 1 as being the foundation of routine discourse interpretation, when a suitable knowledge base already exists in long-term memory. When the routine process of interpretation meets an impasse, then system 2 comes into operation, albeit often briefly, before system 1 can resume interpretation. On the other hand, some impasses may require substantial conceptual learning, or argument between the parties to the discourse, and in this case resumption won't be so quickly achieved.

When discussing the phenomenology of reasoning, we distinguish between literate and illiterate people; the classical results of Luria and Scribner have exhibited considerable phenomenological differences in reasoning styles in these subgroups, and it is useful to discuss these differences from our interpretive perspective.

5.3.1 The Literate Wild: System 1 Processes

We have argued that much of the psychology of reasoning is (albeit unwittingly) about interpretation, and that we should reinterpret an important subset of system 1 processes as automatic, but defeasible, reasoning to interpretations. We further claim that much *planning* is an important system 1 process subserving interpretation. For the construction of discourse models this has been shown in [282], and chapter 7 will establish the formal relation between planning and reasoning. Here we stay at the phenomenal level, and discuss what forms planning can take in the wild. Before we start out, a distinction must be made.

We perhaps tend to think first of conscious deliberate planning – a form of problem solving – rather than the sort of effortless automatic planning involved in, say, planning motor actions. The connection between planning and system 1 is through the latter kind of planning, though relations to the former deliberate kind are important in considering relations between system 1 and system 2. The fundamental *logical* connection between interpretation and planning is that both are defeasible. When we plan (deliberately or automatically) we plan in virtue of our best guess about the world in which we will have to execute our plan. We may plan for what to do if we miss the bus, but we don't plan for what to do if the bus doesn't come because the gravitational constant changes, even though that is a logical possibility. If we used classical logic throughout our planning, we would have to consider all logically possible worlds, or at least make explicit exactly what range of worlds we consider. This necessity is what gives rise to the notorious frame problem in AI [223].

Closed–world reasoning (as introduced in chapter 2) is a particular logic for planning designed to overcome the frame problem.[2] It does so with a vengeance: it is now sufficient for a *single* model of the discourse to be maintained at every point of its development. Maintaining a single model of our best guess about the current situation and its relevance to current goals is a very much more plausible biological function than reasoning about all logically possible models of our current assumptions. As we briefly mentioned in chapter 2, and will see in greater detail in chapter 8, along with biological plausibility of function comes efficiency of computation – the model is derived from the repre-

---

2. For this reason, planning logics are also used in robotics for planning motor actions (see, e.g., [246]).

sentation of the assumptions in linear time. Focusing on biologically plausible automatic planning is helpful in connecting this approach to other cognitive processes. In particular, we may call an automatic process such as planning an instance of closed–world *reasoning* if it can be viewed as the construction of a (representation of a) model from which conclusions are read off.

The neuropsychological literature on "executive function" has much to offer to understanding planning, and, obliquely, also reasoning too. Lots of categories of patients have planning problems, often to do with inhibiting prepotent responses,[3] managing goals and subgoals, balancing top-down and bottom–up influences, and so forth. This literature straddles automatic and deliberative planning and control. In chapter 9 we shall see how these planning problems are related to peculiarities in reasoning often found in autistic people; but there are many other disorders to which the approach may have something to contribute: a substantial set of psychiatric conditions – anxiety, depression, schizophrenia, attention–deficit disorder, obsessive-compulsive disorder – are now seen as being accompanied by problems of executive function. These problems may or may not be central causes, and they may be different problems in different disorders, but it seems that understanding executive function and dysfunction has a contribution to make.

Perhaps the moral of this literature of most current relevance here is that although human system 1 processes include our biological heritage from nonhuman cognition, system 1 is also distinctively changed in humans. Our system 1 not only keeps a model of our best interpretation of our current real-world circumstances but can also maintain models of our best interpretation of, at the other extreme, completely fictional discourses where relation to the real world is totally unspecified, and any number of situations in between. It is understanding such fictional discourses in the laboratory that provides the data that we began by discussing, as well as the new data discussed in chapter 7. It is always a salutary exercise to rehearse the many levels of fiction involved in laboratory experiments, right down, for an example from the selection task, to the fact that turning the diagram of the cards yields a blank piece of paper. Even this has been shown to affect subjects' reactions, relative to considering real cards on the table in front of the subject. On the account of the nature of system 1 processes as defeasible automatic reasoning to an interpretation, they have of course already received considerable attention in a range of psychological literatures. Closest to reasoning is the psycholinguistics literature [93]. Here the whole enterprise is to ask how subjects defeasibly derive interpretations for discourses, culminating in successful understanding.[4] Psycholinguistics has recently branched out beyond the interpretation of purely linguistic input to treat

---

3. The prepotent response is the response which is strongest when stimuli with different, conflicting, responses occur together.
4. Studies of the evolution of human language and cognitive skills also exploit this relation between planning and language skills [3], [107], [256].

situations in which visual perception of the nonlinguistic world goes on in parallel with linguistic interpretation of relevant utterances [275]. Indications are that linguistic and nonlinguistic interpretations are about as integrated as it is possible to be. Visual evidence can be used "immediately" to resolve linguistic choices in interpretation. This should serve to remind us that defeasible processes modelled by closed–world reasoning are not particularly linguistic.

One thing that is special about interpreting discourse (as opposed to present perceptual circumstances) is that it requires reasoning about others' intentions and meanings. One sees this made concrete in pragmatic frameworks, such as Grice's [108], where credulous interpretation of discourse involves assumptions of cooperativeness, knowledge, and ignorance, for example. The "theory of mind" reasoning that has been studied in the developmental literature provides further examples. In chapter 2 we have seen how "theory of mind" can be analysed as closed world reasoning. The key idea here is to analyse communications, perceptions, and beliefs, as causes and consequences of a specific kind, and the reasoning as a variety of causal reasoning. In chapter 9 we will study how breakdown of this system leads to failures on "false–belief tasks."

Conscious *deliberate* planning has been studied in normal subjects in the context of problem solving, and indeed it is strange that this literature is regarded as so separate from the psychology of reasoning literature. When subjects have to solve a Tower of Hanoi problem [199], reasoning seems to be what is called for. This, at first experience, evokes system 2 planning. But the surprising outcome of Simon and Newell's empirical studies and theoretical conclusions was that expertise resulted in system 2 processes "going underground" and being compiled into system 1 skills. The expert chess player or physician has to a large extent automated the planning process and indeed may have done so to the extent that the skill is no longer accessible to reflective analysis – a hallmark of system 1 processes. This change was indeed conceptualized by Simon and Newell as the acquisition of very large databases of "productions" – conditional rules.

This same turn toward the study of learning and acquisition of reasoning skills has not happened in the psychology of reasoning. As long as the goal is characterization of the fundamental human reasoning mechanism, learning, acquisition, and even skill are deemed irrelevant, and as processes which are "educational," rather than part of the nature of human cognition in the wild. Stenning [258] shows how differences between subjects' reasoning and learning can be explained in terms of their representational strategies, developed by slow deliberate system 2 learning. It is a fine irony that professors, of all people, should come to the view that conceptual learning is not a part of human nature, but merely a cultural oddity.

Summary

The standard laboratory tasks for reasoning embody a prejudice inherited from classical logic, that reasoning is a conscious process starting from explicitly given premises. Taking a wider view of what reasoning consists in, by incorporating certain automatic processes as well, provides one with a much better vantage point from which to study the *grandeur et misère* of classical reasoning.

5.3.2   The Literate Wild: System 2 Processes

A breakdown of mutual interpretation in credulous processing interrupts a discourse if the hearer's interpretation yields an interpretational impasse. Here, however much the hearer is willing in general to accept the speaker's assertions, a contradiction or other divergence of new utterances from the hearer's model of the speaker's intentions to this point, means that no model can be found, and no model means no "intended model." The hearer now has to engage in repair, and may interrupt the speaker to find out how to repair understanding. Such repair of contradiction is based on interludes of skeptical reasoning *from* interpretations (or broken attempts at interpretation), embedded in credulous reasoning *to* interpretations.

On this story, classical logic is a good account of some reasoning that does occur in the wild under particular circumstances – the circumstances of "adversarial" communication (in a technical sense of adversarial to be made clear in what follows). The credulous interpretation of discourse assumes a certain asymmetry of authority between speaker and hearer. The hearer accepts that speaker's authority for the truth of the discourse, at least for the purposes of the current episode of communication. The purest case is where a speaker tells a novel fictional story to the hearer who patently accepts he has no grounds for disagreement. But as we have just seen, this acceptance of asymmetry of authority breaks down when contradiction is encountered, and can only be restored by repair. The discourses of adversarial communication are cases where breakdown of mutual interpretation is much more widely spread.

In full-fledged argument, the parties may be unwilling to accept offered repairs. They may explore for reinterpretations of the explicitly stated assumptions on which they can agree, or they may resort to less communicative tactics. Here it is plausible that the logic governing the derivations from assumptions is classical – demanding that conclusions be true in all logically possible interpretations of the assumptions. Here is what lies behind the statement of Ryle [239] quoted above on page 23, and repeated here for convenience:

> There arises, I suppose, a special pressure upon language to provide idioms of the [logical] kind, when a society reaches the stage where many matters of interest and importance to everyone have to be settled or decided by special kinds of talk. I mean, for example, when offenders have to be tried and convicted or acquitted; when treaties and

contracts have to be entered into and observed or enforced; when witnesses have to be cross-examined; when legislators have to draft practicable measures and defend them against critics; when private rights and public duties have to be precisely fixed; when complicated commercial arrangements have to be made; when teachers have to set tests to their pupils; and ... when theorists have to consider in detail the strengths and weaknesses of their own and one another's theories.

One of the hallmarks of formal adversarial communication is that reasoning is intended to proceed from the *explicit* assumptions negotiated to define the 'admissible evidence' (usually as written down). Introduction of extraneous assumptions not formally entered in the record is strictly impermissible. This making explicit of what is assumed for reasoning classically from interpretations contrasts with the vagueness of what long-term knowledge is in play in defeasible reasoning *to* interpretations. In adversarial communication, reasoning is not defeasible, at least when the rules are followed literally, and finding some interpretation which makes the premises true and the opponent's desired conclusion false is sufficient to defeat it. What combination of classical or defeasible logics provides the best model of how real legal and parliamentary practice works is a complex question, but an albeit highly idealized core of adversarial legal reasoning arguably provides one model for classical logical reasoning in the wild. A purer example of adversarial communication involving skeptical classical reasoning is the discourse of mathematical proof. Yet another example of adversarial communication is argument about the correct interpretation of religious texts – the context which seems to have been particularly important in the emergence of Indian logical theory. Of course, we assume that capacities for skeptical reasoning preceded these theories of it.

Conceptual learning in educational dialogue has many of the same features. Teacher and student start out, by definition, conceptually misaligned – the teacher knows some concepts that the student doesn't. The abstract concepts of secondary and tertiary education are not teachable by ostension, and require teaching indirectly through rehearsal of their axioms and applications of those axioms in argument. For example, to teach a student to differentiate the physical concepts of amount, weight, density, volume, and mass it is no good pointing at an instance of one, because any instance of one is an instance of all the others. Instead one has to rehearse the transformations which leave them invariant and the ones that change them. For example, compression changes density and volume but not weight or mass. Going to the moon changes weight but not mass. (Stenning [261] discusses the close analogy between learning abstract physical concepts and learning logical concepts such as truth, validity, consequence, inference rules, etc.). The relation between adversarial communication and logic was traditionally very much the focus of late secondary and tertiary education, at least of the elites who were trained for performance in law court and parliament (and later scientific laboratory). We have already made reference to legal reasoning on page 23. The tasks of the psychology of reasoning are directly taken from, or derived by small extensions from, the curriculum of this tradition of education [258].

Summary

On this account, classical deductive reasoning is important not because an implementation of it is the "universal deductive reasoning mechanism," but rather because classical reasoning is important for aligning and repairing mutual interpretation across some gulf of understanding or agreement, and that learning more explicit control over system 2 processes, and their relation to system 1 processes, can have a large impact on many students' interpretation, learning and reasoning processes. The skills of skeptical reasoning are then one extremely important set of concepts and skills for learning to learn.[5]

5.3.3   The Relation between System 1 and System 2

System 1 and system 2 processes work together from early on in human development. The relevant parts of system 1 processes are rather direct implementations of a range of nonmonotonic logics. System 2 processes start as repair processes when a system 1 process meets an impasse and gradually shade into full blown adversarial discourses, perhaps with their underlying logic being classical.

Questions arise at two different levels about the relation between systems 1 and 2. At the level of ontogeny there are questions about how the two systems develop and the role of formal education in these relations. At the evolutionary level, there are questions about the history of the two systems: did the cognitive capacities for system 2 reasoning come into being at some point roughly coincident with the advent of developed societies and the first formulations of theories of system 2 reasoning (i.e., with the development of logical theory), or did the system 2 processes exist long beforehand? At the educational level, there are questions about the level of transfer of the learning of classical logic to the students' reasoning practices. We approach these issues through what is known about reasoning in less developed societies among illiterate subjects, and then move on to consider evolutionary questions in chapter 6.

5.4   The Illiterate Wild

It has sometimes been maintained that logical reasoning, if not exactly a party trick, is an ability acquired only in the course of becoming literate, for instance by going to school, or worse, by attending a logic class. This is grist to the

---

5. For ease of exposition we have in the above more or less identified skeptical and classical reasoning. For a more subtle approach, the reader may consult Dung, Kowalski, and Toni [67].

mill of those who believe that, evolutionarily speaking, logical reasoning is
not a basic human ability. It is indeed true that the fundamental fact to be
explained about reasoning in illiterate subjects is their obstinate refusal to draw
conclusions from premises supplied by the experimenter, as in Luria's famous
example [177,p. 108]:

> *E.* In the Far North, where there is snow, all bears are white. Novaya Zemlya is in the Far
> North and there is always snow there. What color are the bears there?
> *S.* I don't know what color the bears are there, I never saw them.
> *E.* But what do you think?
> *S.* Once I saw a bear in a museum, that's all.
> *E.* But on the basis of what I said, what color do you think the bears are there?
> *S.* Either one-colored or two-colored ... [ponders for a long time]. To judge from the
> place, they should be white. You say that there is a lot of snow there, but we have never
> been there!

Here Luria is talking to an illiterate peasant from Kazakhstan. He attributed
the peasant's refusal to answer, to an overriding need to answer from personal
knowledge only, interfering with the deductive inference.

A careful analysis of this and related data shows, however, that the situation
is considerably more complicated. For one thing, the subject *does* draw the inference when he says "To judge from the place, they should be white'; but he
refuses to consider this an answer to the question posed by the experimenter. It
seems one cannot blame him. Why should someone be interested in truth *relative* to assumptions, instead of absolute truth? There are plenty of circumstances
in our societies where refusing hypothetical reasoning is a common move – one
has only to listen to a politician interviewed. The reason for refusing to answer
may only be because the subject does not know whether the premises are really
true, not because of an inability to draw the correct inference. This point can be
amplified in several ways.

The first thing to observe is that sometimes the refusal to answer may be motivated by a piece of logical (meta-)reasoning, as in Scribner's studies of reasoning among the illiterate Kpelle tribe in Liberia [243,p.112], reprinted from
[244]. Here is a sample argument given to her subjects:

> All Kpelle men are rice farmers.
> Mr. Smith is not a rice farmer.
> Is Mr. Smith a Kpelle man?

Consider the following dialogue with a Kpelle subject:

> *S.* I don't know the man in person. I have not laid eyes on the man himself.
> *E.* Just think about the statement.
> *S.* If I know a man in person, I can answer that question, but since I do not know him in
> person I cannot answer that question.
> *E.* Try and answer from your Kpelle sense.
> *S.* If you know a person, if a question comes up about him you are able to answer. But if

you do not know a person, if a question comes up about him, it's hard for you to answer it.

Under the plausible assumption that in the dialogue "if" means "if and only if," the Kpelle subject actually makes the modus tollens inference in the meta argument (in his second turn) that he refuses to make in the object argument! Luria concluded that subjects' thinking is limited to the concrete and situational, that of which they have personal knowledge: Scribner tended to the conclusion that subjects fail because they don't understand the problem, or what kind of discourse "game" is intended. If this means that subjects do not understand what the experimenter wants from them, one can only agree, as long as this is not taken to imply that there is some deficiency in the subjects' logical reasoning. Many of these examples bear the hallmarks of moral scruples about bearing witness on the basis of hearsay. One may well imagine that these subjects viewed the experimenters as authority figures and perhaps assimilated their questions to those of official inquisitors, and this may explain their scruples.

In line with our analysis of the selection task, we may note here that the experimenter intends the subject to understand the task ("assume only these two premises, nothing more"), the interpretation of the conditional as the material implication, and last but not least to keep in mind the literal wording of the premises. As regards the first, it may very well be that this requires understanding of a discourse genre, roughly that of an exam question, which is not available to the unschooled. Imagine, for example, the confusion the subject gets into if he interprets the experimenter's question as a sincere request for information not already known.

In chapter 2 we have already remarked that the experimenters make the unwarranted assumption that the conditional is material implication. If it is assumed instead to be represented as a rule allowing exceptions, formalized as $p \wedge \neg e \rightarrow q$, then the subject must decide whether Mr. Smith, or Novaya Zemlya, constitutes an exceptional situation, and in the absence of personal information he may not be able to do so. It may also be difficult to memorise the literal wording of the premises instead of the image they convey. Here is another example from Luria [177,p. 108]:

E. Cotton can only grow where it is hot and dry. In England it is cold and damp. Can cotton grow there?
S. I don't know

:*S.* I've only been in Kashgar country; I don't know beyond that.
E. But on the basis of what I said to you, can cotton grow there?
S. If the land is good, cotton will grow there, but if it is damp and poor, it won't grow. If it's like the Kashgar country, it will grow there too. If the soil is loose, it can grow there too, of course.

Luria interpreted this phenomenon as a refitting of the premises according to convention; it seems better to describe it as the construction of a discourse model of the premises using general knowledge ('cold and damp implies poor soil') and solving the task by describing the model, in line with the famous experiments on sentence memory by Bransford et al. [24].

Our student Marian Counihan has recently (2005) done a similar experiment among the Xhosa tribe in South Africa. Although Luria-type answers were not common, she got some, such as the subject's first response:

[Susan, 80 years, illiterate]
E. First story is about a girl, Ntombi. If Ntombi wants to see her boyfriend then she goes to East London. And we know that Ntombi does want to see her boyfriend. Then will she go to East London?
S. How will I know? I don't know.
E. If you just listen to the words, and to the situation they are describing, and [repeats question], will she go then?
S. I don't think she will go because her mother is watching her and not letting her go.

It turned out that Susan lived together with (indeed raised) her granddaughter, whom she forbade to see her boyfriend; her reasoning can be viewed as activating the exception clause in the default with material from her own experience.

The following example from [244,205] by contrast exhibits some classical reasoning in the first exchange, but reasoning with exceptions takes over when classical reasoning becomes counterintuitive:

[Nonkululeko, 56 years, illiterate. Presented material is]
E. All people who own houses pay house tax. Sabelo does not pay house tax. Does he own a house?
S. He doesn't have a house if he's not paying.
E. And now suppose that none of the people in Cape Town pay house tax. Do they own houses or not?
S. They have houses.
E. Why?
S. They can have houses because there are places where you don't pay tax, like the squatter camps.
E. So they can have houses and not pay?
S. They may, they can live at the squatter camps.

Scribner argued that results such as those outlined above do not indicate defective logical skills, but rather point to a tendency not to apply logical skills to familiar material of which the subject has knowledge beyond that stated in the premises. If that knowledge does not suffice to settle the issue, the subject will refrain from giving an answer. By contrast, subjects would have no trouble reasoning from completely new material where they do not have an opportunity to consult their own knowledge. This hypothesis was corroborated in a study by Tulviste [278], who showed that Nganasan[6] children attending primary school

---

6. A tribe in Northern Eurasia.

failed on logical reasoning tasks involving daily activities, but did well on tasks involving typical school material (his example featured the metal molybdenum, with which the children would have little acquaintance). Leevers and Harris [169] provide a comparable example where 4–year–old European subjects can be induced to reason hypothetically when given a science fiction context.

5.4.1 Excursion: Electroconvulsive Therapy and Syllogistic Reasoning

Evidence suggestive of effects of this kind of detachment, or the lack of it, from context, this time from a clinical population, was obtained by an experiment involving electroconvulsive therapy (ECT) performed by Deglin and Kinsbourne [61]. Bipolar disorder and schizophrenic patients were given arguments of the form $\forall x(Ax \rightarrow Bx), Aa/?Ba?$[7] to solve, after having received ECT to one of the hemispheres only. Sometimes the premises were familiar, sometimes unfamiliar, and sometimes plainly false. Here are some examples:

[familiar] All rivers contain fish.
The Neva is a river.
Does the Neva contain fish?

[unfamiliar] All countries have flags.
Zambia is a country.
Does Zambia have a flag?

[false] All countries have flags.
Quetzal is a country
Does Quetzal have a flag?

The pattern of results was consistent. When the right hemisphere is suppressed, subjects calmly accepted the premises and affirmed that the conclusion follows, sometimes showing irritation at being asked such a simple question. When the left hemisphere was suppressed,[8] however, the experimenters obtained answers such as

There used to be lots of fish in the Neva, but the river is now so polluted it is completely dead!

Is there really such a state, Zambia? Where is it? Who lives there?

How can I know? I don't even know that country [i.e., Quetzal]!

---

7. This type of material is customarily called a "syllogism," although it is not a syllogism in the Aristotelian sense. We shall follow custom here.
8. Since subjects could still comprehend natural language, the suppression cannot have been total.

Note that for these Russian subjects from St. Petersburg, the Neva is part of their autobiographical experience, whereas Zambia and Quetzal are not. So the first example constitutes a rejection of the premise's truth, whereas the second and third represent expressions of ignorance. The authors conclude from this that the left hemisphere is capable of performing formal logical operations independent of truth-value; in contrast, the right hemisphere seems incapable "of the willing suspension of disbelief" and in any case unable to abstract from truth-value. Note the similarity of the answers of the lefthemisphere-suppressed patients to those given by subjects in Luria's and Scribner's experiments. This study is perhaps to be interpreted with some caution since it is far from clear how patients with ECT suppression of their left hemisphere were able to respond verbally.

Our interpretation of the data from illiterate reasoners makes us skeptical of the idea that system 2 reasoning arrives with literacy and formal schooling. The range of relations between discourse and world may greatly expand with formal schooling, but we believe that even the least developed societies provide enough scope and demand for interpretive capacities to require system 2 reasoning in some contexts. Indeed, as soon as human system 1 discourse interpretation capacities became capable of interpreting discourses about situations distant in time or space, there would have been a need for system 2 capacities to reason about breakdowns of mutual interpretation. We think it very unlikely that system 2 had to wait for the advent of societies with formal schooling. The division of labour which is, after all, one of the driving forces behind the institution of formal education, vastly expands the need for system 2 supervision of system 1 interpretations, but it does not create that need from scratch. Once the question is approached from this perspective, evidence does emerge of system 2 reasoning in traditional societies. Perhaps some of the best examples can be found in Hutchins's work on legal reasoning in Polynesia [136]. This perspective might also help to resolve the puzzle posed by anthropological observations such as that of Evans-Pritchard [79] of the great sophistication displayed, for example, by Azande cosmology, coupled with the refusal to reason hypothetically or theoretically about other matters.

This leaves the ontogenetic question: what part does formal schooling play in the arrival of system 2 reasoning capacities? Answers to the evolutionary and the ontogenetic questions tend to correlate. If one thinks of the advent of system 2 as happening in historical time with the arrival of the social institutions of debate, then it is natural to think of system 2 as dependent in ontogeny on formal education. The correlation also tends to be true of how the content of educational practices is viewed.

If the very capacities required for reasoning in something approaching classical logic are acquired in formal education, the mental processes acquired tend to be thought of as implementations of patterns of reasoning explicitly taught –

implementation of a novel formalism of "Ps and Qs," or mnemonics for valid syllogisms, say. If system 2 is thought of as pre-dating formal education, then it is more natural to think of effective education as operating at a more semantic and pragmatic level where the skill of detecting misalignments of communication is central. Certainly the traditional teaching of logic at some times in history focused on teaching students the skill of detecting equivocations in arguments – cases where the same word is used in different interpretations.

There are several well-known empirical studies of the teaching of (classical) formal logic which show little transfer to general reasoning ability [38, 170]. However, Stenning [258] reviews these studies as seeking transfer at inappropriate levels, and presents empirical evidence from real classroom logic learning that logic teaching can transfer to improvements of general reasoning if the teaching objective is transfer at plausible levels. It isn't new inference rules (modus ponens, modus tollens, etc.) that transfer (perhaps because these rules aren't new, being shared with defeasible logics), but the much more general semantic skills of insulating the "admissible evidence" (current assumptions) from "general knowledge" and exploring *all* interpretations rather than just the most plausible ones, along with a much more explicit grasp of (and terminology for) discussing the contrasts between credulous and skeptical stances. Not to speak of the need to unlearn the influences of the information packaging of natural languages designed to focus the credulous interpreter's understanding on the intended model. All this suggests that the reasoning skills involved in system 2 must be viewed (and hence tested!) as strategies for the repair of rapid defeasible conclusions, not as the knowledge of particular argument schemata.

In chapter 1, we noted that Piaget's theory of formal operational thought based on classical logical competences was one of Wason's targets in what he thought was his demonstration that many intelligent undergraduates did not reach the formal operational stage. It should now be evident that the situation is somewhat deeper than Wason originally estimated. His undergraduate subjects, rather analogously to the illiterate subjects just discussed, do not immediately interpret his materials classically, and both sets of subjects have good reason on their side. Of course, Piaget perhaps underestimated how much was involved in flexibly imposing a classical logical interpretation on materials across domains in general as cued by appropriate content, and perhaps underestimated how much young children could be induced to apply system 2 reasoning with suitable contextual support. However, Piaget seems nearer to the mark than Wason. In particular, his hypothesis that it is at adolescence that flexible controlled grasp of system 2 reasoning capacities becomes available for teaching fits suggestively with our proposal that system 2 processes come to the fore when attempting to communicate across substantial misalignments of interpretation.

In summary, system 2 is related to system 1 through the need for repair to interpretations that arises because of the flexibility with which human system 1 interpretive machinery operates. This capacity for reflective reasoning for repair is central to what turned apes into human beings. It is much magnified by the development of the division of labour that came much later, in more complex societies. These societies support the learning of flexible control over system 2 processes in formal education, and they do so by teaching new skills at the level of the semantics of discourse interpretation rather than by implanting new proof-theoretical machinery. This account of where the psychology of reasoning fits into the study of cognition provides a quite different account of where different species of reasoning are important in the wild, and a different view of the evolutionary processes to which we now turn.

6 The Origin of Human Reasoning Capacities

The last chapter set out to shift the focus of the psychology of reasoning from a single derivational apparatus working on an assumed classical logic interpretation of natural language, toward a multiplicity of defeasible logical interpretations necessary for planning action in the world. It argued that this change of focus changed the perceived relations to all the surrounding fields of the study of cognition. It also changed the view of where skeptical reasoning comes to the fore in the wild – in the establishment of mutual interpretation across misalignments in communication. Here classical logic may have a role, but that role can only be understood as it is embedded in the business of credulous interpretation.

In section 5.1.3 we briefly introduced evolutionary psychology's view of logical reasoning: there is no role for (formal, domain–independent) logic in cognition; whenever we appear to reason logically, this is because we have evolved strategies ("Darwinian algorithms") to solve a problem in a particular domain. A particularly important domain is that of "social contracts," infringement of which has to be monitored by an innate "cheater detection module." Evolutionary psychology's claim is that instances of successful reasoning are all due to the action of such modules. Thus, the difference between bad performance on the abstract selection task and good performance on the drinking age rule is hypothesized to be due to the fact that the latter is a social contract which triggers the involvement of the cheater detection module.

Evolutionary psychology is quite popular, and there are few critical discussions of its founding psychological evidence (as opposed to its biological reasoning) in the literature. This chapter examines that evidence in some detail, starting from the analysis of the selection task given in chapters 3 and 4. The chapter also looks carefully at evolutionary psychology's view of the theory of evolution, a view that will be found wanting. We outline our own view of the evolution of human cognition, and draw out its implications for the study of reasoning. Part II of the book then studies these implications in much greater detail, both in terms of experiments and of formal models.

But the arguments of the evolutionary psychologists about the selection task are not the only applications of biology to cognition which strike us as unbiological. When cognitive scientists discuss evolution they often do so in terms of processes of adaptation through the addition of innate modules. This picture is profoundly at odds with modern views of evolutionary processes. What has come to be known as the "evo devo" movement in biology sees evolution in terms of the tweaking of old modules by changes to the controlling genetic "switches" that alter the timing and spatial expression of cascades of genes, and thus change developmental processes (see [31] for a highly readable introduction). This relation between development and evolution is central to understanding human cognitive evolution but hardly seems to have impinged on cognitive science's big picture.

We start our evolutionary excursion with some prehistory, before sketching a more biological approach and returning to reassess evolutionary psychology.

6.1   Crude Chronology

Many of the problems of explaining human evolution stem from the briefness of the particular evolutionary episode which split us off from the apes. Nonetheless, the tale of human evolution goes back a long way, and long-standing trends in primate evolution are a key to the particularities of the final steps of the human case.

Mammals are distinguished by their heavier investment in a smaller number of young, and the consequent expense of offspring has far-reaching effects on mammals' social organization, and even, as we shall see, on their molecular genetics. The following chronology of primate social evolution (adapted and condensed from Foley [83]) sets the story in its large–scale context:

- 35M years – primate sociality;

- 25M years – social space and kinship as bases of matrilocal[1] social organization;

- 15M years – male kin bonding in catarrhines (old-world monkeys);

- 5M years – out of the trees, bipedal locomotion, patchy resources, and the origin of group breeding;

- 2M years – expensive offspring, eating of meat, larger brains;

- 300K years – use of fire, increase in social group size, phatic functions of language[2], helpless kids, delayed maturity;

---

1. "Matrilocal" here means that spatially cohesive groups contain genetically related females and genetically unrelated males. The phenomenon is almost certainly not continuous with the anthropological concept of social organization of some modern humans.

2. The term phatic is due to the anthropologist Malinowski and designates speech, utterances, etc., that serve to establish or maintain social relationships rather than impart information or communicate ideas.

- 100K year – geodispersal and population increase but little behavioral change, loss of skeletal and dental robustness, then the emergence of art, intensified inter-group conflict, and territoriality;

- 30K year – "end" of genetically based evolution.

Somewhere between old world monkeys and apes, primates switched from matrilocal to patrilocal social organization, probably because of changes in the evenness of distribution of resources. This had fundamental implications for issues of social coordination. The following quotation is a nice encapsulation of this long–term trend in the evolution of primate social organization:

> The paradox of hominid evolution is that the context in which very expensive offspring have evolved is a social environment where females do not live in female kin-bonded groups and therefore one where their options for recruiting female kin-bonded allo-mothers and helpers is limited. The major question that arises is how have females been able to cope? (Foley [83,p. 111])

Many researchers agree that many human cognitive innovations are adaptations to pressures of the increasing social complexity that results from increasing group size [133]. Big brains support big social groups. The nutritional consequences of big brains may demand meat, which simultaneously allows small guts (the other energy–hungry tissue), and big social groups enable various cooperative activities such as big–game hunting, warfare, division of labour, but big social groups also demand more social coordination and communication. There are various positive feedback loops. These are the kinds of backdrops to the commonly held theory that language is the central human innovation, and that all else follows from that. This is also a form of adaptationism, now with regard to a language module. Closer inspection suggests that different views of language yield very different ideas about what is in this module.

To put some flesh on this alternative adaptation-as-module approach we take Hauser, Chomsky and Fitch [119] who propose a framework for studying the evolution of the 'broad language faculty' which distinguishes three subfaculties and three issues for research. The three capacities are: the peripherals (acoustic processors, motor control specializations, etc.), the "conceptual-intentional system" (what one might think of as mentalizing capacities and for which "theory of mind" is a useful shorthand), and the "narrow language faculty." This last is, negatively characterized, the broad language faculty minus the other two. Its positive characterization is as "recursion." The three issues for research for each capacity can be paraphrased as: whether the capacity is shared with ancestors or whether it is unique to modern humans (continuity in function across species); gradual vs. saltational in arrival (continuity in time); and whether it is an adaptation or an exaptation (continuity of selection pressure).

Several aspects of this doubly tripartite scheme are striking. The "conceptual intentional" capacities are already imported *within* the broad language faculty.

If this is intended to reflect the fact that these are necessary capacities underpinning language, then that is a useful marker that meaning is important. But talk of them as a (sub)faculty rather strongly suggests that conceptual-intentional capacites are novel and modular – reasons for skepticism on both counts will come shortly. But the real purpose of the scheme is to place syntax at the heart of human evolutionary innovation (which is of course where it *may* belong, though again, more skepticism presently).

A generic problem with such explanations is that since they almost always pick changes to the adult phenotype as their focal innovation, they explain, if anything, cognitive adaptations to the adult. These adaptations would then have to travel backward down the developmental sequence to explain the modern human infant. We can be confident that mammoth hunting just isn't something human infants ever did. Warfare similarly. This is particularly true of explanations by sexual selection – language as the peacock's tail [119]. Darwin already marshaled formidable evidence that sexually selected characters appear at sexual maturity. And if they later migrated all the way down the developmental sequence to where we find them in today's infants, there wasn't a lot of time for that to happen. Babies don't seem to wait for adolescence to get stuck into language.

One importance of Foley's paradox is that it turns attention to a different part of the life cycle and a different set of selective pressures – the old mammalian problem of investment in the next generation, only now greatly magnified by circumstances. Pressure on female investment in child rearing as a focus of human innovation has the great advantage that it may also get the peacock's tail of language attached to the right sex. As well as emphasizing how individual cognitive changes brought about changed circumstances of mother-infant communication, the paradox also focuses attention on changes in social organization required to cope with group breeding. We will return to this presently when we sketch our specific proposals, but first we revisit the basics of evolutionary theory in order to stand on firmer ground when discussing modularity and the twin problems of identifying bases of continuity and innovation.

6.2   Evolutionary Thinking: From Biology to Evolutionary Psychology

We assume the reader is familiar with the broad outlines of the theory of evolution. To state precisely what the theory of evolution is immediately involves us in a number of conceptual puzzles. For instance: what is selected? Genes, cells, traits,[3] organisms (phenotypes), groups of organisms? Evolutionary psychologists believe that human cognition is in toto a product of adaptation. This claim

---

3. A "trait" is an aspect of an organism's phenotype, particularly an aspect that can have effects in the environment, and interesting traits especially have effects which have an influence on reproductive success.

may seem counterintuitive at first sight, since humans have impressive learning abilities. Certainly evolutionary psychologists would claim that learning abilities are also the result of adaptation and that they are composed of specialized learning abilities rather than generalized ones. The evolutionary psychologists' view is that human cognition consists of a number of adaptations, which have been useful for survival at one stage or another of the environment of evolutionary adaptation (EEA), the Pleistocene, when (proto-)humans lived in small bands as hunter-gatherers. Since this time period is much longer than the agricultural period (which started some twelve thousand years ago), such traits as humans have must have evolved either as part of their common ancestry with primates or in the EEA. This "adaptationist" view of evolution means that two concepts are critical in assessing their claims – *modularity* and *innateness*.

6.2.1   Analogy and Disanalogy with Language

In this respect the hotly debated issue of the origin of language is of particular interest. As is well–known, Chomsky advanced the *poverty of the stimulus* argument in support of his view that the language capacity must somehow be innate. In outline, the argument is this: children reach grammatical competence in language very quickly, at about age 8. This competence includes complicated constructions of which they will have heard few examples; more importantly, the recursive nature of language cannot be inferred only from the linguistic data presented to the child. But if that is so, some construction principles (universal grammar) must be innate; the role of the linguistic input is to set some parameters in universal grammar (hence principles and parameters). Chomsky wishes to remain agnostic about the possible evolutionary origins of universal grammar. Some followers (Pinker, more recently Jackendoff) have been less inhibited and have argued that humans must have evolved a specific "language module," a genetically determined piece of wetware specifically dedicated to the processing of language. They argue that Chomsky should have followed his own argument to its logical conclusion, by identifying "innate" with "genetically determined." This leads us into two interesting issues: (1) is the identification of "innate" with "genetically determined" really unproblematic? and (2) what is this notion of a "module"?

6.2.2   Innateness

We should make it clear that we have no doubt that humans are the product of evolution; that many if not most cognitive structures are at least partially genetically determined; and that the implementations of human cognitive abilities are organized in at least a somewhat modular fashion. Our substantive argument here is that the evidence presented for particular modularizations is defective evidence in a large number of ways; that adaptations have to be distinguished from exaptations, with substantial implications for methodology; and that innateness is not a concept current in modern biology, for good reason.

Talk of the innateness of traits cannot be related to talk of genetic determination of traits without relativizing to an environment. Modern geneticists understand that the heritability of phenotypic traits can be radically different in different environments. The classical example is Waddington's demonstration [293] that patterns of wing veining in *Drosophila* are 0% genetically determined in one environment and 100% determined in another (the relevant environmental dimension here is humidity). It is also often forgotten that, as far as the calculation of heritability of a trait by a target gene or genes goes, all the other genes are part of the environment. As heritability is used in biological research, it is usefulness is understood as highly contextually determined. Innateness is a fixed property of a trait in an organism. This picture of apportioning the determination of the cognitive phenotype between a percentage caused by genetic factors and a percentage caused by other factors, across all environments, is defective – and has been assigned to the dustbin of history by modern biology.

Of course, innate might not be taken to mean "under total genetic control," or even "under total genetic control in environment X." Innate might just be intended to mean "present in 100% of the population," or "developing without rote learning," or "developing as a result of common experiences shared by the whole population." But if we are going to talk evolution, then none of these senses of "innate" are going to be useful in relating phenotypic traits to genetic control in whatever environments. Innateness is a prescientific concept preserved in the discourse of psychology by unacknowledged ideological needs.

Chomsky's argument from the poverty of the stimulus about language acquisition was historically extremely important. Faced with extreme theories holding that all behavior consists in rote-learned conditioned reflexes, Chomsky's argument cleared space for cognitive scientists to consider a wide range of other causes of behavior. But Chomsky's use of "innate" is adequately served by the negative characterization – "not learned by conditioning." Chomsky was careful not to claim that "innate" meant "genetically determined" in all environments. Chomsky's argument now stands in need of reappraisal in the resulting more catholic environment. For example, the demonstration of abstract structure in language raises the question to what degree development of language relies on structure in the environment, or structure in other knowledge and behaviors.

Remember that none of this is an argument against the involvement of genes in the causal determination of behavior. We firmly believe that genes are as involved in the determination of behavior as they are in the determination of morphological traits. Behavioral traits pose much more severe problems of specification than morphological ones, as we shall see when we consider "language" as a human phenotypic trait (see section 6.3.4 for discussion of the general problem of identifying insightful phenotypic descriptions). But the difficulty of finding the right specification does not militate against genetic influences. Few interesting traits are known to be either 0% or 100% controlled by any combination of genes in every environment (remember that for calculations of heritability, other nontarget genes *are* environment). The situation has been further complicated in the last 10 years by the proliferation of epigenetic[4] factors now understood to control the expression of genes. Among these genetic "imprinting" is of particular relevance, to which we return in chapter 9. The job of the biologist or the evolutionary cognitive scientist ought to be to account for how genes and environment interact to bring about phenotypic traits and their development in evolution.

6.2.3   Adaptationism and its Discontents

Evolutionary psychologists tend to hold that all traits of interest, including cognitive traits, are adaptations. In fact, they claim that only an evolutionary perspective can give cognitive science theories of any explanatory power, where "evolution" is taken to be tantamount to "adaptation to the pressures of natural selection." Accordingly, they advocate that cognitive science's methodology should proceed as follows:

1. analyse the information processing task (in the sense of Marr) that corresponds to a particular cognitive trait;

2. find the highly specialized mechanism that is able to execute this task;

3. explain how this mechanism came about as an adaptation.

A quotation from [50,p. 72-83] gives the flavor:

> An organism's phenotypic structure can be thought of as a collection of "design features"– micro-machines such as the functional components of the eye and the liver. The brain can process information because it contains complex neural circuits that are functionally organized. The only component of the evolutionary process that can build complex structures that are functionally organized is natural selection. And the only kind of problems that natural selection can build complexly organized structures for are adaptive problems, where "adaptive" has a very precise, narrow technical meaning. Natural selection is a feedback process that "chooses" among alternative designs on the basis of how well they function. By selecting designs on the basis of how well they solve adaptive problems, this process engineers a tight fit between the function of a device and its structure. [Cognitive] scientists need to realize that while not everything in the designs of organisms is the product of selection, all complex functional organization is.

---

4. Epigenetic factors are environmental influences on the expression of genes. As an example, *imprinting* is a phenomenon whereby the alleles of genes of one parent are suppressed (often by the process of methylation).

This "radical adaptationism" of evolutionary psychologists is not typical of biologists, and was indeed rejected by Darwin himself. Unlike most biologists, evolutionary psychologists do not acknowledge the possiblility of structural features of cognition arising by evolutionary accident, only later to become functional (what is known as genetic drift), or under selection pressure for some other original but now obscure purpose (exaptation). Of course exaptations arose as adaptations at some point, but this is not what these evolutionary psychologists need for their arguments. They need the selection pressures to be identifiable from current function, and this is unfortunately not possible. Their picture of the human mind is that of a collection of adaptations (a collection of "design features") more or less hanging together, *tant bien, tant mal*; in a very evocative metaphor: "the mind is a Swiss army knife." These assumptions are critical for the applicability of their methodology. If one cannot simply reason from the current usefulness of some trait to its evolutionary origin from selection pressure for that usefulness, then evolutionary research of course becomes much harder.

Listening to Darwin

This is a view of evolution which was actively opposed by Darwin in his own day. Darwin was acutely aware that evolutionary analysis was a difficult business and that "just so" stories from modern usefulness were easy to imagine and hard to substantiate. In fact, many of Cosmides' arguments (particularly the ones against the idea that we need to be able to detect altruism) are reminiscent of Spencer who was a contemporary of Darwin. Spencer set about justifying recent social changes brought about by the industrial revolution in terms of competition in "nature red in tooth and claw." Darwin already rejected these arguments. It is a salutary reminder that current political contexts are rarely completely irrelevant to developments in the social sciences, and biology too.

Darwin's argument against radical adaptationism was that the impact on reproductive success of the same phenotypic trait could change radically over the course of evolution. The lamprey's gill arch becomes the shark's jaw bone. Chewing is a useful thing for sharks to do, but the lamprey is a more sucky sort of critter. Darwin was well aware that the difficulty of evolutionary analysis was to provide a continuous account of selection pressure through the history of change, even though the selection pressure on the phenotypic trait changes radically. The problem is particularly acute when a modern system is composed of components which are each currently useless themselves without all the others. Each component must be found continual phylogenetic usefulness to preserve it throughout the period before the system was "assembled" and acquired its different modern usefulness.

Human language and reasoning are plausibly perfect cases. For spoken natural languages and their attendant reasoning capacities we need elaborate perceptual and motor abilities (e.g., vocal tract configurations) as well as recursive syntactic apparatus, semantic apparatus for interpreting and reinterpreting representations, pragmatic apparatus for understanding intentions, working memory, episodic long–term memory, and lots else. Some of these components may have obvious usefulness in other cognitive functions, but others do not.

Adaptation and Exaptation   This contrast in traits' relations to selective pressures is captured by the contrast between adaptation and exaptation. An *adaptation* is a trait that has been selected under pressure from natural selection because of its differential effects on reproductive success – the melanic moth's advantage on the blackened tree.[5] An *exaptation* is a trait evolved under one selection pressure which acquires a new (beneficial) effect, without having been selected for that particular effect. Here a prime example is birds' feathers: originally selected for their functions as temperature regulators, they were later exapted for flight. (This is *primary exaptation*. A process of *secondary adaptation* has led to further improvements in the flight-enabling properties of feathers.) A slightly different example is furnished by snails that use a space in their shell to brood eggs. The existence of that space is a necessary consequence of the spiral design of shells – but only the latter can be said to have evolved by selection. Apparently the snails that use the space for brooding eggs evolved after the ones who don't: in this sense the open space is exapted to brooding eggs. (Following Gould and Lewontin [105], such exaptations are often called *spandrels*, an architectural term referring to the open surfaces on the ceiling of a Gothic church, necessarily created by its supporting arches. These surfaces are often decorated with mosaics; but the point is, as argued by Gould and Lewontin, that they were not designed for that purpose. Indeed, the crucial point is that they do not even figure in the description of the function that they were originally selected by – holding up the roof.)

Darwin was adamant that exaptation was important in evolution. We agree with him. We think it is especially likely that in assembling systems as complex and multifaceted as human communicative and reasoning capacities, various component abilities were exaptations of adaptations originally driven by very different selection pressures. In the case of behavioral traits, particularly those related to modern human cognition, it is notoriously hard to know what the shifting selection pressures might have been, and under what phenotypic description those traits emerge. Darwin insisted that his arguments applied to behavior as well as morphology, but he was also aware of the difficulties of analysis posed, the prime one being the extremely wide range of options for de-

---

5. We sketch this classical example of adaptation by natural selection on page 158.

scribing behavioral phenotypes and their functions in the animal's ecology. At the very least, painstaking description of the modern functioning of phenotypic traits is an entry condition for evolutionary analysis.

6.2.4   Massive Modularity

The evolutionary psychologists' point of view has been aptly described as *massive modularity*: the mind is completely composed of domain-specific modules ("Darwinian algorithms").

> [Content-specific mechanisms] will be far more efficient than general purpose mechanisms . . . [content-independent systems] could not evolve, could not manage their own reproduction, and would be grossly inefficient and easily out-competed if they did [49,p. 112].

One can of course agree that the major problem in cognitive evolution is to explain how humans have developed staggeringly more general cognitive abilities than their ancestors. In this context, massive modularity is to be contrasted with Fodorian modularity, which is more of a hybrid architecture. On the one hand, in Fodor's view, there are low-level modules for input and output computations, primarily perception and motor control ("transducers" as Fodor calls them), but these are connected to a central processing unit (CPU), which is able to integrate information from the various low-level modules. As such, the CPU must function in a modality-independent manner, perhaps by symbol processing. That is, one picture of the functioning of the CPU is that the input is first translated into symbols, then processed, then translated back into motor commands.

Evolutionary psychologists claim that Fodorian modularity would be less adaptive (would less lead to reproductive success) than massive modularity; they view the processing that would have to go on in the CPU as so much useless overhead. This inference might be best viewed as an invalid conclusion from the early AI work of Simon and Newell showing that human reasoning cannot be based on "a general logic theorist" because of the intractability of such an architecture. What these authors showed is that guiding the search for theorems in classical logic required the representation of extensive knowledge of the domain. But that is not what evolutionary psychology needs to dissmiss general reasoning. The issue is, of course, about what domain independence means here. Modern logic, computer science, and AI have done more than any other disciplines to show how weak universal reasoning mechanisms are without domain knowledge. So we have no trouble with the notion that reasoning is domain dependent in a certain well-defined sense – domain specific knowledge needs to be encoded so that it can be called on by the procedures which reason about problems in specific domains. But once such specific knowledge is encoded in a way that is compatible with general knowledge, then the procedures that reason over the combination *may* be uniform across domains. We say "may" because there is still the issue whether the general logics that reason over the domains are the same. We have argued not. So we have argued for *logical* domain specificity and against *content* domain specificity. This is not a simple issue of efficiency, but a complex one of qualitative differences.

Modules and Neurogenesis

The ill-defined nature of modules in evolutionary psychology has similar problems when it meets genetics, as innateness has.[6] Evolution does not generally proceed by adding whole new modules, but by tweaking old ones. So identifying cognitive innovations and identifying them with modules in an adaptationist program is a poor way to proceed. Modern genetics tells us that most macrotraits arise by tweaks on control elements which change the operation of a large number of genes already contributing to a module. The classic example from genetics is again due to Waddington [293] who showed that an artificially induced genetic change in *Drosophila* could put an entire new pair of legs onto the head segment of the fly. Many hundreds or thousands of genes may contribute to the production of legs, but a single genetic element which controls the turning on and off of the expression of this complex of genes can produce an extra pair of legs by allowing leg production to go on for one more segment. The control element is not sensibly thought of a gene for legs-on-the-head – though in a sense it is. It is a controller of other genes which work together to produce legs wherever.

X-ray–induced mutations putting extra legs on the heads of fruit flies may seem rather distant from human cognitive evolution, so we will spend a little time on an example nearer to home – the ontogeny and phylogeny of human brain development – as an example where rather few genes can have profound macroscopic effects. Just as the number of genes contributing to *Drosophila* legs is large, the estimations of the number of genes which affect brain development in mammals is of the order of tens of thousands [157]. This is just what one would expect if it is tweaks to old modules that effect macrochanges.

A major source of evidence about the ontogeny of human brain growth comes from the study of a particular sub-type of abnormality – autosomal recessive primary microcephaly (MCPH) [306]. The genetics of this human condition reveals examples of simple control processes having profound consequences on brain size. MCPH results in an adult brain size roughly one third of normal. The surprise is that although this does lead to mild mental retardation, the radically reduced brain seems to function more or less normally. The ontogenetic mechanism of this disorder is beginning to be well understood. By studying families prone to this condition it has been possible to identify at least some

---

6. This section requires some outline knowledge of genetics; readers not so equipped could continue with section 6.3.

of the genes involved. Two important genes are *ASPM* (abnormal spindle-like microcephaly) and *MCPH1* (microcephalin) [78, 77].

The mechanism of the former gene's effect is well analysed, although most of the experimental analysis is of the homologous gene in the mouse. *ASPM* appears to control mitotic spindle orientation in the fetal cells which give rise to the cortex. In one spindle orientation, the progenitor cells divide to give two more progenitors: in the other orientation, mitosis yields one progenitor and one neuron. Obviously, assuming that all progenitors eventually become neurons, the first process is exponential, doubling cell number with each division: the second is linear. *ASPM* controls the exponential process. The mechanism of expression of the second gene (microcephalin) is not yet analysed, but it is a candidate for control of the second linear process through effects on cellular metabolic rate and centrosome structure.

Before these genes had been identified, Rakic [224] had already proposed a model of cortical ontogeny. The huge growth of cortex in mammals, especially in primates, and especially in *Homo*, is overwhelmingly due to an increase in area of the much folded cortex, rather than in its thickness. Rakic proposed that the area of cortex is controlled by a factor with exponential effects and that another factor controls thickness with linear effect. Just a few days' difference in onset and offset of the exponential process will radically alter eventual cortical volume.

In the macaque monkey, with a 165-day gestation, the cells divide in the exponential manner up to embryonic day E40. After E40, there is a gradual switchover to the asymmetric mode of division which gives linear growth. In the monkey, the former phase is 20 days longer than in the mouse, though it has to be taken into account that mouse cells divide about twice as fast as monkey cells. It is possible to calculate that, provided human cell cycle timings are similar to macaque, this phase would only have to be prolonged a few days from the monkey timings to yield the increase in human brain size. In contrast, an increase of 20 days to the second linear process would add only approximately ten cells to each column of cells in the cortex's thickness. Presumably, the mutations occurring in the *ASPM* gene in families with MCPH, alter timings of the exponential process.

This constitutes a genetic model of one major influence on the ontogenetic process controlling cortical size in mammals. (We do not suggest this is the only factor, though it does suggest that there could be rather few major factors.) Of itself, it does not show that the evolutionary process was driven by selection of this gene for brain size. However, it is possible to gauge whether genes have been under selective pressure, at least over evolutionary spans such as these. The method studies the ratio of nonsynonymous to synonymous changes in the proteins produced by the expression of genes – the so-called K_a/K_s ratio. A great many DNA changes do not result in any functional effect. The key idea here is to estimate the proportion of protein changes which do have functional consequences. Dorus et al. [65] studied the K_a/K_s ratio for nervous system related genes (and some control groups of genes) in a range of mammals. They show accelerated evolution of nervous system genes relative to control gene groups, especially in the line leading to *Homo sapiens*. This study identifies a set of genes whose K ratios are particularly outlying. *ASPM* and microcephalin both appear in this set. *ASPM* shows evidence of particularly intense selection pressure in the late stages of our ancestry.

In contrast, another study focusing just on the lineage from chimpanzee to human showed that neural genes have *lower* K_a/K_s ratios than genes expressed outside of the brain between these two species [39, 202]. Perhaps a few neural genes may be targets for positive selection in this period, but neural genes as a whole are here subject to intense negative selection due to the severe disadvantages conferred by mutations that disrupt brain function. We return to this topic below on page 295.

Before leaving issues of neurogenesis, it is worth noting our changing understanding of how long this process continues. From the early twentieth–century studies of Ramón y Cajal, until within the last few decades, it was widely believed that neurogenesis only occurred in embryonic stages of development. Only in the more recent years has it been established that neurogenesis continues in narrowly delineated areas of the adult mammalian brain, chiefly the hippocampus, olfactory bulb, and dentate gyrus [110]. What is more, this process in the hippocampus has been shown to be instrumental in establishing certain kinds of memory [247]. It is even known that there are certain divergences between the patterns and mechanisms of adult neurogenesis in humans as compared to chimpanzees [240]. Some of the cells destined to become new neurons start in the subventricular zone (SVZ) and migrate into their eventual sites by a mechanism called "astrocyte chains." Possibly because the enlargement of the human cortex has greatly increased the distances neuron progenitor cells have to migrate from their starting places in the SVZ, neuronal migration from ventricular walls to eventual positions is not by the ancestral astrocyte-chain mechanism.

There have been controversial reports of adult neurogenesis in neocortex over several years, and more recently studies claiming to show neurons generated in situ in adult human neocortex [60]. Interestingly the contested cells are of a specific type of GABA-ergic inhibitory interneuron. Although these results are controversial, the rate of change of knowledge is enough to make it likely that growth of new structures influenced by experience in the adult brain will be established. As we shall see in chapters 8, this may be of some significance when we come to consider how working memory is to be modelled at a neural level, and even more specifically in abnormalities such as autism and schizophrenia.

So here is a close and rather more cognitively relevant analogy with the extra legs on the heads of *Drosophila*. A large number of genes are involved in producing legs and in producing brains, but a small number of control elements may have profound effects on where legs wind up in fruit flies, and how big mammals' brains grow. Brain size is not everything in human evolution, but the degree of encephalization of *Homo sapiens* is a distinctive feature, and there is evidence that it has played some role in the selection pressures that produced us. It, of course, remains to understand the impact of these brain changes on human functioning, possibly partly through our high–level example of the effects of altriciality (see Chapter 6, section 5), but our point here is that we can only do that as the transformation of old modules by small tweaks. To the extent that cheater detection is a modular function of human cognition, we can only expect to understand it as it grows out of the ancestral functions and structures from which it developed. Cummins [54] provides some preliminary proposals.

Of course, much of the attraction of identifying a cognitive innovation with a new module is that it would make cognitive science so easy. But the wishful thinking backfires. If we think new cognitive functions are new modules, once we hear of the estimate of ten thousand genes affecting brain development, we are likely to throw up our hands about genetics helping to understand cognition. If, on the other hand, we realise that the number of relevant control elements for some critical aspects of brain development may be quite small, then whole new sources of evidence are available and may be useful, and these genetic sources of evidence speak to issues, such as selection pressures, that other sources do not. We return to brain growth when introducing the importance of altriciality in human evolution below, and again when we turn to look at autism in chapter 9.

6.3   What Evolutionary Psychology Has to Say about Reasoning

After this introduction to the biological background, we are now in a position to assess evolutionary psychology's views on logical reasoning. As we have seen in chapter 3 there have been recurrent attempts to oppose form and content as controllers of reasoning, usually to the detriment of the former. The most forceful assault on form is due to the evolutionary psychologist Leda Cosmides, who claims that (1) successful reasoning (according to the canons of classical logic) occurs only in the case of narrowly circumscribed contents, and (2) these contents have been selected by evolution, i.e., they correspond to situations in our environment to which we are especially attuned because they are crucial for survival. "Reasoning" is simply the wrong abstraction: there exists "reasoning" in specific domains, designed to solve a particular adaptive problem, but there is no general overarching innate capacity for reasoning. But by its very definition, logic seems to be content independent: an argument is valid if whatever is substituted for the nonlogical terms, true premises lead to a true conclusion.

Hence logic must be an acquired trick: humans have no special capacity for formal reasoning. Indeed, the difficulty of mastering logic points to its lack of biological roots: the existence of an adaptive module is usually reflected in the ease with which humans learn to use it effectively and quickly.

Cosmides' starting point was reasoning in Wason's selection task as analysed in chapter 3. Originally, Cosmides claimed that all successful reasoning in the selection task involved *social contracts*, in which parties agree to exchange benefits. Recently, the catalogue has been extended to include reasoning about precautions, warnings, etc.[81], supposedly each underpinned by its own neural apparatus, but our discussion will concentrate on the original idea; the same arguments apply to the later claims.[7]

6.3.1 Reassessing Cheater Detection

The research on the Wason task and other reasoning tasks is seen as showing that people reason correctly (according to the norms of classical logic) with material like drinking age rules. Cosmides' argument outlined above proposes that this must be an adaptation, a specific module, responsible for good performance. Cosmides proposed that logically correct reasoning, when it occurs, has its origins in the policing of social cooperation. In particular, she focuses on the domain of social contracts, in which one party is willing to pay a cost to acquire a certain benefit from a second party. In order to ensure survival it would be imperative to be able to check for parties cheating on the contract, i.e., parties accepting the benefit without paying the associated cost. In the crisp summary given by Gigerenzer and Hug:

> For hunter-gatherers, social contracts, that is, cooperation between two or more people for mutual benefit, were necessary for survival. But cooperation (reciprocal altruism[8]) cannot evolve in the first place unless one can detect cheaters [(Trivers [277])]. Consequently, a set of reasoning procedures that allow one to detect cheaters efficiently – a cheater-detector algorithm – would have been selected for. Such a "Darwinian algorithm" would draw attention to any person who has accepted the benefit (did he pay the cost?) and to any person who has not paid the cost (did he accept the benefit?). Because these reasoning procedures, which were adapted to the hunter-gatherer mode of life, are still with us, they should affect present day reasoning performance ([96,p. 3]).

Cosmides ran a number of experiments contrasting social contracts with arbitrary regulations, and contrasting cheater detection with altruism detection.

Figure 6.1 gives her famous experiment on cheater detection in a social contract. Seventy-five per cent of subjects now chose the *did get tattoo* and *Big*

---

7. The purpose of this section is mostly critical. Readers who are more interested in the positive development can continue with section 6.4.

8. Reciprocal altruism is one party behaving altruistically on one occasion on the expectation that this generosity will be reciprocated by the other party at some future time. It is important to note that whether and under what conditions altruism can evolve and to what degree it has to be reciprocal is highly controversial in biology[301]; and even reciprocal altruism requires the ability to detect altruism.

You are an anthropologist studying the Kaluame, a Polynesian people who live in small, warring bands on Maku Island in the Pacific. You are interested in how Kaluame "big men"– chieftains– yield power. "Big Kiku" is a Kaluame big man who is known for his ruthlessness. As a sign of loyalty, he makes his own subjects put a tattoo on their face. Members of other Kaluame bands never have facial tattoos. Big Kiku has made so many enemies in other Kaluame bands, that being caught in another village with a facial tattoo is, quite literally, the kiss of death. Four men from different bands stumble into Big Kiku's village, starving and desperate. They have been kicked out of their respective villages for various misdeeds, and have come to Big Kiku because they need food badly. Big Kiku offers each of them the following deal: "If you get a tattoo on your face, then I'll give you cassava root." Cassava root is a very sustaining food which Big Kiku's people cultivate. The four men are very hungry, so they agree to Big Kiku's deal. Big Kiku says the tattoos must be in place tonight, but that the cassava root will not be available until the following morning. You learn that Big Kiku hates some of these men for betraying him to his enemies. You suspect he will cheat and betray some of them. Thus, this is the perfect opportunity for you to see first hand how Big Kiku wields his power. The cards below have information about the fates of the four men. Each card represents one man. One side of a card tells whether or not the man went through with the facial tattoo that evening and the other side of the card tells whether or not Big Kiku gave that man cassava root the next day. Did Big Kiku get away with cheating any of these four men? Indicate only those card(s) you definitely need to turn over to see if Big Kiku has broken his word to any of these four men.

Cards

did get tattoo	didn't get tattoo	BK gave cassava	BK gave nothing

Figure 6.1   Cosmides' cheater detection task. From [47,p. 211; p.264-5]

Kiku gave nothing cards, a score comparable to that for the drinking age rule. Cosmides interprets this result as falsifying an explanation of the alleged content effect based on familiarity with the rule. As opposed to this, Cosmides claims that unfamiliar content may also elicit good performance, as long as a social contract is involved. It will be clear by now that our explanation of the result is different: Cosmides' rule is of a deontic nature, and hence none of the factors that complicated reasoning in the case of descriptive conditionals are operative here, and so one would expect many competence answers here. Familiarity is important in the postal regulation case (see p.46) because without familiarity with the content, there is nothing to trigger the deontic interpretation of an indicatively stated rule. Familiarity is not necessary in Cosmides material because the scenario is described as requiring deontic interpretation. Note that the drinking age rule is *not* a social contract (nothing is exchanged). Note also that other nonsocial contract deontic examples (such as Wason and Green's inspection rules) were prominent in the literature before Cosmides wrote.

6.3.2 Why Cheater Detection Is Claimed to Override Logical Form

Cosmides, however, has more arguments up her sleeve, and claims that in some cases of reasoning about social contracts, the predictions of logic and cheater detection theory diverge; the experimental results then show that the former are falsified [47,p. 189]. Consider the following social contract:

(1)   If you give me your watch, I give you 20 euro.

According to Cosmides, this contract is equivalent to the following:

(2)   If I give you 20 euro, you give me your watch.

Indeed, both contracts express that the "I" is willing to pay a cost (20 euros) in order to receive a benefit (the watch) from "you." The only difference appears to lie in the ordering of the transactions, in the sense that usually, but not always, the action described in the consequent follows the action described in the antecedent. Now suppose the cards are laid out on the table as in figure 6.2. Then contracts (1) and (2) would, according to Cosmides, both lead

did give watch	didn't give watch	did give 20 euro	didn't give 10 euro

Figure 6.2   Cards in watch transaction.

to the choice "give watch" and "give 10 euro," since "I" have cheated "you" if "I" accept "your" watch while paying "you" less than the 20 euros that we agreed upon. Observe that if the contract is expressed in the form (1), the cards showing "give watch" and "didn't give 10 euros" would correspond with the antecedent and the negation of the consequent of the conditional. If the contract is expressed in the form (2), these cards correspond instead with the consequent and the negation of the antecedent of the conditional. Cosmides now claims that the prediction of propositional logic is different from that of cheater detection, since a falsifying instance would always be of the form "antecedent plus negation of consequent," whereas as we have seen, instances of cheating can take different forms. Thus, if the contract is presented in the form (2), logic and cheater detection would dictate different answers.

Similarly, suppose that the deal proposed by Big Kiku is formulated as a *switched social contract* (figure 6.2).

If I give you cassava root, you must get a tattoo on your face.

Cosmides claims that (a) the original and the switched rule embody the same social contract, therefore in both cases the cards "did get tattoo" and "BK gave nothing" would have to be chosen, and (b) logic dictates that in the case of the switched social contract the following cards would have to be chosen: "BK gave cassava" and "didn't get tattoo." The argument for this is that only these cards can yield counterexamples to the conditional as stated. While we agree to (a), we consider (b) to be another example of the surface form fetishism that has so marred the subject. It is precisely because (a) is true that the logical form of either the original or the switched version is not that of a material conditional. These equivocations brought about by reversing materials with temporal interpretations are common in the psychological literature.

6.3.3 Altruism

Cosmides' second way of arguing that competence reasoning with "if...then" is due only to the activation of cheater detection, and not to the *logical form* of social contracts, is to present an example of reasoning with social contracts in which humans don't excel. Evolutionary theories, according to Cosmides, would not require the existence of "altruists," that is, individuals who are willing to pay a price without taking the corresponding benefit. These individuals would quickly lose out in the struggle for survival, and hence don't exist. But if altruists don't exist, there has been no need for an "altruist detector" to evolve, and accordingly humans should not exhibit a special ability to reason about altruism with respect to a given social contract. The argument outlined here already raises many questions, but let us take it for granted for the moment. We will show that the experiment designed to verify the prediction leaves much to be desired. In figure 6.3 we give Cosmides' instructions, which are for the most part identical to those for the case of cheater detection, until and including the sentence "You suspect he will cheat and betray some of them."

[] However, you have also heard that Big Kiku sometimes, quite unexpectedly, shows great generosity towards others - that he is sometimes quite altruistic. Thus, this is the perfect opportunity for you to see first hand how Big Kiku wields his power. The cards below have information about the fates of the four men. Each card represents one man. One side of a card tells whether or not the man went through with the facial tattoo that evening and the other side of the card tells whether or not Big Kiku gave that man cassava root the next day. Did Big Kiku behave altruistically towards any of these four men? Indicate only those card(s) you definitely need to turn over to see if Big Kiku has behaved altruistically to any of these four men.

Cards

did get tattoo	didn't get tattoo	BK gave cassava	BK gave nothing

Figure 6.3   Cosmides' "altruism" task [48,p. 193ff]

Cosmides claims that in this experiment the "didn't get tattoo" and "Big Kiku gave cassava" cards would have to be turned, with the following argument. Altruists, according to Cosmides, are people ready to pay a price without taking the corresponding benefit; if Big Kiku is an altruist, he wants to pay a price (give cassava root), without demanding his rightful benefit (the tattoo). Hence it would have to be checked whether behind the "didn't get tattoo" card is written "Big Kiku gave cassava" and whether behind the "Big Kiku gave cassava" card is written "didn't get tattoo." Very few subjects made this choice, which led Cosmides to the conclusion that there is no sixth sense for altruism.

Inspection of Cosmides' experiment and argument reveal that her operationalization of the meaning of altruism is random giving. Cursory access to the dictionary suggests this is not a plausible meaning, and as a consequence it becomes unclear what the competence answer should be.

We can see, for instance, that the story about Big Kiku's dealings suggests the opposite of altruism; a truly altruistic person would give that cassava root, no questions asked, without demands. Therefore a conditional promise is not altruistic; only an unconditional promise would count as such. If this is so, then *no* card needs to be turned – one can see immediately that Big Kiku is not an altruist. One arrives at the same conclusion if one argues as follows: "The cards exhibited make plain that at least one of the men did not get cassava. That's not altruistic: a true altruist feeds the hungry. Hence one doesn't have to turn a card to see that Big Kiku is not an altruist." We now have two different predictions, Cosmides', and the "no card" prediction.

A different prediction from these two can be obtained when the subject argues as follows: 'Big Kiku has made a conditional promise. Altruism requires that Big Kiku at the very least keeps his promise, but furthermore displays his generosity. But then all four cards have to be turned.' Hence we have at least three different predictions. It is therefore unclear what follows from the supposed existence of an altruism detector, and hence what counts as a falsification.

Once a more plausible meaning is attached it equally quickly becomes evident that being able to detect acts of altruism is rather an important part of social interaction, whether people who invariably randomly give away their possessions are evolutionarily fit or not.

6.3.4 The Moral, Part 1: The Problem of Phenotypic Description

Our argument has been that Cosmides' phenotypic description is wrong for modern undergraduates. Solubility by cheater detection is not the property that determines difficulty in the selection task, but rather processing differences flowing from differences in logical form. But even if the description were correct, it would be unlikely to be an evolutionarily insightful description. For that one would minimally have to ask questions like: What can undergraduates (and other people) do with conditional sentences outside Wason's task? A large proportion of conditionals are not social contracts yet they persist in the language. What are they for? What could our ancestors do by way of cheating detection? What ancestral capacities evolved into our capacities for cheating detection?

The fundamental problem of applying Darwin's extraordinarily powerful and abstract theory to particular cases is, as he well understood, the problem of phenotypic description and the identification of functionally important traits which are instrumental in evolution. It is worth taking a look at just what is involved in a simple morphological case.

Excursion: To Be a Moth in the Industrial Revolution   *Biston betularia* was a pale brown moth which occurred in the English midlands and lived a beautifully camouflaged life on lichen–covered trees. It was preyed on with only medium success by various birds. Along came the industrial revolution which polluted the Black Country air and killed the sensitive lichens, blackening the trees. The birds had a field day until a melanic (black) form of *B. betularia* rapidly spread throughout the populations in polluted areas. The great majority of *B. betularia* in the still delichened areas is now melanic. This case has all the ingredients of a microstep of evolution by natural selection, and being one of the classical examples of the process actually caught in operation is thoroughly researched. We have a phenotypic description (pale vs. melanic) and this functional property has been shown by field observation of birds' feeding successes to differentially affect reproductive success of the moth *in the natural environment* according to the color of the tree bark as determined by the level of pollution's effect on the lichen. Moreover, it is now known that the melanic form is the result of a single mutant gene, which was present at low levels of occurrence in the original population. As with almost all such cases it is still not known what other phenotypic traits, if any, this same mutant gene controls, nor what range of variability of expression the gene exhibits in the full range of possible environments in which the moth can survive. As with the many single gene traits maintained at low levels in the original population by mutation, this melanic trait has a high heritability in the natural environment, and may have a high heritability in a wide range of environments.

Several points are worth emphasizing. First and foremost, although every description of an animal may be a phenotypic description, vanishingly few such descriptions are evolutionarily significant. Which ones are significant is determined by the environment on the one hand and by the relation between phenotype and genotype on the other. The environment includes the color of the lichens and whether they grow on the trees (in turn determined by sulfur dioxide levels in the atmosphere and the lichens' phenotypic traits of susceptibility to it), and the perceptual sensitivities of the birds and their role in determining their preying behavior, along with much else. The environment also includes all the moth's other genes inasmuch as they affect either the expression of the phenotypic trait in question or the reproductive success of the phenotypic character the target gene controls. Almost all the well-documented cases of evolution in action are cases of traits controlled by few (often one) genes which largely genetically control the relevant trait in the relevant range of environments. For various reasons that need not detain us here, these are often pathological mutations. Most of the characteristics that psychologists want to study are not of this simple kind. This does not argue against genetic involvement, but merely for the difficulty of evolutionary analysis. Blackness from head to tail is a trait which invites a simple description which is transparently related to reproductive fitness in an environment (blackened trees). It doesn't take a lot of other features of the moth to understand how this fits into its pattern of life (and sex and death). The behavior of sitting on trees and being eaten by visually guided birds is more or less enough. The *other* differences between life for a white moth and life for a black moth are also presumably not huge (it might be significant to know if there are mating preferences between varieties).

Compare the trait of turning the P and not Q cards in the drinking age selection task for modern undergraduates. Without a further account of this trait's relation to reproductive fitness it doesn't look to have much of a purchase for selection pressures. Fallacious reasoning about under-age drinking isn't a capital offense, even in America. We need some generalization. Understanding what it is to obey laws (or perhaps conditional commands) sounds perhaps a bit more plausible. But we palpably do not have an insightful characterization of the phenotypic trait involved, in, say, performance of the selection task (any of its variants) which we can relate to more general psychological functioning, let alone the individual variations in performances, let alone reproductive success in our current environment, let alone that of the Pleistocene. (Our proposals in chapter 3 might be a beginning.) Finding more abstract descriptions such as "performing social contract reasoning" is obviously a necessary move if we are to develop insightful phenotypic descriptions of psychological capacities. But we also need evidence to distinguish them from other plausibly more insightful descriptions such as "capacity for generalized natural language communication," or "capacity to distinguish between deontic and descriptive interpretations" and we saw above that the evidence from the selection task is stronger that such descriptions are insightful than anything about social contracts. And however useful such capacities may sound, they need substantial empirical investigation before we should accept them even as candidates for driving evolution.

6.3.5   The Moral, Part 2: What's so Special about Logical Reasoning

We have argued that Cosmides has not presented any evidence that human reasoning is implemented piecemeal by specialized modules. The evolutionary psychologists' arguments for modular specialization, and so against logic, were based on the idea that logic is a general system and that general systems are necessarily inefficient. We have shown that these presuppositions need to be severely modified. Logical reasoning is not domain-independent in the sense envisaged by the evolutionary psychologists; its laws can vary across domains, and reasoning is involved in determining what these laws are.

So the issue must be rather what general skills subjects have for crafting appropriate reasoning systems for localized problems. These are the skills we saw working overtime in the abnormal environment of the descriptive selection task, trying to understand which of the many possible interpretations of the experimenter's intentions might be the one she had in mind.

Although subjects reasoning in Wason's task may be fraught, the overall picture of their reasoning capacities in more familiar situations can hardly be described as specialized or local, especially by the standards of any other creature or system yet known. Human reasoning and communication are surely characterized by amazing, though of course not total, generality relative to any other candidate. The most obvious example is of course human capacities for understanding cooperative communication. The reasoning involved is logically much more complex than the reasoning the experimenters believe they have specified in laboratory "reasoning tasks." For example, computing implicatures and their consequences is more complex than simply computing the logical consequences of material implications. It is very strange to find a group of scientists confronted with this generality who insist that their *first* task is to explain domain dependence [268].

6.4   Modularity with a Human Face

The human mind is modular because organisms are modular. We have argued, however, that finding human cognitive novelties and identifying them with novel modules is not a good approach to analyzing human evolution. It is not a good idea with regard to cheater detectors, nor is it a good idea with a "narrow language" faculty.[9] If the human mind didn't arise through the addition of a large number of new modules, each identified as adding a human innovation, is there some more biologically plausible view of how it might have arisen which stands a chance of explaining the greater generality of human reasoning abilities?

A more biological approach is to seek cognitive continuities with our ancestors, and then against that background of continuity to seek ways to specify innovations and discontinuities. With the giraffe, it is easy to see that necks are the continuity, and the innovation is in length. With cognitive functions, the homologies should not be expected to be so obvious. Specifically, there is no reason to believe that the capacities homologous to modern humans' language capacities should necessarily be capacities for communication. Interestingly, a number of disparate lines of research suggest that we may not need to go much

---

9. Hauser, Chomsky, and Fitch [119] (discussed in section 6.1.) attempt to remain agnostic about whether their faculties are modules, but it is not clear to what extent they succeed.

beyond our analysis of logical reasoning tasks to find some of the relevantly continuous apparatus.

6.4.1   Planning: Continuities with Our Ancestors

Systems of closed–world reasoning are logics of planning. We plan with respect to our expectations of the world, not, as we would have to if we planned using classical logic, with respect to all logical possibilities. Maintaining a model of the current state of the immediate environment relevant to action is a primitive biological function; calculating what is true in all logically possible models of the current sense data is not. These planning logics are just as much what one needs for planning low-level motor actions such as reaching and grasping, as they are for planning chess moves (see Shanahan [246] for examples of such use in robotics).[10]

Recursion is a very important part of planning. We plan with respect to a main goal, and this then creates subgoals and sub–subgoals with respect to which we plan recursively. Our early primate ancestors became planners of much more complex motor actions when they took to the trees and acquired the kind of forward–facing binocular overlap required for doing the depth perception required for complex manipulations. Recursion, and the general complexity of our motor planning, no doubt got a huge boost from our primate ancestors' arboreal habits, and another much more recent but well before language emerged, from the advent of tool–making. Of course all planning does not have to have complete plans before execution. We often plan "reactively," beginning on a course of action and leaving the details to later, taking opportunistic advantage of happenstance as it arrives along the way. But reactive planning of any structured activity requires the holding of goals and subgoals in memory, even if the staging of decision and execution of what turns out to be the plan becomes smeared across time.

It is also well known that apes fail in many planning tasks which we find straightforward. Köhler's chimpanzees fail to fetch the box from next door to climb up to reach the bananas, even though they may use the box if they can see it simultaneously with seeing the bananas out of reach [161]. But the fact that some subgoaling is difficult doesn't mean that apes can't do any subgoaling. What we have in mind is the kind of subgoaling which goes on at a much more implicit level in performing complex motor control – planning a reach for an object through a set of obstacles for example.

As neuroscientists have pointed out, it is intriguing that the motor areas for

---

10. This should remind the reader that there is nothing particularly linguistic about logic, which is one reason why logical analysis may be particularly useful for finding evolutionary continuities between pre– and postlinguistic cognition. Another quite different approach to motor control problems uses continuous models derived form control theory [192] and it would be of great interest to know more about the formal relations between these models and defeasible logical ones.

planning speech are right next to the motor areas for planning action. This hypothesis about the cognitive continuities between primate ancestors and man has been elaborated by many researchers [3, 107]. Approaching from the direction of the syntactic and semantic analysis of temporal expressions of natural languages also directs attention to planning as underlying our faculties for language [256, 282]. More generally, a main human brain innovation is the increase in neocortex, and specifically in frontal areas of neocortex. These frontal areas are involved in planning and "executive functions," among other things.

Another striking demonstration of unexpected continuities in planning in internal mental functions is provided by work on monkeys' working memory. *Cebus appella* has been shown to have hierarchical planning capabilities with respect to their working memories remarkably similar to the hierarchical chunking strategies that are evidenced in human list recall.[11] When humans are given a suitably categorized list of words, the animal words all come out clustered together, followed by the vegetable words etc. McGonigle et al. [189] trained monkeys on a touchscreen task requiring that they touch each of a set of hierarchically classifiable icons exhaustively. Of course, if the positions of the icons remain constant between touches, very simple spatial sweep strategies suffice. So the icons are spatially shuffled after each touch. The monkeys have to remember, with no external record, just which icons they have already touched, and they still succeed. McGonigle et al. showed that the monkeys were then capable of efficiently exhausting an array of nine items, but more interestingly that they did so by touching all the icons of one shape, followed by all of those of another, just as humans' recall sequence is clustered. Here is recursive hierarchical planning in individual (rather than socially expressed) working memory, in the service of strategic planning of action sequences.

Seeing such sophisticated strategic planning with respect to a private memory function in monkeys is rather suggestive of the hypothesis that human innovations may have more to do with introducing the social expression of recursive planning in communication than with any lack of recursion in our ancestors' individual mental capacities[12] This is a good example of the problem of phenotypic description – whether "recursion" is novel depends on whether we confine our search to communicative behaviors, or cast the net more broadly. Planning provides a good basis for understanding cognitive continuities at various timescales in our evolution. At least some of the simpler versions of closed–world reasoning, unlike classical logic, carry out the biologically primitive function of maintaining a model of the current environment, and, as will be explored in

---

11. These monkeys are of the order of 25 million years diverged from their last common ancestor with humans.

12. This approach contrasts with Chomsky's belief that recursion is what is novel about human language. But at a deeper level it is closely aligned with his own preference for the hypothesis that language may have evolved as a private "language of thought" whose function is internal mental "calculation," and only rather recently has become expressed as a medium of social communication.

chapter 8, are demonstrably neurally implementable in an extremely efficient manner.

6.4.2   Discontinuities

If externalization of planning, and plan recognition abilities, are one candidate area for what is special about human cognition, what does closed–world reasoning have to offer as a framework for understanding the transition to modern humans? In our discussion of causal reasoning, and attribution of beliefs and intentions, we suggested that reasoning about beliefs can be viewed as an extension of causal reasoning in which perception is a kind of causal effect on beliefs. Then there is still more complex reasoning about false beliefs, and about intentions for intentions to be recognized.

Without pretending to have a full cognitive account of reasoning about minds in terms of closed–world reasoning, we would claim that this is a good potential basis for understanding the cognitive discontinuities of our reasoning capacities as well as the continuities. It is a good framework because it offers many gradations of reasoning and implementation. Notice that this approach takes the capacities provided by the conceptual-intentional subfaculty postulated by Hauser, Chomsky, and Fitch [119] to be novel (if continuous) with earlier ancestral capacities (recursion, working memory, plan recognition, defeasible reasoning, etc.) but is entirely agnostic about the degree to which they are modular. The relations between system 1 interpretive capacity and system 2 "supervision-of-interpretation" capacity belong among the innovations here.

For example, we saw above that closed–world reasoning is a whole family of modes which can model many qualitative changes in what can be achieved. The psychological literature on reasoning about mental states indicates the need for such gradations. It is at present controversial in human development at what stage "theory of mind" abilities emerge. False-belief tasks were proposed as diagnosing a lack of these abilities in normal 3-year-olds and their presence in normal 4-year-olds [172]. Others have proposed that irrelevant linguistic demands of these tasks deceptively depress 3-year-olds' performance. For example, in the false belief task, the child sees the doll see the sweet placed in one box, and then the child but not the doll sees the sweet moved to another. Now if the child is asked, "Where will the doll look for the sweet *first*?" instead of "Where will the doll look for the sweet?" then children as young as 2 can sometimes solve the problem [248]. Intriguingly, this might be read as evidence of the 3-year-olds in the original task adopting a deontic reading of the question (Where *should* the doll look?) rather than a descriptive one (Where will the doll look first?).[13] Clement and Kauffman [40] offer evidence that children's

---

13. There are of course other possibilities. Another, which also echoes a problem in the selection task, is that the younger children's problem may be with sequencing contingencies in their responses.

capacity to reason about the relation between the actual world and some discrepant 'ideal' state (the capacity underlying false-belief reasoning and many other kinds) develops much earlier in deontic reasoning. It would be hardly suprising if children's grasp of the discrepancy between what someone did and what they were supposed to do loomed early and large in children's reasoning.

Onishi and Baillargeon [207] use data from nonverbal expectation of looking in infants of only 15 months to argue for the beginnings of effective reasoning about false beliefs at this age. Although these data can, as the authors point out, alternatively be interpreted in terms of more superficial strategies of looking for things where they were last seen, even this requires the child to preserve distinctions between who last saw the object and where. Nevertheless, all these arguments push reasoning about mental states earlier in ontogeny. Above we raised the possibility that some theory–of–mind failures might be more perspicuously described as failures of reasoning about possibilities (rather than specifically about mental states), so there is a great need for a more analytical classification of these reasoning tasks. An approach based on the variety of logics and their contextual triggers offers a gradation of models of performance which can plausibly explain such developmental sequences whereas posing a theory-of-mind module itself offers little help.

This approach through continuities and discontinuities of function still needs to be supplemented by a much more biological grounding. We will end this chapter by illustrating what one highly speculative grounding might look like.[14] Our purpose here is to provide an example of how the different levels of evidence – from cognitive function to genetics – might actually come together in a biological account of human speciation[15] that does justice to the large–scale innovations of the human mind and the far greater generality of our reasoning.

6.5 Out of the Mouths of Babes and Sucklings

One of the great biological distinctions of the species *Homo sapiens* is the immature state of its offspring at birth, and the lengthened period of their maturation (known in biology as *altriciality*). We will take this example of a biological innovation and trace out some of its consequences and how it relates evidence at many levels. Here is an indisputable novel biological feature which engages both with our social reorganization into a group-breeding species – intensified by the cost of rearing altricial infants – and with the distinctive cognitive changes that enable language and culture in such a group-breeding species. Remember that the purpose of our example is to provide a contrast with the kinds of stories on offer which identify cognitive innovations as modules. Altriciality is an example that shows how one adaptation, plausibly driven by relatively

---

14. Developed from the argument of Stenning [257].
15. Human speciation is the process which gave rise to *Homo sapiens* from its ape ancestors.

few selection pressures, could give rise to changes in large numbers of other modular systems. It is an excellent illustrative example of biological grounding because it brings together effects at so many levels. Evolution does not, by and large, proceed by adding new modules, but by retiming the control of developmental processes of old ones. Altriciality is just such a process where few control elements might retime macromodules in development.

Evolutionary stories must begin with a characterization of selection pressures. A prime candidate for the driving force behind human altriciality is that constraints on growth rates of neural tissue along with maternal anatomy may mean that altriciality was the only way to develop a big-brained narrow-hipped species of biped. Whatever the pressure for larger brains, larger brains would have forced more altricial birth, given constraints on maternal pelvic dimensions – "Get out while you can!" being the wise human infant's motto. There may even be a positive feedback loop here – more altricial birth means greater dependence and more pressure for social coordination in order to group-rear infants. But social coordination is one candidate for driving the need for bigger brains, and so it goes round.

It is easy to see that altriciality has radically affected the data to which human learning mechanisms are exposed, and the sequence of exposure. Maturational mechanisms which previously occurred in utero now happen in the external environment. Humans are, for example, unique in the amount of postnatal neural growth they exhibit. The human changes in the duration and sequencing of brain development, which constitute an important part of altriciality, are prime candidates for being one cause of the kind of widespread modular repurposing which took place in human speciation and subsequent evolution.

6.5.1   Altriciality and Social Behavior

We hypothesise that the intensification of humans' focus on reasoning about the intentions of conspecifics, and particularly their communicative intentions, arose as an outgrowth of existing capacities for reasoning in other kinds of planning. One very important contribution of altriciality to human cognitive evolution is its pressures toward cooperation – first between mother and infant, then between adults in small groups, and outward to larger societies. Hare and Tomasello [116] have pointed to the predominantly competitive interactions between chimpanzees as being a major brake on the development of their mind–reading abilities. Even domestic dogs are superior in this regard, and, interestingly, domestic dogs are altricial in respect of a number of critical behavioral characteristics with regard to their wolf ancestors. For example, mammalian young engage in play, which involves suspension of aggression, along with intense cooperation in coordination, and social signaling of group comembership through greeting. Altricial domestic dogs continue these infantile behavioral traits into adulthood. Whereas adult wolves may greet once daily, domestic dogs may repeat their greetings on a 10 minute separation. Humans may continue play into old age.

There are good general reasons for believing that the social coordination required for the establishment and preservation of language conventions requires a highly cooperative setting such as that which altriciality provides. For example, Davidson's arguments for the "principle of charity" in interpretation [57] provide just such reasons. If we were really so focused in our earliest social dealings on whether we are being cheated or lied to, it seems unlikely that human communication would ever have got off the ground. Reasoning about interpretations is quite hard enough under assumptions of cooperation, and the evidence of misalignment all too easy to come by once one expects deliberate misalignment. Policing of contracts may be important at the margins, but is not a plausible explanation of the initial establishment of cooperation. Furthermore, it is far from clear that our ancestors were in general incapable of detecting cheating on social regulations in say food-sharing cliques—no effort on the part of those who propose cheating detectors as novel modules seems to have gone into studying the ancestral precursors. Almost certainly it is the capacity for creating and dissolving the regularities we call social contracts which is novel and that has more to do with communication and the formation of trust than the negative detection of cheating.

Views of altruism in the several literatures which have cause to study it seem to have undergone a recent marked transformation. Economists, for example, have started to acknowledge that when players consider themselves to be members of a team, immediate cooperative play in the Prisoner's Dilemma game, without the expectation of repeated play, is often observed [6]. Study of the Ultimatum game and other non-zero sum games clearly illustrate that *Homo economicus* is a rare species possibly largely confined to economics departments [98]. This has immediate implications for the possibility of group selection and non-Spencerian evolutionary theory. Such cooperative possibilities were, of course, pointed out by the early users of game theory [242], but seem to have been dismissed, as far as one can tell, on ideological grounds. Human social organization, relative to that of our immediate ancestors, is characterized by hugely decreased within-group aggression (with, it may be argued, greatly increased between-group aggression) [32].

Quite apart from a generalized increased pressure for cooperation arising from altriciality, we should expect some more specifically cognitive impacts. Dumping an immature brain out into the external world exposes its learning mechanisms to quite different inputs and outputs than retention in utero. Learning is closely related to what can be controlled. Human infants have little control over their physical environment for an extended period from birth. In round figures, human infants take 9 months to reach the state of motor development of a newborn chimpanzee. However, in the extended period of their development, they have considerable access to social control, mainly through voice but also through facial expression. Screaming brings one set of effects, cooing another, and a little later, smiling yet different effects. Bruner has emphasized the development of taking turns in primitive preverbal exchanges between mother and infant. The development of this predictable shifting pattern of authority and control is clearly an important precursor of discourse and possibly of the self as the locus of control. This flexibility of assignment of authority is another rather biologically distinctive human pattern of behavior. Most animals have pecking orders which determine patterns of authority with limited contextual flexibility. Along with this change goes substantial changes in eye movement patterns: in most animals eye contact tends to be aggressive; in humans it often signals social bonding and its refusal can be agonistic, though there is evidence the change in this pattern already began in our ape ancestors.

One might speculate that this shift of emphasis from physical control to social control may have widespread implications for human cognition. Learning social control requires developing intentional concepts. It has long been observed by philosophers of science that our common grasp of even physical causality has many intentional aspects. More exotically, philosophers, at least since Nietzsche, have argued that our capacity for anthropomorphism (and with it the basis of religion) stems from our earliest experiences of causality and control being of social rather than physical control. Stenning [257] develops some implications for the origins of human cognition.

6.5.2   Altriciality and Neurogenesis

If altriciality is a good candidate adaptation for driving widespread cognitive innovation, what are the biological details of altricial development patterns and when did they happen in evolution? Focus on the changes in the temporal profile of human development reveals some complicated and controversial patterns. Strict neotony (continuation of an infantile state of some trait into adulthood) does not appear to be the best model of, for example, human brain growth. Once a more general class of multiphasic growth models are considered, it has been shown that the best fit to human brain growth timing is provided by a four-phase nonlinear model, with breakpoints at 4.4, 9.3, 13.8, 18.2, and 114 conception months [292] (see figure 6.4). The final phase has a zero growth parameter and a large estimation error (error bar on the last point: 38-288). When compared to the chimpanzee model, the human growth rate parameter has remained fixed, and each phase has been lengthened by a factor of about 1.3. So at least for brain growth, this is not neotony – rather lengthening of the same pattern. Nevertheless altriciality, at a descriptive level, is indisputable. Other characteristics can, of course, show either no changes in timing, or different changes in developmental scheduling.

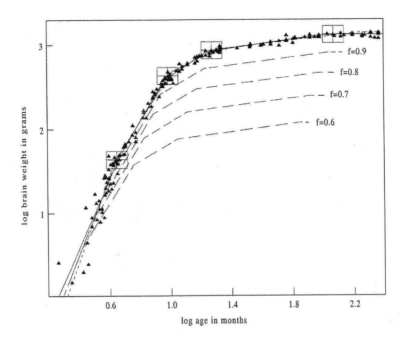

Figure 6.4   Multiphasic regression of human log ages and log brain weights. Reprinted from [292,p. 232] by permission of Elsevier Inc.

Above we already introduced Rakic's model of brain growth (see page 150), which describes an exponential process of expansion of neuron progenitor numbers, placed in the first half of the first phase (up to 4.4 conception months). This is the phase critical for the eventual brain size. It has been calculated that during this phase, on average about 225,000 cortical neuron progenitors are generated per *minute*. What has been referred to as the "brain growth spurt" roughly corresponds to the second phase. It starts near the beginning of midgestation with multiplication of glial cells and growth and myelination of neurons, which continue until the end of the second postnatal year or later. The third phase, the "cerebellar phase," starts prenatally and proceeds especially rapidly soon after birth. Phase 4 may be underestimated in current data and is not so easily identified with a dominant process.

Normal brain growth works by producing a very large number of interconnections between neurons early on, and then subsequently pruning many of these out. This pruning is assumed to be associated with less active usage. So the connections that are reinforced (and which are presumed to be functionally active in the individual's processing) survive, but those not used die out – use it or lose it as a kind of natural selection among neurons. The timing of the major phases of synaptic pruning are currently contentious though probably start within the first year of postnatal life.

We will revisit this temporal profile when we turn to autism is chapter 9. Brain growth is, of course, only one much–studied example of evolutionarily changed temporal profile in development. Nor is it clear what part brain size plays in human cognitive evolution—whether size matters. We merely offer it as on example which is probably cognitively relevant. Scerif and Karmiloff-Smith [241] review evidence that several genetically based behavioral disorders (e.g., Williams syndrome are to be at least partly understood as distortions of relative developmental phasing of different systems.

6.5.3   Altriciality in the Evolution of *Homo*

One immediate evolutionary question about the changes in the temporal profile of human development is just when they happened in phylogeny. Until recently, it was widely assumed that the pressures for altriciality from obstetric problems must have arisen with the origins of bipedalism – that is fairly far back in our divergence from our ape ancestors. More recently, a variety of kinds of evidence point to a much later date for the major changes in the timing of development.

Although australopithecine bipedal walking evolved around 5 million years ago, there were 2.5 to 3 million years of walking before distance running evolved [23]. A secondary narrowing of the pelvis to facilitate the mechanics of efficient running is claimed by these authors not to occur in *Homo erectus* but to arrive in *Homo sapiens*. The tall human body with a narrow trunk, waist, and pelvis creates more skin surface for our size, permitting greater cooling during running. It also lets the upper and lower body move independently, which allows us to use the upper body to counteract the twisting forces from the swinging legs. If distance running was a factor in narrowing the pelvis, then we can assume that this would have increased the selection pressure on obstetric problems arising from large fetal heads.

Studies of the evolution of the mechanics of human birth show that it evolved in several stages [234]. The early australopithecines' shift to bipedalism brought some of the innovations invoked by the changes in human shoulders, but not the problems due to brain size. Australopithecines probably displayed one of two part rotations which modern human infants perform on passing through the pelvis, but not both. Martin [184] proposes that pelvic size began to constrain brain size only around 1.5 miilion years ago, and by 100,000 years ago we reached essentially the modern arrangements, although even these exert considerable selection pressure on the systems of development and delivery. This time scale certainly overlaps with the emergence of modern human cognition.

Study of the skull openings in a single well-preserved skull of *Homo erectus* from Java [46] provides some information on this issue. These authors argue from estimates of the skull's age (1.8 million years) and age at death (0.5 to 1.5 years), that this it is more ape-like than modern *Homo sapiens*-like in its degree of development at birth. They conclude that secondary altriciality (the extension of brain growth after birth) was a late innovation in the mutual ancestor of *Homo sapiens* and *Homo neanderthalensis*. They comment that both displayed enlarged brains and reduced pelvic inlet sizes. To give some idea of the scale of the long-term changes, whereas macaque newborns have 70% of their adult brain volume, in humans the figure is 25% (then after first year it's 50% and after 10 years, 95%). Apes are intermediate (40%) at birth.

A completely different kind of evidence comes from molecular clock comparisons between human, chimpanzee, gorilla, and baboon which have been used to estimate when human generation length extended. It turns out that human and chimpanzee are much more similar in clock speed than the gorilla and baboon. Humans' molecular clock speed is about 10% slower than the gorilla and 3% slower than the chimpanzee's. The significant 3% slowdown of humans from chimpanzees is taken to indicate that the human slowdown is recent. Making the simplifying assumptions that all the difference is due to generation lengthening and the change was instantaneous, the estimate is of a change about 1 million years ago [70]. This is a little earlier than the other sources of evidence.

All these diverse sources of evidence place changes in the timing of human development as possibly being active not too far from the period of the emergence of modern human cognition starting around 1 million to half a million years ago, an important motivator for choosing an intensification of the long-term trend to altriciality as an organizing adaptation. Altriciality illustrates how the impact of a single well-established coherent biological change can ramify throughout the biology of a species, altering a myriad of ancestral functions, each itself already modularized in complex ways. Existing machinery is exapted for dealing with the resulting new situations. Secondary adaptations are required to live with these exaptations.

6.6 Conclusion: Back to the Laboratory (and the Drawing Board)

In summary, our sketch of an answer to how human cognition became so much more general than that of our immediate ancestors is a variant of the traditional one that communication through language (suitably understood) is central. But it is a variant with considerable twists. Humans gained the ability to plan and reason about the complex intentions involved in communication, and so to process the multiple interpretations in the multiple logics required for natural language use. Considerable planning in thought may have been possible before it could be externalized in communication. The languages of thought led to the languages of expression.

These conjectures send us back to the laboratory. If reasoning developed out of planning, it is worth investigating reasoning tasks which somehow activate the planning system. In the following two chapters several such tasks – suppression task, box task, false–belief task, counterfactual reasoning task – will be discussed. As the reader can see from this list, it concerns tasks which have been around for a considerable time, having been used for quite different purposes. Formal modeling in nonmonotonic logic will be applied to show that these tasks all embody aspects of planning. This opens up the possibility to establish a correlation between failures on verbal reasoning tasks and nonverbal planning tasks, and the chapter on autism will show that such correlations indeed exist.

In this chapter we have proposed altriciality as an example of an important development in human evolution which can serve as *one* organizing principle for thinking about phenomena at many different levels. We do not propose that it is the only, nor even the best, example. However, it is sufficient to illustrate how fundamental biological concepts such as modularity, heritability, adaptation, and exaptation have been mistreated in discussions of cogntive evolution. Biology's new "evo devo" insights lead us to expect that an important theme in human evolution is the retimings of modular development under the influence of relatively few control elements. This model virtually guarantees that exaptation will be as important as adaptation – when complex modules develop in different contexts, their behavior will change in complex ways, exposing them to repurposing. This means that phenotypic description, and especially cognitive phenotypic description, is hard because the identification of selection pressures from current function is fraught with difficulty. Since innovation does not happen by the arrival of new modules, our method must be to identify both continuity and discontinuity with our ancestors.

PART II

Modeling

The preceding chapters have introduced a perspective on human reasoning which emphasizes the large variety of logical systems not only available, but actually necessary for, describing human reasoning behavior. If classical logic is taken as the norm, irrationality seems to abound, but on a wider conception of reasoning which also involves assigning logical form, apparent irrationality may turn out to be compliance with a different norm, or the impossibility of imposing any logical form whatsoever. Indeed, in chapter 4 we have seen how a variety of contexts supporting subjects in imposing classical logical form in the selection task considerably improve their performance vis– à– vis even the classical criterion.

After the detailed information about parameter setting in the selection task obtained from tutorial dialogues and presented in chapter 3, it might seem that the selection task is an ideal task for studying the process of assigning logical form. However, the great variety of possible parameters, and the complexity of the logical forms associated to each of these parameters, create considerable problems; the number of combinations is simply too large for a first attempt. We therefore need a task in which parameter setting is apparently more constrained, in order to yield information both about parameter setting and about consistency with the parameters thus set.

Another problem with the selection task is that the rule is such a compressed discourse that the subjects' interpretive efforts are narrowly focused, and hard to elicit. A further problem is that what is at issue is clearly the communication between the experimenter and the subject, and the information is intended to be insulated from general knowledge or a larger population of cases. A better task would more obviously invoke interpretation of a more extended discourse with the focus on using general knowledge to resolve the absent speaker's intentions rather than on the experimenter's. In chapter 7 we turn to the so-called "suppression task" which fulfills these requirements. We outline the results obtained and describe a family of defeasible logical theories of closed-world reasoning as a framework for modeling the course of discourse interpretation in this task. We make some premilinary observations of the range of interpretations that occur and the degree of subjects' success in maintaining consistency. We also consider some probabilisitic approaches that have been taken to similar tasks, and argue that these approaches still need to distinguish the process of constructing a (probabilistic) interpretation, and the process of deriving consequences from that interpretation.

If defeasible logics are our framework for specifying what function is computed when we interpret discourses, we can then consider how these logics are implemented in the brain. In chapter 8, we show that this logic, unlike classical logic, is readily implementable in neural networks. In fact, it is possible to account not only of the computations within networks but also to at least outline how such networks might be constructed anew as discourse processing proceeeds. This is something that few neural accounts even attempt. These neural implementations have certain computational properties which are psychologically suggestive – their rules are, for example, unlike classical ones, asymmetric in the amount of computation for forward and backward reasoning.

Rather than leave this as an abstract implementation of general reasoning within albeit particular logics, we illustrate what the availability of logic and implementation can offer to the analysis of particular behavioral syndromes. Since our logic is "planning logic," an obvious choice is an area where "executive function" has figured prominently in psychological analyses, and in chapter 9 we choose autism as a developmental disorder where this is true. Our study of autism also leads us to extend our earlier sketch of the evolutionary basis of cognition.

In the final chapter of part II, we turn our new tools back onto the other heartland task of the psychology of reasoning – the syllogism. We present evidence that credulous interpretation of syllogisms is an important interpretive factor in this task too. Employing exploratory empirical methods, a combination of the credulous/skeptical dimension, with features of the expression of information structure in this simple logical fragment, is used to reveal groups of subjects approaching the syllogism in qualitatively different fashion. This raises the bar on empirical investigations of reasoning.

By this time we would claim to have outlined a broadly based interpretive approach to human reasoning which provides an alternative to what has been on offer in this field. Interpretation is a substantial process, to be distinguished from derivation. It has well–understood logical models which relate long–term general knowledge to episodic information arriving in discourse. These logics can be given interesting neural implementations. The combination can be applied to behavioral phenomena such as autism to reveal hidden continuities and contrasts between diverse behaviors and theories of the condition. This approach also suggests very different accounts of the biological and evolutionary grounding of cognition. Above all, the approach takes seriously the contributions both of psychological experimentation and of formal studies of cognition in logic and linguistics.

7 Planning and Reasoning: The Suppression Task

Before we introduce the reasoning task which will play the lead role in the coming three chapters, we start with a preamble explaining its wider significance. The evolutionary considerations of chapter 6 suggested that instead of thinking of reasoning as an adaptation to a specific environmental pressure (e.g., the necessity to detect cheaters), it is more fruitful to view it as an exaptation, a new use of an older capacity. We proposed the following evolutionary sequence

1. Language exapted the planning capacity, both for syntax and for semantics, and in particular discourse interpretation

2. Discourse interpretation involves *credulous* reasoning by the hearer, that is to say the hearer tries to accommodate the truth of all the speaker's utterances in deriving an intended model

3. Credulous reasoning itself is best modelled as some form of nonmonotonic logic

4. Classical logic arose from conscious reflection on the outcome of (often automatic) credulous reasoning.

With reference to 4, it may be noted that there are various reasons why classical first–order logic is not a very plausible candidate for a "natural" reasoning process, operative also in the absence of schooling. The first reason is that classical logic requires an *extensional* representation of concepts as sets, hence inter alia assumes that it is fully determined whether an object falls under the concept or not. It is much more plausible to assume that concepts are represented cognitively as algorithms which test whether or not the object falls under the concept, that is, *intensionally*, not extensionally. (For an early defense of this idea, see [194].) At the very least the logic describing such concepts is three-valued Kleene logic (see chapter 2) because the algorithm may be undecided on some inputs. If, moreover, the algorithm operates by comparing the input to a prototype, the logic is doubtlessly more complicated, although it is not fully clear what it should be. (Compare, for example, [153] and [90, 91].)

The second reason why classical logic may have to be laboriously learned instead of coming naturally is that the definition of validity underlying classical logic creates computational problems for working memory (when unaided by external devices such as pen and paper). Viewed semantically, one has to go through all models of the premises and check for each of these whether the conclusion holds. One needs a routine to search through all models, and keep track of where one is in the search. The point can be illustrated by asking the reader to determine without use of paper and pencil whether the syllogism

$$\neg \exists x (Ax \wedge Bx),\ \exists x (Bx \wedge Cx)/\ \exists x (Ax \wedge \neg Cx)$$

is valid or not. Classroom experience shows that even students with some logic training find this difficult.[1] Logics which are computationally less taxing for working memory may well precede, both phylogenetically and ontogenetically, those logics which require conscious computation. Note that this complexity is a *mathematical* feature of classical logic and as such independent of a "rules" or "models" representational format. The claim of the next three chapters is that (a) such less taxing logics exist, and (b) it can be tested whether subjects actually reason consistently with such a logic. In this chapter we will first introduce the pertinent reasoning task, then the associated logical form, and lastly some data relevant to the assignment of logical form.

As an introduction to the reasoning task to be discussed in this chapter consider the following two examples. The first is from a boarding card distributed at Amsterdam's Schiphol Airport, where we read

> If it's thirty minutes before your flight departure, make your way to the gate.
> As soon as the gate number is confirmed, make your way to the gate.

The traveler looking at the screen and seeing the gate number confirmed 2 hours before flight departure might well be in a quandary: Can I wait for another hour and a half, or do I proceed to the gate immediately? But his dilemma pales beside that of the hapless visitor who sees it's 30 minutes before departure and is thus told to go the gate, which is, however, as yet undisclosed.

The second example[2] is from a notice explaining the alarm signal button in trains of the London underground.

> If there is an emergency then you press the alarm signal button.
> The driver will stop if any part of the train is in a station.

Here the second sentence, taken literally, on its own, does not even make sense: the train could never leave the station. However, its intended meaning does make sense:

---

1. Clearly, algorithms like semantic tableaux do help in these simple cases, but they are available only to the initiated.
2. Brought to our attention by R.A. Kowalski. See also his [163].

> The driver will stop the train if someone presses the alarm signal button *and* any part of the train is in a station.

Similarly, in the first example, the intended meaning is likely to be

> If it's thirty minutes before your flight departure and the gate number is confirmed, make your way to the gate.

Rigid adherence to classical logic would have little survival value in these cases. Instead there seems to be a reasoning process toward a more reasonable interpretation, in which the antecedents of the conditionals become conjoined. But why this interpretation, and how is it computed? Surprisingly, there is considerable experimental and theoretical information about this question. This is because the very same problem was studied in an entirely different context: the so-called *suppression task* in the psychology of reasoning.

Suppose one presents a subject with the following innocuous premises:

(1)   *If she has an essay to write she will study late in the library.*
       She has an essay to write.

In this case roughly 90% of subjects draw the conclusion She will study late in the library. Next, suppose one adds the premise

(2)   *If the library is open, she will study late in the library.*

In this case, only 60% conclude She will study late in the library. However, if instead of (2) the premise

(3)   *If she has a textbook to read, she will study late in the library.*

is added, then the percentage of She will study late in the library conclusions is comparable to that in (1).

These observations are originally due to Ruth Byrne [28], and they were used by her to argue against a rule-based account of logical reasoning such as found in, e.g., Rips [228]. For if valid arguments can be suppressed, then surely logical inference cannot be a matter of blindly applying rules; and furthermore the fact that suppression depends on the *content* of the added premise is taken to be an argument against the role of logical *form* in reasoning.[3]

While we believe Byrne's interpretation of the results is mistaken, we agree that the task connects to deep issues in the psychology of reasoning. In this chapter we give a logical analysis of the various answer patterns observed. We have distinguished in the previous chapters between two main kinds of logical reasoning: reasoning *from* a fixed interpretation of the logical and nonlogical terms in the premises, and reasoning *toward* an interpretation of those terms.

---

3. Note that the percentages refer to population averages of endorsement; they provide no information about an individual subject's behavior. In section 7.4 we will present some data which bear on this issue.

Here we show that Byrne's interpretation of her data (a "failure" to apply classical logic) follows only if experimental subjects in her task reason from a fixed interpretation. If what they are doing is reasoning to a consistent interpretation of the experimental materials, their answers can be shown to make perfect logical sense, albeit in a different logic. This is where closed–world reasoning, which has been touched upon repeatedly in the preceding chapters, comes to the fore. We provide an extended introduction to this form of reasoning and show how the deviation from classical logical reasoning found in Byrne's data and those of others (e.g., Dieussaert et al. [63]) can be accounted for in the proposed formalism. Here, we will look not only at "binary" data on whether or not a particular inference is suppressed but also consider data from tutorial dialogues, which give some clue to the interpretational processes involved. Chapter 8 will then show that closed–world reasoning has an efficient neural interpretation. In chapter 9 we show that the logic behind the suppression task is the common logical core behind several benchmark tests for autism, such as the false–belief task, unexpected contents task, and box task. This leads one to expect that people with autism show a consistently different answer pattern on the suppression task, a hypothesis that was corroborated in an experiment.

7.1   The Suppression Task and Byrne's Interpretation

As mentioned in the introduction to this chapter, if one presents a subject with the following premises:

(4a)   *If she has an essay to write she will study late in the library.*
(4b)   She has an essay to write.

In this case roughly 90% of subjects[4] draw the conclusion She will study late in the library (we will later discuss what the remaining 10% may be thinking). Next, suppose one adds the premise

(5)   *If the library is open, she will study late in the library.*

and one asks again: what follows? In this case, only 60% conclude She will study late in the library.

However, if instead of the above, the premise

(6)   *If she has a textbook to read, she will study late in the library*

---

4. The figures we use come from the experiment reported in [63], since the experiments reported in this study have more statistical power than those of [28].

is added, then the percentage of She will study late in the library conclusions is around 95%.

In this type of experiment one investigates not only modus ponens (MP), but also modus tollens (MT), and the "fallacies" *affirmation of the consequent* (AC), and *denial of the antecedent* (DA), with respect to both types of added premises, (5) and (6). In table 7.1 we tabulate the relevant data, following Dieussaert et al. [63].

Table 7.1   Percentages of Dieussaert's subjects drawing target conclusions in each of the four argument forms *modus ponens* (MP), *modus tollens* (MT), *denial of the antecedent* (DA), and *affirmation of the consequent* (AC), in two–premise and three–premise arguments: conditional 1 is the same first premise in all cases. In a two-premise argument it is combined only with the categorical premise shown. In a three-premise argument, both are combined with either an alternative or an additional conditional premise.

Role	Content
Conditional 1	If she has an essay to write, she will study late in the library
Categorical	She has an essay to write
Conclusion	She will study late in the library (MP 90%)
Alternative	If she has a textbook to read, she will study late in the library
Conclusion	She will study late in the library (MP 94%)
Additional	If the library stays open, she will study late in the library.
Conclusion	She will study late in the library (MP 60%)
Conditional 1	If she has an essay to write, she will study late in the library.
Categorical	She will study late in the library
Conclusion	She has an essay to write (AC 53%)
Alternative	If she has a textbook to read, she will study late in the library
Conclusion	She has an essay to write (AC 16%)
Additional	If the library stays open, then she will study late in the library.
Conclusion	She has an essay to write (AC 55%)
Conditional 1	If she has an essay to write, she will study late in the library
Categorical	She hasn't an essay to write
Conclusion	She will not study late in the library (DA 49%)
Alternative	If she has a textbook to read, she will study late in the library
Conclusion	She will not study late in the library (DA 22%)
Additional	If the library stays open, she will study late in the library
Conclusion	She will not study late in the library (DA 49%)
Conditional 1	If she has an essay to write, she will study late in the library.
Categorical	She will not study late in the library
Conclusion	She does not have an essay to write (MT 69%)
Alternative	If she has a textbook to read, she will study late in the library
Conclusion	She does not have an essay to write (MT 69%)
Additional	If the library stays open, then she will study late in the library.
Conclusion	She does not have an essay to write (MT 44%)

We start with Byrne's explanation in [28] of how mental models theory[5] explains the data. Mental models assumes that the reasoning process consists of the following stages:

1. The premises are interpreted in the sense that a model is constructed on the

---

5. Section 10.6 in chapter 10 will give a more detailed exposition (and criticism) of mental models theory in the context of syllogistic reasoning.

basis of general knowledge and the specific premises.

2. An informative conclusion is read off from the model.

3. This conclusion is checked against possible alternative models of the situation.

In this particular case the model for the premises $p \rightarrow q$, $r \rightarrow q$ that is constructed depends on the content of p and r, and the general knowledge activated by those contents. If r represents an alternative, the mental model constructed is one appropriate to the formula $p \vee r \rightarrow q$, and the conclusion q can be read off from this model. If, however, r represents an additional condition, that model is appropriate to the formula $p \wedge r \rightarrow q$, and no informative conclusion follows. The conclusion that Byrne draws from the experimental results is that

> in order to explain how people reason, we need to explain how premises of the same apparent logical form can be interpreted in quite different ways. The process of interpretation has been relatively neglected in the inferential machinery proposed by current theories based on formal rules. It plays a more central part, however, in theories based on mental models [28, p. 83].

Byrne thus sees the main problem as explaining "how premises of the same apparent logical form can be interpreted in quite different ways."

We would question the accuracy of this formulation, and instead prefer to formulate the main issue as follows: it is the job of the interpretive process to *assign* logical form, which cannot simply be read off from the given material. In other words, the difference between Byrne (and others working in the mental models tradition) and ourselves appears to be this: whereas she takes logical form to be more or less given, we view it as the end result of a (possibly laborious) interpretive process.

Before we embark on our modeling exercise, however, some preliminary remarks on what we mean by "modeling" are in order. Since we view task understanding as an integral component of reasoning, the model must include both reasoning to an interpretation – setting crucial parameters – and reasoning from the interpretation so defined. This goal places constraints on the kind of data most revealing of appropriate models. As we saw in our discussion of the selection task in chapter 3, even within a group of subjects which exhibit the same final answer pattern, the underlying parameter settings can be very different, thus leading to qualitatively different models of what subjects are doing and why. The contrast is most blatant when the stark "outcome data" of four binary card choices are contrasted with the rich processes revealed in the socratic dialogues.

With the suppression task, we see this contrast repeated. Cross–sectional statistical information about proportions of groups of subjects suppressing or not is a poor and indirect foundation for discriminating the different interpretations which are behind these choices. As long as the investigation remains focused on the spurious contrast between models and rules, the investigators have remained content with cross–sectional proportion analyses. If we want to know what subjects are doing (deriving a variety of interpretations) we need to know at least what a single subject does on the sequence of inferences MP, MT, AC, and DA, with or without an extra conditional premise of one or other of the two types—additional or alternative. One can then hope to build up a picture of subjects' setting of the various logical parameters critical for understanding their reasoning.

But what if the trajectory through a sequence of interpretational choices is actually a random walk? What if the subject's answer pattern is not consistent with any parameter setting? The analysis of logical form may still not be fine-grained enough, in the sense that additional parameters can be identified which have a causal role in determining the subject's behavior. Still another possibility is that the subject is learning while doing a task, and so changing earlier settings. There is ample opportunity for this, as lots of items are necessary to achieve statistical significance. If none of these possibilities appear to be the case, in a dialogue situation the experimenter can still probe the subject's assignment of logical form and point out to him that some of his inferences do not conform to the logical form assigned. There is a clear educational moral in this: rather than impose a formal system upon a student, it is preferable to teach the assignment of logical form, and the value of being consistent with the form assigned.

7.2   Logical Forms in the Suppression Task

Chapter 2 has given a lengthy introduction to the notion of logical form; here it suffices to repeat what are the main parameters to be set.

1. $\mathcal{L}$ a formal language into which $\mathcal{N}$ (the natural language) is translated,

2. the expression in $\mathcal{L}$ which translates an expression in $\mathcal{N}$,

3. the semantics $\mathcal{S}$ for $\mathcal{L}$,

4. the definition of validity of arguments $\psi_1, \ldots, \psi_n/\varphi$, with premises ψ_i and conclusion φ.

As in the selection task, the cardinal parameter to be fixed is the form of the conditional. Byrne assumed that the conditional can be represented by a material implication, in all circumstances. We believe, on the contrary, that the logical form is the endpoint of an interpretation process, which may be the material implication, but may also be entirely different.

We claim that one meaning of the conditional that naturally occurs to the subject in the suppression task is that of a law-like relationship between antecedent and consequent. An example of a law expressed by means of a conditional is

(7)   If a glass is dropped on a hard surface, it will break.

or

(8)   If a body is dropped, its velocity will increase as gt^2.

What is common to both examples is that the antecedent hides an endless number of unstated assumptions: in the first case, e.g. that the glass is not caught before it falls, etc., in the second case, e.g., that there are no other forces at work on the body, etc.[6] This implies that there may very well be exceptions to the law; but these exceptions do not falsify the law. [7]

We will therefore give the general logical form of law-like conditionals "if A, then B" as

(9)   If A, *and nothing abnormal is the case*, then B.

where what is abnormal is provided by the context. This characterization is, however, incomplete without saying what "if ... then" means in (9).

We contend that the conditional is often not so much a truth–functional connective, as a license for certain inferences.[8] One reason is the role of putative counterexamples, i.e., situations where A and not-B; especially in the case of law-like conditionals, such a counterexample is not used to discard the conditional, but to look for an abnormality; it is thus more appropriate to describe it as an exception. Thus, one use of the conditional is where it is taken as given, not as a statement which can be false, and we claim that this is the proper way to view the conditionals occurring in the suppression task, which are after all supplied by the experimenter.[9] Having posited that, in the present context, the conditional is rather a license for inferences than a connective, what are these inferences? One is, of course, modus ponens: the premises φ and "if φ then B" license the inference that B. The second type of inference licensed is what we have dubbed closed–world reasoning in chapter 2: it says that if it is impossible to derive a proposition B from the given premises by repeated application of modus ponens, then one may assume B is false. This kind of reasoning is routinely applied in daily life: if the timetable doesn't say there is a train

---

6. For a recent defense of the idea that this is how scientific laws must be conceptualized, consult [307].
7. As we shall see in section 7.5, several authors have tried to explain the suppression effect by assuming that the conditional expresses a regularity rather than a material implication, and feel forced to consider a probabilistic interpretation of the conditional. But the fact that the conditional, viewed as a law, in a sense represents an uncertain relationship, does not thereby license the application of probability theory. "Uncertainty" is a multifaceted notion and can be captured by probability only in very special circumstances.
8. A connective differs from a license for inference in that a connective, in addition to licensing inferences, also comes with rules for inferring a formula containing that connective as main logical operator.
9. The preceding considerations imply that the conditional cannot be iterated. Natural language conditionals are notoriously hard (although not impossible) to iterate, especially when a conditional occurs in the antecedent of another conditional – "If, if conditionals are iterated, then they aren't meaningful, then they aren't material" is an example; one more reason why "if ... then" is not simply material implication.

from Edinburgh to London between 5 pm and 5:10 pm, one assumes there is
no such train. Closed world reasoning is what allows humans to circumvent the
notorious frame problem (at least to some extent): my reaching for a glass of
water may be unsuccessful for any number of reasons, for instance because the
earth's gravitational field changes suddenly, but since I have no positive information that this is likely to happen, I assume it will not. We hypothesise that
closed–world reasoning plays an important part in reasoning with conditionals;
in particular, the suppression effect will be seen to be due to a special form of
a closed–world assumption. We now recast the preceding considerations as a
formal definition in the branch of logic known as logic programming.

7.2.1 Logic Programming and Planning: Informal Introduction

In chapter 6, we defined *planning* as setting a goal and devising a *sequence* of
actions that will achieve that goal, taking into account events in, and properties
of the world and the agent. In this definition, "will achieve" cannot mean:
"*provably* achieves" because of the notorious frame problem: it is impossible
to take into account all eventualities whose occurrence might be relevant to the
success of the plan. Therefore the question arises: what makes a good plan? A
reasonable suggestion is: the plan works to the best of one's present knowledge.
In terms of models, this means the plan achieves the goal in a "minimal model"
of reality, where, roughly speaking, every positive atomic proposition is false
which you have no reason to assume to be true. In particular, in the minimal
model no events occur which are not forced to occur by the data. This makes
planning a form of nonmonotonic reasoning: the fact that

"goal G can be achieved in circumstances C"

does not imply

"goal G can be achieved in circumstances $C + D$."

The book by van Lambalgen and Hamm [282] formalises the computations performed by our planning capacities by means of a temporal reasoner (the event
calculus) as formulated in a particular type of nonmonotonic logic, namely
first-order constraint logic programming with negation as failure. Syntactically,
logic programming is a good formalism for planning because its derivations are
built on backward chaining (regression) from a given goal. Semantically, it corresponds to the intuition that planning consists in part of constructing minimal
models of the world. The purpose of [282] is to show that the semantics of tense
and aspect in natural language can be formally explained on the assumption that
temporal notions are encoded in such a way as to subserve planning. For our
present purposes we may abstract from the temporal component of planning,
and concentrate on the skeleton of the inference engine required for planning,

namely propositional logic programming. Planning proceeds with respect to a model of the world and it is hypothesized that the automatic process of constructing a minimal model which underlies planning also subserves discourse integration. We present our analysis of the suppression task as evidence for this hypothesis.

Nonmonotonic logics abound, of course,[10] but logic programming is attractive because it is both relatively expressive and computationally efficient.[11] In chapter 8 we shall see that logic programming also has an appealing implementation in neural nets, and that it may thus shed some light on the operation of working memory. Taken together, the proven merits of logic programming in discourse processing [282] and its straightforward implementation in neural networks suggest to us that it is relevant to cognitive modeling. We are not aware of any other nonmonotonic logic which has this range of features, but definitely do not claim that there cannot be any such logic.[12]

7.2.2   Logic Programming and Planning Formally

Logic programming is a fragment of propositional (or predicate) logic with a special, nonclassical, semantics embodying closed–world reasoning. For the sake of clarity we start with the fragment of logic programming in which negation is not allowed.

Definition 2 *A positive clause* is a formula of the form $p_1, \ldots p_n \rightarrow q$, where the q, p_i are proposition letters; the antecedent may be empty, in which case q is referred as a fact.
In this formula, q is called the head, *and* $p_1, \ldots p_n$ *the* body *of the clause.*
A positive program is a finite set of positive clauses.

Until further notice, we assume that propositions are either true (1) or false (0); but the semantics is nonetheless non-classical. The only models to be considered are those of the following form

Definition 3 *Let P be a positive program on a finite set L of proposition letters. An assignment* $\mathcal{M}$ *of truth-values* $\{0, 1\}$ *to L (i.e., a function* $\mathcal{M} : L \longrightarrow \{0.1\}$*) is a* model *of P if for* $q \in L$,

---

10. See Pelletier and Elio [210] for a plea for more extensive investigations into the psychological reality of nonmonotonic logics.
11. This is because it does not involve the consistency checks necessary for other nonmonotonic logics, such as Reiter's default logic [226]. This point is further elaborated in chapter 8.
12. Consider for instance the defeasible planner OSCAR developed by Pollock (see, e.g., [221]). This planner is built on top of a theorem prover for classical predicate logic, and is thus more expressive than logic programming. But the gain in expressiveness is paid for by less pleasing computational properties, since such a system cannot be interpreted semantically by iterations of a fixed–point operator, a prerequisite for an efficient neural implementation.

1. $\mathcal{M}(q) = 1$ *if there is a clause* $p_1, \ldots p_n \rightarrow q$ *in* P *such that for all* i, $\mathcal{M}(p_i) = 1$.

2. $\mathcal{M}(q) = 0$ *if for all clauses* $p_1, \ldots p_n \rightarrow q$ *in* P *there is some* p_i *for which* $\mathcal{M}(p_i) = 0$.

The definition entails that for any q not occurring as the head of a clause, $\mathcal{M}(q) = 0$. Furthermore, if q occurs in a single formula of the form $p \rightarrow q$ and p does not occur as the head of a clause, also $\mathcal{M}(q) = 0$. More generally, the model $\mathcal{M}$ is minimal in the sense that any proposition not forced to be true by the program is false in $\mathcal{M}$; this is our first (though not final) formulation of the closed–world assumption.

We now present a generalization of this definition in terms of a three-valued semantics. This is necessary for the following reasons:
(i) Since the proposed notion of conditionals requires negation, we have to liberalise the preceding definitions and allow negation in the body of a clause, and this will be seen to entail a move to a different semantics[13].
(ii) It is useful to have some freedom in deciding to which propositions we want to apply closed–world reasoning; the above definition applies it to all propositions, whereas it is more realistic to remain agnostic about some.
We first generalize the definition of clause.

Definition 4 *A* definite clause *is a formula of the form* $(\neg)p_1 \wedge \ldots \wedge (\neg)p_n \rightarrow q$,[14] *where the* p_i *are either proposition letters,* $\top$ *or* $\bot$,[15] *and* q *is a propositional variable.* Facts *are clauses of the form* $\top \rightarrow q$, *which will usually be abbreviated to* q. *Empty antecedents are no longer allowed. A* definite logic program *is a finite conjunction of definite clauses.*

The intuitive meaning of negation is what is known as "negation as (finite) failure": $\neg\varphi$ is true if the attempt to derive φ from the program P fails in finitely many steps. To make this precise requires specifying in detail the notion of derivability, which we shall not now do; but see section 7.2.3. Instead we give a semantic characterization, which will allow the reader to see the connection with closed–world reasoning. The proper semantics for definite programs requires a move from two-valued semantics to Kleene's strong three-valued semantics (introduced in chapter 2), which has the truth–values *undecided* (u), *false* (0), and *true* (1). The intuitive meaning of *undecided* is that the truth–value can evolve toward either true or false (but not conversely). This provides us with the notion of a three-valued model. It is an important fact that the models of interest can be captured by means of the following construction.

---

13. For instance, the program clause $\neg p \rightarrow p$ is inconsistent on the above semantics.
14. $(\neg)p$ means that p may, but need not, occur in negated form.
15. We use $\top$ for an arbitrary tautology, and $\bot$ for an arbitrary contradiction.

Definition 5 *(a) If q is a proposition letter occurring in a program P, the definition of q with respect to P is given by:*

1. *take all clauses $\varphi_i \rightarrow q$ whose head is q and form the expression $\bigvee_i \varphi_i \rightarrow q$;*

2. *if there is no such φ_i, then the expression $\bot \rightarrow q$ is added;*

3. *replace the $\rightarrow$'s by $\leftrightarrow$'s (here, $\leftrightarrow$ has a classical interpretation given by: $\psi \leftrightarrow \varphi$ is true if ψ, φ have the same truth–value, and false otherwise).*

(b) The completion of a program P, denoted by $comp(P)$, is constructed by taking the conjunction of the definitions of atoms q, for all q in P.
(c) More generally, if S is a set of atoms occurring in P, the completion of P relativized to S, $comp_S(P)$, is obtained by taking the conjunction of the definitions of the atoms q which are in S.
(d) If P is a logic program, define the nonmonotonic consequence relation $\approx\!\!\!\mid$ by

$$P \mathrel{\mid\!\!\!\approx_3} \varphi \text{ iff } comp(P) \models_3 \varphi,$$

where $\models_3$ denotes consequence with respect to three–valued models.[16] *For $comp(P)$ one may also read $comp_S(P)$; in which case one should write, strictly speaking, $P \mathrel{\mid\!\!\!\approx_3^S} \varphi$.*

Here are some examples.

1. Let the definite program P consist of $p \rightarrow q$ and $\bot \rightarrow p$. In this case the completion $comp(P)$ is $p \leftrightarrow q, \bot \leftrightarrow p$, which implies that both p and q are false.

2. Take the same program, but restrict the completion to q. In this case the completion $comp_{\{q\}}(P)$ is $p \leftrightarrow q$, which is true on all models in which p and q have the same truth–value.

3. Let P be the program $\{p; p \wedge \neg ab \rightarrow q\}$. closed–world reasoning for abnormalities can be viewed as forming the completion $comp_{\{ab\}}(P)$, which in this case equals $\{\top \leftrightarrow p; \bot \leftrightarrow ab; p \wedge \neg ab \rightarrow q\}$, which is equivalent to $\{p; p \rightarrow q\}$. We thus have $comp_{\{ab\}}(P) \models q$.

4. Suppose the program P equals $\{\bot \rightarrow p; p \wedge \neg ab \rightarrow q\}$. If we form the completion $comp_{\{ab,p\}}(P)$, we obtain $\{\bot \leftrightarrow p; \bot \leftrightarrow ab; p \wedge \neg ab \rightarrow q\}$, from which nothing can be concluded in the sense of $\models_3$. A conclusion becomes possible, however, if the completion $comp_{\{ab,p,q\}}(P)$ is considered instead, because now

$$comp_{\{ab,p,q\}}(P) \models_3 \neg q.$$

---

16. $\Gamma \models_3 \psi$ means that every three-valued model of Γ is a model of *psi*. The subscript will be dropped when there is no danger of confusion.

Thus closed–world reasoning can be analyzed in rather fine detail using this procedure.

If $P \hspace{1pt}\approx_3 \varphi$, we say that φ *follows from P by negation as failure*, or by *closed–world reasoning*. The process of completion is also referred to as *minimization*.[17] Using the terminology introduced above, our main hypothesis in explaining Byrne's data as conforming to the logical competence model of closed–world reasoning can then be stated as

a. the conditionals used in the suppression task, far from being material implications, can be captured much more adequately by logic programming clauses of the form $p \wedge \neg ab \rightarrow q$, where ab is a proposition letter indicating that something abnormal is the case;

b. when making interpretations, subjects usually do not consider *all* models of the premises, but only *minimal* models, defined by a suitable completion.

The readers who wish to see some applications of these notions to the suppression task before delving into further technicalities may now jump ahead to section 7.3, in particular the explanations with regard to the forward inferences MP and DA. The backward inferences MT and AC require a slightly different application of logic programming, which will be introduced in the next subsection. The final subsection will look at the construction of models, which is necessary for the connection with neural networks.

7.2.3 Strengthening the Closed–World Assumption: Integrity Constraints

So far we have applied the closed–world assumption to atomic formulas (for instance, ab) and their negations: if ab is not in the database, we may assume it is false. We now extend the closed–world assumption to cover program clauses as well: if we are given that q and if $\varphi_1 \rightarrow q$, $\ldots$, $\varphi_n \rightarrow q$ are all the clauses with nontrivial body φ_i which have q as head, then we (defeasibly) conclude that q can only be the case *because* one of φ_1, $\ldots$, φ_n is the case. We therefore do not consider the possibility that q is the case because some other state of affairs ψ obtains, where ψ is independent of the φ_1, $\ldots$, φ_n and such that (unbeknownst to us) $\psi \rightarrow q$. This kind of reasoning might be called "diagnostic" or "abductive" (see [151]); we will also call it "closed–world reasoning for rules."

---

17. Readers who recall McCarthy's use of an abnormality predicate *ab* may wonder why we do not use circumscription [185] instead of logic programming, since circumscription also proceeds by minimizing the extension of *ab*. There is a technical reason for this: circumscription cannot be easily used to explain the fallacies; but the main reason is that logic programming, unlike circumscription, allows incremental computation of minimal models, and this computation will be seen to be related to the convergence toward a stable state of a neural network. This shows why model construction can here proceed automatically.

This notion of closed–world is not quite expressed by the completion of a program. For in the simple case where we have only a clause $p \to q$ and a fact $\top \to q$ is added, the completion becomes $(p \vee \top) \leftrightarrow q$, from which nothing can be derived about p. What we need instead is a principled way of adding q such that the database or model is updated with p. The proper technical way of achieving this is by means of so-called *integrity constraints*. To clarify this notion, we need a small excursion into database theory, taking an example from Kowalski [164,p. 232].

An *integrity constraint* in a database expresses obligations and prohibitions that the states of the database must satisfy if they fulfil a certain condition. For instance, the "obligation" to carry an umbrella when it is raining may be formalized (using a self-explanatory language for talking about actions and their effects) by the integrity constraint

$$Holds(rain, t) \;\to\; Holds(carry\text{-}umbrella, t) \tag{7.1}$$

The crucial point here is the meaning of $\to$. The formula (7.1) cannot be an ordinary program clause, for in that case the addition of $Holds(rain, now)$ would trigger the consequence $Holds(carry\text{-}umbrella, now)$ which may well be false, and in any case does not express an obligation.

A better way to think of an integrity constraint is to view the consequent as a constraint that the database must satisfy if the antecedent holds. This entails in general that the database has to be *updated* with a true statement about the world. The relevant notions are most easily explained in terms of the derivational machinery of logic programming.

Derivations in Logic Programming

We first need a piece of terminology.

Definition 6 *A* query *is a finite (possibly empty) sequence of proposition letters denoted as* $?p_1, \dots, p_m$. *Alternatively, a query is called a* goal. *The empty query, canonically denoted by* $\square$, *is interpreted as* $\bot$, *i.e., a contradiction.*

Operationally, one should think of a query $?q$ as the assumption of the formula $\neg q$, the first step in proving q from P using a reductio ad absurdum argument. In other words, one tries to show that $P, \neg q \models \bot$. In this context, one rule suffices for this, a rule which reduces a goal to subgoals.

Definition 7 Resolution *is a derivation rule which takes as input a program clause* $p_1, \dots p_n \to q$ *and a query* $?s_1, \dots, q, \dots, s_k$ *and produces the query* $?s_1, \dots p_1, \dots p_n, \dots, s_k$.

Given a goal $?q$ several clauses may match with q, so we need a *choice rule* to provide a unique choice. Since we choose only one clause, derivations become linear. A linear derivation starting from a query $?A$ can be pictured as the acid rain-affected tree depicted in figure 7.1. A linear derivation starting from a

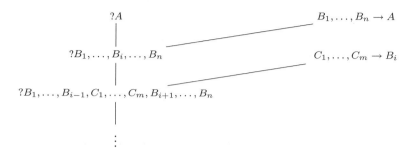

Figure 7.1 An illustration of a linear derivation with resolution.

query $?q$ is *successful* if it ends in the empty query (i.e., $\bot$); if the derivation is finite but does not end with the empty query it is said to *fail finitely*.

If one does not use a choice rule but executes all possible resolution steps simultaneously one obtains a (rather more healthy–looking) derivation *tree*. The tree is successful if one branch ends in the empty query; if there is no such branch and all branches are finite, it is said to fail finitely.

Finite failure is important in providing the operational semantics for negation: a query $?\neg\varphi$ is said to succeed if $?\varphi$ fails finitely. The relation between derivations and semantics is given by

Theorem 2 *A query $?\varphi$ succeeds with respect to a program P, if $P \approx_3 \varphi$, i.e., if φ is entailed by the completion of P in the sense of $comp(P) \models_3 \varphi$. Likewise, a query $?\varphi$ fails with respect to a program P, if $P \approx_3 \neg\varphi$, i.e., $comp(P) \models_3 \neg\varphi$.*

Integrity Constraints and Derivations

An integrity constraint is a query used in a very particular way. Let $?\varphi$ be a query, and P a program, then one may or may not have $P \approx_3 \varphi$. In the latter case, the integrity constraint

$$?\varphi \text{ succeeds}$$

means that P must be transformed by a suitable update into a program P' such that $P' \approx_3 \varphi$. In principle, the way to do this is to take a finitely failed branch in the derivation tree and update P with the leaves on the branch.

A conditional integrity constraint of the form

$$\text{if } ?\psi \text{ succeeds, then } ?\varphi \text{ succeeds}$$

then means the following: If a program P be given, and P' an extension of P such that $P' \approx_3 \psi$, then also $P' \approx_3 \varphi$.

To return to our example, the integrity constraint which was formulated as (7.2)

$$Holds(rain, t) \rightarrow Holds(carry\text{-}umbrella, t) \qquad (7.2)$$

must be interpreted as[18]

$$\text{if } ?Holds(rain, t) \text{ succeeds,} \qquad (7.3)$$
$$\text{then } ?Holds(carry\text{-}umbrella, now) \text{ succeeds}$$

Suppose that observation has shown that it rains, leading to an update of the database with $Holds(rain, now)$. It follows that the antecedent of the integrity constraint is satisfied, and the agent is now required to satisfy the consequent. The database will contain a name for the action $take\text{-}umbrella$, linked to the rest of the database by

$$Initiates(take\text{-}umbrella, carry\text{-}umbrella, now),$$

and there will be a general clause to the effect that taking an umbrella now leads to

$$Holds(carry\text{-}umbrella, t),$$

for $t \geq now$. In order to make the query

$$?Holds(carry\text{-}umbrella, now)$$

succeed, the agent reasons backward from this query using the clauses in the database to conclude that he must take an umbrella. Once he has informed the database that he has done so, the query succeeds, and integrity is restored.

Readers who wish to see applications to the suppression task may now jump ahead to the second part of section 7.3, which treats the backward inferences MT and AC. The next (and final) subsection is only essential for the neural implementation discussed in chapter 8.

7.2.4 Constructing Models

In this last subsection of section 7.2, we explain how minimal models of a definite logic program can be efficiently computed. As above we start with the simpler case of positive programs. Recall that a positive logic program has clauses of the form $p_1 \wedge \ldots \wedge p_n \rightarrow q$, where the p_i, q are proposition letters and the antecedent (also called the body of the clause) may be empty. Models of a positive logic program P are given by the fixed–points of a monotone operator.[19]

---

18. Here, t must be interpreted as a constant.
19. Monotonicity in this sense is also called continuity.

Definition 8 *The operator T_P associated to P transforms a model $\mathcal{M}$ (viewed as a function $\mathcal{M} : L \longrightarrow \{0, 1\}$, where L is the set of proposition letters) into a model $T_P(\mathcal{M})$ according to the following stipulations: if v is a proposition letter,*

1. $T_P(\mathcal{M})(v) = 1$ *if there exists a set of proposition letters C, true on $\mathcal{M}$, such that $\bigwedge C \to v \in P$;*

2. $T_P(\mathcal{M})(v) = 0$ *otherwise.*

Definition 9 *An ordering $\subseteq$ on (two-valued) models is given by: $\mathcal{M} \subseteq \mathcal{N}$ if all proposition letters true in $\mathcal{M}$ are true in $\mathcal{N}$.*

Lemma 1 *If P is a positive logic program, T_P is monotone in the sense that $\mathcal{M} \subseteq \mathcal{N}$ implies $T_P(\mathcal{M}) \subseteq T_P(\mathcal{N})$.*

This form of monotonicity would fail if a body of a clause in P contains a negated atom $\neg q$ and also a clause $\neg q \to s$: one can then set up things in such a way that s is true at first, and becomes false later. Hence we will have to complicate matters a bit when considering negation, but this simple case illustrates the use of monotone operators. Monotonicity is important because it implies the existence of so called *fixed–points* of the operator T_P.

Definition 10 *A fixed point of T_P is a model $\mathcal{M}$ such that $T_P(\mathcal{M}) = \mathcal{M}$.*

Lemma 2 *If T_P is monotone, it has a least and a greatest fixed point. The least fixed point is the minimal model with respect to the ordering of definition 9.*

Monotonicity is also important because it allows incremental computation of the minimal model. This is achieved through *iteration* of T_P, as follows. One starts from the 'empty model' $\mathcal{M}_0$ in which all proposition letters are false. One then constructs a sequence $\mathcal{M}_0 \subseteq T_P(\mathcal{M}_0) \subseteq T_P(T_P(\mathcal{M}_0)) \subseteq \ldots \subseteq T_P^n(\mathcal{M}_0) \subseteq \ldots$, where the inclusions follow from lemma 1. It can then be shown that the least fixed point, i.e., the minimal model, can be written as $\bigcup_n T_P^n(\mathcal{M}_0)$. As noted above, other formats for default reasoning such as circumscription do not give this computational information. Computability is a consequence of the syntactic restrictions on logic programs.

The logic programs that we need must allow negation in the body of a clause, since we model the natural language conditional 'p implies q' by the clause $p \wedge \neg ab \to q$. As observed above, extending the definition of the operator T_P with the classical definition of negation would destroy its monotonicity, necessary for the incremental approach to the least fixed point. Our preferred solution is to replace the classical two-valued logic by Kleene's strong three-valued logic, for which see figure 2.2 in chapter 2. We also define an equivalence $\leftrightarrow$ by assigning 1 to $\varphi \leftrightarrow \psi$ if φ, ψ have the same truth–value (in $\{u, 0, 1\}$), and 0 otherwise.

We show how to construct models for definite programs, as fixed points of a three-valued consequence operator T_P^3. We will drop the superscript when there is no danger of confusing it with its two-valued relative defined above.

Definition 11 *A three-valued model is an assignment of the truth–values $u, 0, 1$ to the set of proposition letters. If the assignment does not use the value u, the model is called* two-valued. *If $\mathcal{M}, \mathcal{N}$ are models, the relation $\mathcal{M} \leq \mathcal{N}$ means that the truth–value of a proposition letter p in $\mathcal{M}$ is less than or equal to the truth–value of p in $\mathcal{N}$ in the canonical ordering $\leq$ on $u, 0, 1$ (i.e., $u \leq 0, 1$; $0, 1$ are incomparable in the ordering).*

Definition 12 *Let P be a program.*

a. *The operator T_P^3 applied to formulas constructed using only $\neg$, $\wedge$, and $\vee$ is determined by the above truth–tables.*

b. *Given a three-valued model $\mathcal{M}$, $T_P^3(\mathcal{M})$ is the model determined by*

    (a) *$T_P^3(\mathcal{M})(q) = 1$ iff there is a clause[20] $\varphi \to q$ such that $\mathcal{M} \models \varphi$,*

    (b) *$T_P^3(\mathcal{M})(q) = 0$ iff there is a clause $\varphi \to q$ in P and for all such clauses, $\mathcal{M} \models \neg\varphi$,*

    (c) *$T_P^3(\mathcal{M})(q) = u$ otherwise.*

The preceding definition ensures that unrestricted negation as failure applies only to proposition letters q which occur in a clause with nonempty antecedent, such as $\perp \to q$; proposition letters r about which there is no information at all (not even of the form $\perp \to r$) may remain undecided.[21] This will be useful later, when we will sometimes want to restrict the operation of negation as failure to ab. Once a literal has been assigned value 0 or 1 by T_P, it retains that value at all stages of the construction; if it has been assigned value u, that value may mutate into 0 or 1 at a later stage.

Here are two essential results, which will turn out to be responsible for the efficient implementability in neural networks.

Lemma 3 *If P is a definite logic program, T_P is monotone in the sense that $\mathcal{M} \leq \mathcal{N}$ implies $T_P^3(\mathcal{M}) \leq T_P^3(\mathcal{N})$.*

Lemma 4 *Let P be a definite program.*

1. *The operator T_P^3 has a least fixed point, obtained by starting from the model $\mathcal{M}_0$ in which all proposition letters have the value u. The least fixed point of T_P^3 can be shown to be the minimal model of P.*

---

20. Recall that according to definition 4, empty clauses are not allowed.
21. This parallels the similar proviso in the definition of the completion.

2. *The least fixed point of T_P is reached in finitely many steps ($n + 1$ if the program consists of n clauses).*

3. *All models $\mathcal{M}$ of $comp(P)$ are fixed points of T_P^3, and every fixed point is a model.*

These notions can be elucidated by means of some simple examples.

1. Let the definite program P consist of the single clause $p \rightarrow q$. The initial model $\mathcal{M}_0$ assigns u to p and q. Inspection of definition 12 shows that $\mathcal{M}_0$ is the least fixed point of T_P^3. The models which make both p and q true (resp. false) are also fixed points.

2. Let the definite program P consist of the clauses $p \rightarrow q$ and $\perp \rightarrow p$. Then $\mathcal{M}_1(p) = T_P^3(\mathcal{M}_0)(p) = 0$, $\mathcal{M}_1(q) = T_P^3(\mathcal{M}_0)(q) = u$. In the next iteration we get $\mathcal{M}_2(p) = T_P^3(\mathcal{M}_0)(p) = 0$ and $\mathcal{M}_2(q) = T_P^3(\mathcal{M}_0)(q) = 0$, and this is the least fixed point.

3. Let the definite program P consist of the single clause $\neg p \rightarrow q$. The initial model $\mathcal{M}_0$ is the least fixed point.

4. Let the definite program P consist of the clauses $\neg p \rightarrow q$ and $\perp \rightarrow p$. Then $\mathcal{M}_1(p) = T_P^3(\mathcal{M}_0)(p) = 0$, $\mathcal{M}_1(q) = T_P^3(\mathcal{M}_0)(q) = u$, whence $\mathcal{M}_1(\neg p) = 1$. In the next iteration therefore $\mathcal{M}_2(q) = T_P^3(\mathcal{M}_0)(q) = 1$, and this is the least fixed point.

The last two examples illustrate the semantic effect of closed–world reasoning. If for a proposition letter p, the program P contains the clause $\perp \rightarrow p$ this means (via the completion $comp(P)$) that p represents a proposition to which closed–world reasoning can be applied. If P does not contain $\perp \rightarrow p$, nor any other clause in which p occurs as head, p's initial truth–value (u) may never change.

Recall (from definition 5) that the nonmonotonic consequence relation $P \mid\approx_3 \varphi$ is given by "$comp(P) \models_3 \varphi$," or in words: all (three-valued) models of $comp(P)$ satisfy φ. The relation $\mid\approx$ is completely determined by what happens on the least fixed point. Larger fixed points differ in that some values u in the least fixed point have been changed to 0 or 1 in the larger fixed point; but by the monotonicity property (with respect to truth–values) of Kleene's logic this has no effect on the output, in the sense that an output value 1 cannot be changed into 0 (or conversely).

7.3 How Closed–World Reasoning Explains Suppression

The suppression task sets subjects the problem of finding an interpretation which accommodates premises which at least superficially may conflict. It therefore provides a good illustration of how closed–world reasoning can be used to model human interpretation and reasoning. It is one of the benefits of formalization that it reveals many aspects of the data which are in need of clarification and suggests how finer-grained data might be found, as well as how the formalism may be modified to account for richer data. As the literature review and the sample of new data below will reveal, there are several prominent interpretations subjects may adopt. All that is attempted in this section is to provide an illustrative model of one important interpretation subjects adopt.

The explanation of the suppression effect will be presented in two stages, corresponding to the forward inferences (MP and DA) and the backward inferences (MT and AC).

7.3.1 The Forward Inferences: MP and DA

We will represent the conditionals in Byrne's experiment as *definite clauses* of the form $p \land \neg ab \to q$, where ab is a proposition which indicates that something abnormal is the case, i.e., a possibly disabling condition. These clauses are collected together as programs.

Definition 13 *In the following, the term* program *will refer to a finite set of conditionals of the form* $A_1 \land \ldots \land A_n \land \neg ab \to B$, *together with the clauses* $\bot \to ab$ *for all proposition letters of the form* ab *occurring in the conditionals. Here, the* A_i *are proposition letters or negations thereof, and* B *is a propositional letter. We also allow the* A_i *to be* $\top$ *and* $\bot$. *Empty antecedents are not allowed.*[22]

In the following we will therefore represent (10a) as (10b)

(10a)   If she has an essay, she will study late in the library.
(10b) $p \land \neg ab \to q$.

and (11a) and (11b) both as formulae of the form (11c)

(11a)   If the library is open, she will study late in the library.
(11b)   If she has a textbook to read, she will study late in the library.
(11c) $r \land \neg ab' \to q$.

It is essential that the conditionals are represented as being part of a definite logic program, so that they function as licenses for inference rather than truth–functional connectives. We show that on the basis of this interpretation, the forward inferences MP and DA *and* their "suppression" correspond to valid argument patterns. in this nonmonotonic logic. The main tool used here is the completion of a program, as a formalization of the closed–world assumption

---

22. As mentioned before, this definition is formulated because we do not necessarily want to apply closed–world reasoning to *all* proposition letters, although always to proposition letters of the form ab.

applied to facts. We emphasize again that in virtue of lemmas 3 and 4, the completion is really "shorthand" for a particular model. Thus, *what we will be modeling is how subjects reason toward an interpretation of the premises by suitably adjusting the meaning of the abnormalities.* Once they have reached an interpretation, reasoning from that interpretation is trivial.

The backward inferences (MT and AC) require the closed–world assumption as applied to rules, and will be treated separately, in section 7.3.2.

MP for a Single Conditional Premise

Suppose we are given a single conditional $p \wedge \neg ab \rightarrow q$ and the further information that p (i.e., $\top \rightarrow p$ – to economise on notation we will usually write the shorter form in spite of the strictures of definition 13.). The full logic program for this situation is $\{p; p \wedge \neg ab \rightarrow q; \perp \rightarrow ab\}$. Closed–world reasoning as formalized in the completion gives the set $\{p; p \wedge \neg ab \leftrightarrow q; \perp \leftrightarrow ab\}$, which is equivalent to $\{p; p \leftrightarrow q\}$, from which q follows. This argument can be rephrased in terms of our distinction between two forms of reasoning as follows.

Reasoning to an interpretation starts with the general form of a conditional,[23] and the decision to apply nonmonotonic closed–world reasoning. The former gives the logic program $\{p; p \wedge \neg ab \rightarrow q\}$; the latter extends this program to $\{p; p \wedge \neg ab \rightarrow q; \perp \rightarrow ab\}$, and constructs the completion $\{p; p \wedge \neg ab \leftrightarrow q; \perp \leftrightarrow ab\}$. As a consequence, one derives as the logical form of the conditional $p \leftrightarrow q$. Reasoning from an interpretation then starts from this logical form and the atomic premise p, and derives q.

There are, however, also subjects who refuse to endorse MP, and in the tutorial dialogues we conducted we found that this was because the subject could think of exceptional circumstances preventing the occurrence of q even when p. Such subjects combine the enriched representation of the conditional with a refusal to apply closed–world reasoning to the abnormality.

A "Fallacy": DA for a Single Conditional Premise

Suppose we are again given a conditional $p \wedge \neg ab \rightarrow q$ and the further information $\neg p$.[24] Reasoning to an interpretation starts from the program $\{\neg p; p \wedge \neg ab \rightarrow q; \perp \rightarrow ab\}$ and the closed–world assumption. As above, the end result of that reasoning process is $\{\neg p; p \leftrightarrow q\}$. Reasoning from an interpretation

---

23. There is nothing sacrosanct about this starting point. It may itself be the consequence of a reasoning process, or a different starting point, i.e., a different interpretation of the conditional may be chosen. The formalization chosen is a first approximation to the idea that natural language conditionals allow exceptions. For other purposes more complex formalizations may be necessary.

24. Strictly speaking $\neg p$ is not an allowed clause, but we may interpret $\neg p$ as obtained from the allowed clause $\perp \rightarrow p$ by closed–world reasoning.

then easily derives $\neg q$.[25]

A considerable number of subjects do not endorse DA, usually with the motivation that the protagonist may have other reasons for going to the library. This can be viewed as a refusal to apply closed–world reasoning to q, i.e., as defining the completion only with reference to the set $\{p, ab\}$ (see definition 5 and the examples which illustrate it).

MP in the Presence of an Additional Premise

As we have seen, if the scenario is such that nothing is said about ab, minimization sets ab equal to $\bot$ and the conditional $p \wedge \neg ab \rightarrow q$ reduces to $p \leftrightarrow q$. Now suppose that the possibility of an abnormality is made salient, e.g., by adding a premise "if the library is open, she will study late in the library" in Byrne's example. This leads to an extension of the set of clauses with the clause $r \wedge \neg ab' \rightarrow q$. We furthermore propose that the set of clauses is extended with the clause $\neg r \rightarrow ab$ connecting the two conditionals, because the possibility of an ab-normality is highlighted by the additional premise.[26] Although this is not essential, the situation may furthermore be taken to be symmetric, in that the first conditional highlights a possible abnormality relating to the second conditional. The circumstance that the library is open is not a sufficient incentive to go and study there; one must have a purpose for doing so.[27] This means that the further condition $\neg p \rightarrow ab'$ for ab' is added. That is, reasoning toward an interpretation starts with the set

$$\{p; p \wedge \neg ab \rightarrow q; r \wedge \neg ab' \rightarrow q; \bot \rightarrow ab; \bot \rightarrow ab'; \neg r \rightarrow ab; \neg p \rightarrow ab'\}.$$

Applying closed–world reasoning in the form of the completion yields

$$\{p; (p \wedge \neg ab) \vee (r \wedge \neg ab') \leftrightarrow q; (\bot \vee \neg r) \leftrightarrow ab; (\bot \vee \neg p) \leftrightarrow ab'\},$$

which reduces to $\{p; (p \wedge r) \leftrightarrow q\}$. Reasoning from an interpretation is now stuck in the absence of information about r. Here we see nonmonotonicity at work: the minimal model for the case of an additional premise is essentially different from the minimal model of a single conditional premise plus factual information.

As will be seen in section 7.4 there are many reasons why nonsuppression occurs, but one hardly if ever sees nonsuppression because of the application of classical logic to conditionals interpreted as material implication. Instead,

---

25. We wrote "fallacy" in quotes in the section heading, because, contrary to beliefs often expressed in the psychology of reasoning, whether or not an argument pattern such as DA is invalid cannot be determined from its syntactic form alone without recourse to the interpretation. There are no absolute fallacies.

26. Obviously, this is one place where general knowledge of content enters into the selection of appropriate logical form. Nothing in the *form* of the sentence tells us that the library being open is a boundary condition on her studying late in the library.

27. Evidence for such symmetry can be found in experiment 1 of Byrne et al. [29].

nonsuppression seems to be due to forms of closed–world reasoning not yet taken account of here.

DA for an Additional Premise

Now suppose we have as minor premise $\neg p$ instead of p. Reasoning toward an interpretation derives as above the set $\{\neg p; (p \wedge r) \leftrightarrow q\}$. Since $\neg p$ implies $\neg(p \wedge r)$, reasoning from an interpretation concludes $\neg q$. One may therefore expect that those subjects who endorsed DA in the two-premise case will not suppress it here. Our data furthermore show that subjects who did not endorse DA in the two-premise case did not endorse it here, and for the same reason.

This derivation hides the assumption of symmetry made above, culminating in the condition $\neg p \rightarrow ab'$ and its completion. In the case of MP this assumption does not make a difference, but here it does. One possibility is that no content for ab' is envisaged, which means that whenever the library is open, the protagonist can be found there. This is called the "strengthening interpretation" in section 7.4.5 below. In this case the second conditional reduces to $r \rightarrow q$, in which case one expects suppression. Another possibility is that ab' is given more content than just $\neg p \rightarrow ab'$, for instance $\neg p \wedge \neg s \wedge \neg t \rightarrow ab'$ for contextually salient s, t. Closed–world reasoning then yields the combined conditional $(r \wedge p) \vee (r \wedge s) \vee (r \wedge t) \rightarrow q$, which again leads one to expect suppression of DA. This matter will be taken up again in section 7.4.2.

MP for an Alternative Premise

The alternative conditional is again formalized as $r \wedge \neg ab' \rightarrow q$, but the manner of connection of the conditionals differs. The difference between this case and the previous one is that, by general knowledge, the alternatives do not highlight possible obstacles. This means that the clauses $\neg r \rightarrow ab; \neg p \rightarrow ab'$ are lacking. Reasoning to an interpretation thus starts with the set

$$\{p; p \wedge \neg ab \rightarrow q; r \wedge \neg ab' \rightarrow q; \bot \rightarrow ab; \bot \rightarrow ab'\}$$

closed–world reasoning converts this to

$$\{p; (p \wedge \neg ab) \vee r \wedge \neg ab') \leftrightarrow q; \bot \leftrightarrow ab; \bot \leftrightarrow ab'\},$$

which reduces to $\{p; (p \vee r) \leftrightarrow q\}$. Reasoning from an interpretation then easily derives q: no suppression expected.

DA for an Alternative Premise

We interpret $\neg p$ again as obtained from $\bot \rightarrow p$ by closed–world reasoning. The completion then becomes $(p \vee r \leftrightarrow q) \wedge (p \leftrightarrow \bot)$, and reasoning from an interpretation is stuck: suppression. Indeed, in Byrne's study [28] DA for this type of problem was applied by only 4% of the participants. However, in the study of Dieussaert et al. [63], 22% applied DA in this case. This could be a consequence of applying negation as failure to r as well (that is, including $\bot \to r$ in the program), instead of only to abnormalities. Reasoning to an interpretation also decides to what propositions negation as failure must be applied.

7.3.2   The Backward Inferences: MT and AC

As we have seen, the forward inferences rely on the completion, that is, the closed–world assumption for facts. We propose that the backward inferences rely in addition on the closed–world assumption for rules. When we come to discuss the neural implementation of the formalism we will see that this explains to some extent why backward inferences are perceived to be more difficult. This section uses the material on integrity constraints introduced in section 7.2.3.

AC for a Single Conditional Premise

Suppose we have a single conditional premise $p \wedge \neg ab \to q$ and a fact q. closed–world reasoning about facts would yield the completion $\{((p \wedge \neg ab) \vee \top) \leftrightarrow q; ab \leftrightarrow \bot\}$, from which nothing can be concluded about p. Thus this form of closed–world reasoning, like classical logic, does not sanction AC.

But now assume that reasoning to an interpretation sets up the problem in such a way that AC is interpreted as an integrity constraint, that is, as the statement

```
if ?q succeeds, then ?p ∧ ¬ab succeeds.
```

In this case, closed–world reasoning for rules can be applied and we may ask what other atomic facts must hold if $?q$ succeeds. Since the only rule is $p \wedge \neg ab \to q$, it follows that $?p \wedge \neg ab$ must succeed. For $\neg ab$ this is guaranteed by closed–world reasoning about facts: the query $?ab$ fails finitely. The truth of p must be posited, however, meaning that the database must be updated with p. In this sense AC is valid.

MT for a Single Conditional Premise

For MT, the reasoning pattern to be established is

```
if ?q fails, then ?p ∧ ¬ab fails.
```

One starts from the integrity constraint that the query $?q$ must fail. This can only be if at least one of $?p$ and $?\neg ab$ fails. Since in this situation we know that $\neg ab$ is true (by closed–world reasoning for facts), we must posit that $?p$ fails. Here is a subject who refuses to apply closed–world reasoning to ab. Occasionally one observes this type of reaction with MP as well, but it is much more frequent in the case of MT.

> *Subject 7*[28]
> *S*: Either she has a very short essay to write or no essay. Maybe she had to write an essay but didn't feel like going to the library, or that it was so short that she finished it on time, so she didn't have to stay.

AC for an Additional Premise

In the case of an additional premise such as

> If the library is open, she will study late in the library.

the program consists of

$$p \wedge \neg ab \to q, r \wedge \neg ab' \to q, \neg p \to ab', \neg r \to ab.$$

If the reasoning pattern is AC, one starts with the integrity constraint that the query $?q$ succeeds. It follows that at least one of $?p \wedge \neg ab$, $?r \wedge \neg ab'$ must succeed. But given the information about the abnormalities furnished by closed–world reasoning for facts, namely the completions $\neg r \leftrightarrow ab$ and $\neg p \leftrightarrow ab'$, in both cases this means that $?p$ and $?r$ must succeed, so that AC is supported.

MT for an Additional Premise

Now consider MT, for which we have to start from the integrity constraint that $?q$ must fail. The same reasoning as above shows that at least one of p, r must fail – but we don't know which. We thus expect suppression of MT.[29]

AC for an Alternative Premise

In the case of AC, an alternative premise such as

> If she has a textbook to read, she will study late in the library.

leads to clear suppression (from 55% to 16%). It is easy to see why this must be so. closed–world reasoning for facts reduces the two conditional premises to $p \to q$ and $r \to q$ by eliminating the abnormalities. Given that $?q$ must

---

28. In the experiment conducted by Borensztajn et al. [22].
29. Dieussaert et al. [63] observed that in the case of MT for an additional premise, 35.3% of subjects, when allowed to choose compound answers, chose $\neg p \wedge \neg r$, whereas 56.9% chose $\neg p \vee \neg r$. The second answer has just been explained. The first answer can be explained if subjects actually interpret the additional premise as alternative, or in other words interpret the conditional premises as independent. With these aggregate data it is hard to tell; section 7.4 contains some data relevant to choice of interpretation.

succeed, closed–world reasoning for rules concludes that at least one of $?p$, $?r$ must succeed – but we don't know which. It is interesting at this point to look at an experiment in Dieussaert et al. [63] where subjects are allowed to give compound answers such as $p \wedge q$ or $p \vee q$.[30] For AC, 90.7% of subjects then chose the nonmonotonically correct $p \vee r$. In our own sample, those who don't cite refusal to endorse closed–world reasoning for rules as a reason.

MT for an Alternative Premise

Turning to MT, we do not expect a lower rate of endorsment than in the two-premise case, because of the following argument. If $?\neg q$ succeeds, $?q$ must fail finitely. This can only happen if all the branches in the derivation starting from $?q$ fail finitely, which means that both $?p$ and $?r$ must fail finitely. In the data of Dieussaert et al. for MT, 96.3% of the subjects, when allowed to choose compound answers, indeed chose $\neg p \wedge \neg r$.

7.3.3   Summary

Let us retrace our steps. Byrne claimed that both valid and invalid inferences can be suppressed, based on the *content* of supplementary material; therefore, the *form* of sentences would determine only partially the consequences that people draw from them. Our analysis is different. Consider first the matter of form and content. We believe that logical form is not simply read off from the syntactic structure of the sentences involved, but is assigned on the basis of "content" – not only that of the sentences themselves but also that of the context. In this case the implied context – a real-life situation of going to a library – makes it probable that the conditionals are not material implications but some kind of defaults. We then translate the conditionals, in conformity with this meaning, into a formal language containing the ab, ab', ... formulas; more importantly, in this language the conditional is a special, noniterable non-truth-functional connective. However, translation is just the first step in imposing logical form. The second step consists in associating a semantics and a definition of validity to the formal language. For example, in our case the definition of validity is given in terms of minimal models, leading to a nonmonotonic concept of validity. Once logical form is thus fixed (but not before!), one may inquire what follows from the premises provided. In this case the inferences observed correspond to valid

---

30. These authors correctly argue that Byrne's experiment is flawed in that a subject is allowed to judge only for the antecedent or for consequent of the first conditional whether it follows from the premises supplied. This makes it impossible for the subjects that draw a conclusion which pertains to both conditional premises. Accordingly, the authors also allow answers of the form $(\neg)A(\wedge)(\vee)(\neg)B$, where A, B are atomic. Unfortunately, since they also require subjects to choose only one answer among all the possibilities given, the design is flawed. This is because there exist dependencies among the answers (consider, e.g., the set $\{p \vee q, p \wedge q, p, q\}$) and some answers are always true (e.g., $p \vee \neg p$). Thus, the statistics yielded by the experiment are unfortunately not interpretable.

inferences, given the assignment of logical form. Hence we would not say that content has beaten form here, but rather that content contributes to the choice of a logical form appropriate to content and context. There are many different ways of assigning logical form, and that of classical logic is not by any means the most plausible candidate for commonsense reasoning; indeed systems for closed–world reasoning can provide formal explanations for the variety of reasoning behavior observed.

7.4 Data from Tutorial Dialogues

The previous sections have introduced the formal machinery of closed–world reasoning and have shown how suppression of inferences can be a consequence of applying a form of closed–world reasoning to an enriched representation of the conditional as a ternary logical connective: "if p then q" is formally represented as $p \wedge \neg ab \rightarrow q$, which can be viewed as a single connective with arguments p, q, ab. However, we view this formal model as the starting point, not the endpoint, of empirical investigations. A host of empirical questions are left open by the data obtained by Byrne and others, such as

1. Do individual subjects exhibit consistent patterns of suppression and non-suppression, across materials and across inference patterns?[31]

2. Is the second conditional premise always assigned to one of the categories "additional" or "alternative," or are there other possibilities?

3. More generally, to what type of discourse is the subject assimilating this peculiar material?[32]

4. Is there evidence that (suppressing) subjects indeed view the conditional as exception tolerant?

5. More generally, what is the interpretation of the conditional assumed by the subject?[33]

6. Is there a uniform description of what nonsuppressing individuals are doing? In particular, are they all applying classical logic to conditionals interpreted as material implication?

---

31. That is, suppression of, say, MP in one kind of material leads to suppression of MP for other materials; suppression of MP leads to suppression of MT in those cases where it is endorsed, etc.

32. Peculiar, because it is hard to imagine a single person uttering these sentences in a single discourse act. The sentences would seem to be more natural when uttered by different participants in a discourse.

33. e.g., the running example "if she has an essay, she will study late in the library" can be interpreted as a generic (referring to a habit), or as pertaining to an individual occasion. This difference becomes important when incorporating the contribution of the second conditional.

These questions and others will be discussed using dialogue data obtained by our students. Our principal sources here are two experiments conducted by our students, A. Lechler [168] and G. Borensztajn et al. [22].

7.4.1   Suppression of MP Exists

But in the dialogues it is usually formulated positively: the conclusion holds if the antecedent of the second (additional) conditional holds. This does not seem to be a simple repetition of the second conditional, but rather the inference of the conclusion when the antecedent of the second conditional is added to the premises.[34] We present two examples of this phenomenon.[35] The reader can see from the first excerpt that the experimenter tried to mitigate the pragmatic infelicity of the discourse by assigning the sentences to different participants in a conversation.

> *Subject* 25.
> *E*: Again three sentences: If the green light is on, the rabbit is in the cage. If the door is closed, the rabbit is in the cage. I can see that the green light is on. So, imagine that's a conversation, you hear these sentences, what can you conclude now?
> *S*: What I conclude? If the cage door is shut, then the rabbit is in the cage. Again, you've met one of the two criteria for the rabbit being in the cage. The green light is on, the rabbit is in the cage. Um, but we don't know whether or not the door is open or not. If the door's shut, then that's it, we got it for sure, the rabbit is definitely in the cage.
> *E*: So, you are not sure now?
> *S*: I'm not sure because I don't know whether the door is open or not. The point about the door being open or not hasn't been cleared up to my satisfaction. The point about the green light has been cleared up to my satisfaction, but not the point about whether the door is open or not. If the door is open, I'm not sure the rabbit's in the cage, it's probably somewhere else by this time.

The following excerpt shows the same type of answer, which then mutates into a conditional of the form $p \wedge r \rightarrow q$.

> *Subject* 2.
> *S*: Ok yeah I think it is likely that she stays late in the library tonight, but it depends if the library is open... so perhaps I think [pauses]. yeah, in a way I think hmm what does it say to me? I mean the fact that you first say that she has an essay to write then she stays late in the library, but then you add to it if the library stays open she stays late in the library so perhaps she's not actually in the library tonight, because the library's not open. I don't think it's a very good way of putting it.
> *E*: How would you put it?
> *S*: I would say, if Marian has an essay to write, and the library stays open late, then she does stay late in the library.

These answers can be accounted for in a straightforward manner by the formal model: the addition of the premise r licenses the inference that q.

---

34. Compare the analogous difference in classical logic between the implication $\varphi \rightarrow \psi$ and the entailment $\varphi \models \psi$.
35. Similar data have been obtained by Dieussert et al. [63].

7.4.2 Evidence for the Involvement of Closed–World Reasoning in Suppression

This heading covers a number of issues, namely

1. evidence for the conditional as an exception-tolerant construct $p \wedge \neg ab \rightarrow q$,

2. evidence for closed–world reasoning with respect to exceptions, including redefining ab,

3. evidence for closed–world reasoning with respect to arbitrary propositions not of the form ab.

The reader may wonder why we cared to separate (2) and (3). There is a clear theoretical motivation for the distinction, since the abnormalities play a special role in the system, e.g., because they occur negatively, and because their definitions can change. On the empirical side there appears to be some form of "double dissociation" between the two reasoning styles, in the sense that suppression of MP and MT for an additional premise (which requires (2)) appears to be independent of the suppression of AC and DA for an alternative premise (which requires (3)). In chapter 9 we will see that people with autism tend to be good at (3) but bad at (2). Conversely, we have data[36] showing that a high degree of suppression of MP (99% ⇓ 55%, i.e., from 99% down to 55%) and MT (86% ⇓ 48%) for an additional premise is compatible with a very low rate of endorsement of AC (19%) in the two-premise case.

As to the question what "evidence" means here: we mean something stronger than "behavior in accordance with the predictions of the model." Ideally the subject's reasoning in the dialogue should reflect some of the considerations that are formalized in the closed–world computation, for instance, in an utterance of the form: "I can see there are such and such exceptions possible, but since nothing is said about these here I assume ...." Such utterances are rare, but they do occur.

> *Subject* 7.
> *S*: ... that she has to write an essay. because she stays till late in the library when she has to write an essay, and today she stays till late in the library.
> *E*: Could there be other reasons for her to stay late in the library?
> *S*: That could be possible, for example, maybe she reads a very long book. *But as I understand it she stays late in the library only if she has to write an essay.*

The italicized phrase seems to point to closed–world reasoning. Evidence for (1) can be found particularly in subjects who hesitate to endorse two-premise MT (i.e., MT with one conditional and one categorical premise). To repeat a quotation given earlier:

---

36. These were obtained by Judith Pijnacker at the F.C. Donders Centre for Neuroimaging , Nijmegen, Netherlands.

Subject 7.

S: Either she has a very short essay to write or no essay. Maybe she had to write an essay but didn't feel like going to the library, or that it was so short that she finished it on time, so she didn't have to stay.

The subject envisages abnormalities such as "didn't feel like going," but does not at first apply closed–world reasoning to it. Now look at the continuation of this conversation:

E: But if you look again at the first sentence...
S: So she doesn't have to write an essay today, because she doesn't stay in the library till late.

Prompting by the experimenter thus leads to closed–world reasoning, eliminating the exceptions that the subject originally explicitly entertained.

Evidence for the manipulation of abnormalities can also be found in the context of DA for three premises, where the second conditional is of the additional type. In section 7.3 we showed that, given a certain definition of the abnormalities involved, DA is not suppressed, in conformity with the data of Byrne and others. However, our own data[37] show considerable suppression in this case (42% $\Downarrow$ 19%). We explained in section 7.3 that this is likely to be due to a different definition of the abnormalities. Indeed we find a subject who does precisely this, in an explicit manner.

Subject 1.

S: Marian doesn't have an essay to write, which means she would not stay late in the library, but the second condition says that if the library stays open that she will stay late in the library, but it doesn't say dependent or independent of the essay that she might have to write, so she could still stay late in the library if it's open to do something else.
E: So you're saying that ...
S: that there could be another reason for her to go to the library and to stay late in the library ...
E: ...and the fact that she doesn't have an essay to write...
S: doesn't mean that she won't go to the library and stay there till late.
E: OK, so she doesn't have an essay to write, then normally you'd say she wouldn't stay late in the library.
S: Well, it doesn't really say because the second condition is that *if the library is open, she stays late in the library; so apparently there could be another reason for her to stay in the library.*
E: And that being ...
S: a book she might want to read, some research she has to do, maybe she fancies someone there.
E: And if you had to reformulate the text the way you understood it, as text for a following experiment?
S: You could give other reasons for her to stay in the library, or you could indicate whether there are other reasons for her to stay late in the library.

---

37. See footnote 36.

The italicized phrase says that the additional conditional suggests that "she" might have a reason to go the library, different from having an essay, and these reasons are detailed in the subject's next utterance. The subject thus rejects the completion of $\neg p \rightarrow ab'$, but in the process she highlights the fact that there is a hidden $\neg ab'$ in the second conditional about which some clarity must be obtained first.

To conclude, we give a lovely excerpt showing the discourse role that closed–world reasoning plays.

Subject 2.
S: OK, it's likely that she has to write an essay; it's also possible that she's staying late in the library because she has something else to do. so I'm not sure that she has to write an essay, but it's likely.
E: If you had to describe this situation to someone else, would you describe it in a different way?
S: Well, if I would say it like this, in this order, I would suggest or I would mean to suggest with the second sentence that she has to write an essay, that she is writing an essay and I could leave out the second sentence. *It does suggest that she is writing an essay, because otherwise why would you bother saying the first sentence? You could just say she's staying late in the library.*
E: But if you were just thinking about Marian in real life you see her studying late in the library, what might you think then?
S: Oh, then I think she must have some deadlines coming up.
E: But not necessarily that she has an essay to write?
S: From this? [pointing to card]
E: You know this information (someone has told you this information) and you see Marian studying late in the library.
S: Oh, then I think she's probably writing an essay.
E: So, you don't think she might be doing something else?
S: Well, yeah, of course it's possible, but because I was told this, I'm more likely to take this as a first option.

The italicized phrase says it all: the only point of using the conditional whose antecedent is confirmed is to make the hearer infer the antecedent via closed–world reasoning (cf. the last sentence).

7.4.3   Is there a Role for Classical Logic?

In the normal population, nonsuppression because of strict adherence to classical logic appears to be rare.[38] The following excerpt appears to be an instance, although only after some prompting by the experimenter.

Subject 12.
S: [reading] If John goes fishing, he will have a fish supper. If John catches fish, he will have a fish supper. John is almost always lucky when he goes fishing. John is going fishing.

---

38. In chapter 9 we shall see that the situation is markedly different in a population of autistic people.

E: So, what follows here?

S: There's a good chance of having a fish supper.

E: What could prevent him here from having a fish supper?

S: If he doesn't catch a fish.

E: Okay, so what...

S: Well, ah, not, not necessarily actually, he is going fishing, so he might have bought fish supper.

E: So, do you think... So, if you know that he catches fish, do you know then for sure that he will have a fish supper?

S: Well, it says of John: if he goes fishing, he WILL have a fish supper, so he may have fish supper, even if he doesn't catch fish.

E: Which information do you need to be sure that he will have a fish supper?

S: Um..., that he is going fishing, I don't know.

At first the subject suppresses the MP inference in the sense of qualifying it by "a good chance," noting that not catching a fish is a disabling condition, but he then decides to stick to the literal wording of the conditional (see the emphasis on "will"), and invents a reason why John might still have a fish supper if he doesn't catch a fish.

A clearer instance is given in

> *Subject* 8.
> *S*: The second [conditional] again has no function. If you suppose that it is always the case that when she has an essay to write, she studies late in the library, then of course she now stays late in the library.

7.4.4   Nonsuppression Comes in Different Flavors

Contrary to first impressions, nonsuppression may also be a consequence of closed–world reasoning; it need not be stubborn adherence to classical logic. In the next excerpt, the experimenter is reading the experimental material aloud, so that the experiment becomes partly a recall task.

> *Subject* 2.
> *E*: ...?If she has an essay to write, she will be in the library. If she has to train for a competition, she will be in the gym. If the library stays open, then she will be in the library. Oh, I remember her telling me that she has to hand in an essay next week.? So, where would you look for her now?
> *S*: In the library.
> *E*: Why?
> *S*: Because, you said: if she has an essay to write then she will be in the library, and it stays open.
> *E*: Okay, so, do you know that it stays open?
> *S*: *Didn't the guy just say that it stays open? While it stays open.*
> *E*: It says: if the library stays open, she will be in the library.
> *S*: Okay, then I would go to the library, I would bet that the library is open.
> *E*: Okay. Could you think of any situations where she has an essay to write, but she isn't in the library?

S: Just random ones, like if she was going to the library, and then she saw her boyfriend and they decided to go out for coffee instead [laughing]....

Although the situation that the library is open was presented as hypothetical (since it occurs as the antecedent of a conditional), the subject's recall is that of a fact. This is a form of credulous reasoning; it is assumed that all the conditions necessary for the first conditional to apply in fact hold, and that the antecedent of the second conditional is one such condition. It is easy to model this type of reasoning as an instance of closed–world reasoning. Suppose the premise set is formalized as $\{p; p \wedge \neg ab \rightarrow q; r \wedge \neg ab' \rightarrow q\}$, then the second conditional again contributes the premise $\neg r \rightarrow ab$, but the credulousness now has to be represented[39] as the integrity constraint $?\neg ab$ succeeds. That is, $?ab$ must fail finitely, from which it follows (using $\neg r \rightarrow ab$) that $?r$ must succeed. Note that this form of credulousness does not make the abnormality in the representation of the conditional superfluous: the abnormality still has an essential role in integrating the necessary conditions into the first conditional. The argument given is also a form of closed–world reasoning, in that the abnormality is connected only to the necessary condition explicitly introduced. Note, however, that subject 2 could open up his world when prompted to do so by the experimenter.[40]

Looking back to our closed–world analysis of suppression, we can see the similarities and differences between the two forms of credulousness. What is common is that the first conditional is not taken as false after the second (additional) conditional has been digested, as a skeptical stance would require. Suppression is, however, due to a residue of skepticism, in which the subject remains agnostic on the abnormality. Nonsuppression is then a consequence of also eradicating this residue.

7.4.5   Different Roles of the Second Conditional

Byrne originally distinguished between alternative and additional conditionals and assumed that her experimental material is classified by all subjects in the same way. This is not true: often additional conditionals are interpreted as alternatives, and in isolated cases alternatives can be interpreted as additionals as well.[41] In these circumstances rough statistical data on how many subjects do or do not suppress are meaningless. Subjects may fail to suppress because

---

39. This is not ad hoc, but the standard "dynamic" way of treating presupposition accommodation.

40. The interpretation of "the library is open" as presupposition provides interesting indirect support for the present analysis of integration of premises, using abnormalities. At least, according to the theory of presuppositions, the use of "if ... then" cancels possible presuppositions of its arguments; "the library is open" now functions as a presupposition because of its link to the abnormality.

41. Here is an extreme case of this phenomenon. The two conditionals are *If Bill has AIDS, he will make a good recovery* and *If Bill has cholera, he will make a good recovery*. One subject interpreted this as saying *If Bill has AIDS and cholera, he will make a good recovery.*

they interpret the additional premise as an alternative, or take the antecedent of the additional premise to be true, as above. Compounding the difficulty is that sometimes the interpretation of the second conditional fits in neither category. An example is furnished by

> *Subject* 10.
> *S*: She is late in the library. Actually I can conclude she has no life because she will study late in the library as long as it is open. I wonder what she should do if she has an essay and the library is closed.

> *Subject* 23.
> *E*: Hm, hm. Then you read the next message, which says: If the library is open, she'll be in the library.
> *S*: Um, yeah, then I think it was getting increasingly likely that she was there.
> *E*: What do you think that person meant?
> *S*: Um, just exactly what she, exactly what they said, really. That she can be found most of the time in the library, um, she's hard-working.

The additional premise is thus interpreted as strengthening the first one, by saying something like "in fact she's such a diligent student, she'll be in the library whenever it is open."

Formally, this means that the abnormality in the representation of the second conditional, $r \wedge \neg ab' \to q$, is set to $\bot$: no circumstance (such as not having an essay) is envisaged in which the protagonist is not in the library. The premise set then reduces to $\{p; p \wedge r \to q; r \to q\}$, which is equivalent to $\{p; r \to q\}$. Thus we get suppression of MP (and MT); but also of AC and DA, unlike the case where the additional conditional leads to the inclusion of the clause $\neg r \to ab$.

It is also possible to interpret the second conditional as denying the first one. For example, with the conditionals introduced in footnote 41, one can imagine that the first one is said by a novice medical student, the second by an experienced professor, correcting the student. Again we have suppression of MP, in this case because of a skeptical reading.

> *Subject* 16.
> *E*: You have a medical student saying: If Bill has AIDS, he will make a good recovery. And the situation is: Bill has AIDS.
> (...)
> *E*: If you also had a professor of medicine saying: If Bill has cholera, he will make a good recovery?
> (...)
> *E*: What do you think why the professor is saying that, in this situation?
> *S*: The "if cholera" part?
> *E*: Yeah.
> *S*: I think he's saying you can't recover from AIDS. But if he had cholera, then he'd have a chance to recover.

7.4.6 Suppression is Relative to Task Setup

As mentioned in section 7.3 it was noticed by Dieussaert et al. [63] that suppression of inferences can be observed only if the experimenter's questions relate to the antecedent and consequent of the first conditional. If a more liberal answer set is supplied, for example including "$\neg p \vee \neg r$" in the case of MT (i.e., when given $\neg q$), most subjects are willing to conclude something. Strictly speaking the results in [63] were vitiated by a flaw in the design of the response choice offered, or answer set, but the idea is suggestive. Redoing the experiment with a better design (on ten subjects) showed the pattern exhibited in table 7.2 (taken from [22]). Many phenomena alluded to earlier can also be seen in this table. The main difference with the earlier table 7.1 is that subjects could choose from a more liberal answer set; the table lists the answers most frequently given.

Table 7.2   Data from [22].

Role	Content
Conditional 1	If she has an essay to write, she will study late in the library.
Categorical	She has an essay to write.
Conclusion	She will study late in the library. (MP 100%)
Alternative	If she has a textbook to read, she will study late in the library.
Conclusion	She will study late in the library. (MP 100%)
Additional	If the library stays open, she will study late in the library.
Conclusion	She will study late in the library. (MP 40%)
Conclusion	The library is open (presupposition to previous conclusion 30%)
Conclusion	If the library is open, she will study late in the library. (MP[42] 70%)
Conditional 1	If she has an essay to write, she will study late in the library.
Categorical	She will study late in the library.
Conclusion	She has an essay to write. (AC 50%)
Alternative	If she has a textbook to read, she will study late in the library.
Conclusion	She has an essay to write *or* she has a textbook to read. (AC 80%)
Additional	If the library stays open, then she will study late in the library.
Conclusion	The library is open. (AC 80%)
Conditional 1	If she has an essay to write, she will study late in the library.
Categorical	She doesn't have an essay to write.
Conclusion	She will not study late in the library. (DA 30%)
Alternative	If she has a textbook to read, she will study late in the library.
Conclusion	If she has no textbook to read, she will not study late in the library. (DA 70%)
Additional	If the library stays open, she will study late in the library.
Conclusion	She will not study late in the library. (DA 10%)
Conditional 1	If she has an essay to write, she will study late in the library.
Categorical	She will not study late in the library.
Conclusion	She doesn't have an essay to write. (MT 80%)
Alternative	If she has a textbook to read, she will study late in the library.
Conclusion	She doesn't have an essay to write. (MT 100%)
Additional	If the library stays open, she will study late in the library.
Conclusion	She doesn't have an essay to write or the library is closed. (MT 70%)

Of the four subjects who continue to draw the MP inference, three do this because of the credulous inference that the library is closed. As we have seen in section 7.4.3, there is one subject who adheres strictly to classical logic, but the remaining six state their inference in conditional form, the formal rationale of which was explained in section 7.4.1. In the case of DA for an alternative premise, seven subjects choose a conditional formulation; it is interesting that closed–world reasoning is much more in evidence here than in the other two forms of DA. Lastly, the answers to MT and AC show that allowing disjunctions greatly increases subjects' tendency to give an answer.

The enlarged answer sets thus provide strong evidence that most subjects represent the effect of an additional premise formally as $p \wedge r \rightarrow q$ and that of an alternative premise formally as $p \vee r \rightarrow q$. There are probably few subjects who reason completely classically, that is, who adopt the uniform interpretation $p \vee r \rightarrow q$ for the premise set and who endorse neither DA nor AC; in this sample there were none. The term "suppression effect" for this phenomenon is something of a misnomer, since few subjects say that there is no valid conclusion. This observation directs the spotlight away from inference and toward interpretation.

7.4.7   The Consistent Subject: a Mythical Beast?

The question arises, therefore, whether these subjects have consistent interpretations. It is impossible to answer this question definitively based on the data that we have, because those same data suggest that there are so many possibilities. We therefore make a reasoned choice among the possibilities, based on our theoretical understanding of the main interpretive mechanisms: the meaning of the conditional and the choice of logical form. Among the former we count the interpretation of the (intended) additional conditional as strengthening; the latter includes, for example, the precise form of closed–world reasoning, e.g., whether it applies only to abnormalities or across the board. With these distinctions in mind we consider the data of [22]. Here seven out of ten subjects behave in a manner predicted by strengthening and closed–world reasoning with respect to abnormalities. The remaining three subjects endorse MP in the case of an additional premise, but suppress MT. This is hard to make sense of: the presupposition interpretation as illustrated in section 7.4.4, which works well to explain nonsuppression of MP, would seem to predict that MT is also not suppressed, unless negative contexts do not trigger presupposition accommodation.

Of the seven subjects who behaved consistently with strengthening and closed–world reasoning with respect to abnormalities, six also behaved more or less as predicted by full closed–world reasoning, in the following sense: closed–world reasoning is not very much in evidence for two premises (one conditional, one categorical), but becomes prominent when a second conditional premise is added. This can be formulated as a form of closed–world reasoning in its own right, but we need not do so here. Suffice it to say that although a much larger data set is needed to get statistical significance, the available results show that the majority of subjects are consistent to a considerable extent.

7.5   Probabilities Don't Help as Much as Some Would Like

After this excursion to the data, which showed a great variety of possible interpretations, we return to the literature and tackle one particular proposal for a monolithic interpretation of the suppression phenomenon. A number of authors believe that the main problem with the "mental models" account of the suppression effect lies in its assumption of an absolute connection between antecedent and consequent, and propose that this should be replaced by a form of conditional probability, either qualitative or quantitative. We discuss these views here because they furnish a good example of why probabilistic methods in the study of cognition cannot stand on their own, but have to be supplemented by an account of how the probabilistic interpretation is set up in the first place.[43]

As a preliminary, consider the work of Chan and Chua [33], who correctly upbraid both the "rules" and "models" camps for their failure "to give a principled account of the interpretive component involved in reasoning." Chan and Chua propose a "salience" theory of the suppression task, according to which antecedents are more or less strongly connected with their consequents – "operationalized as ratings of perceived importance [of the antecedent in the second conditional premise] as additional requirements for the occurrence of the consequent [33,p. 222]." Thus Chan and Chua adopt a "weak regularity" interpretation of the conditional (somewhat like a conditional probability) instead of the material implication, and they assume their subjects do too. They correctly argue that both the "rules" and the "models" theories do not fit this interpretation, because

> [W]e believe that in the suppression experiments, the way subjects cognise the premise "If R then Q" may be more fine-grained than merely understanding the antecedent as an additional requirement or a possible alternative [33,p. 222].

Their main experimental manipulation accordingly varies the strengths of the connections between antecedents and consequents, and shows that the magnitude of the suppression effect depends upon such variations. In principle such results can be modelled in the framework presented here, if one equates the strength of the connection between antecedent and consequent with the (inverse of the) number of preconditions (i.e., r such that $\neg r \rightarrow ab$) that have to

---

43. This section assumes the reader is acquainted with probability theory, and knows the basics of Bayesian networks.

be fulfilled. The more preconditions, the weaker the connection.

A full-fledged probabilistic account of the suppression effect is presented in Stevenson and Over [270], who performed four experiments designed to support the idea that subjects interpret the materials of Byrne's experiment in terms of conditional probabilities. Two quotations give a flavor of their position. In motivating the naturalness of a probabilistic interpretation they argue that

> it is, in fact, rational by the highest standards to take proper account of the probability of one's premises in deductive reasoning [270,p. 615].

> ...performing inferences from statements treated as absolutely certain is uncommon in ordinary reasoning. We are mainly interested in what subjects will infer from statements in ordinary discourse that they may not believe with certainty and may even have serious doubts about [270,p. 621].

How are we to interpret claims that subjects' interpretations are "probabilistic"? First there is a technical point to be made. Strictly speaking, of course, one is concerned not with the probability of a premise but with a presumably true statement about conditional probability. The authors cannot mean that subjects may entertain doubts about their own assignments of conditional probabilities; or if they do, the formalism becomes considerably more complicated. In fact, in this and other papers on probabilistic approaches to reasoning there is some ambiguity about what is intended. At one point we read about "probability of one's premises," only to be reminded later that we should not take this as an espousal of the cognitive reality of probability theory: "Even relatively simple derivations in that system are surely too technical for ordinary people [270,p. 638]." So there is a real question as to how we are to interpret occurrences of the phrase "conditional probability."

In our opinion, at least two issues should be distinguished here – the issue of the role that knowledge and belief play in arriving at an interpretation, and the issue whether the propositions which enter into those interpretations are absolute or probabilistic. We agree that subjects frequently entertain interpretations with propositions which they believe to be less than certain. We agree that subjects naturally and reasonably bring to bear their general knowledge and belief in constructing interpretations. And we agree that basing action, judgment or even belief on reasoning requires consideration of how some discourse relates to the world. But we also believe that subjects can arrive at both absolute and less than absolute interpretations only by some process of constructing an interpretation. Stevenson and Over need there to be a kind of discourse in which statements are already interpreted on some range of models known to both experimenter and subject within which it is meaningful to assign likelihoods. Most basically, hearers need to decide what domain of interpretation speakers intend before they can possibly assign likelihoods.

The most important point we want to make about probabilistic interpretations is this: probabilistic and logical interpretations share an important characteristic in that they necessarily require the same interpretive mechanisms. For instance, as designers of expert systems well know, it is notoriously difficult to come up with assignments of conditional probabilities which are consistent in the sense that they can be derived from a joint probability distribution. This already shows that the probabilistic interpretation may face the same problems as the logical interpretation: both encounter the need to assure consistency.

Now consider what goes into manipulating conditional probabilities of rules, assuming that subjects are indeed able to assign probabilities.[44] Recall that an advantage of the probabilistic interpretation is supposed to be that conditional probabilities can change under the influence of new information, such as additional conditionals. What makes this possible? Let the variable Y represent the proposition "she studies late in the library," X the proposition "she has an essay," and Z: "the library is open." These variables are binary, with outcomes in $\{0, 1\}$. We first study MP. We are then given that $X = 1$. Probabilistic modus ponens asks for the a posteriori probability $P(Y = 1)$, and by Bayes' rule this equals the a priori probability $P(Y = 1 \mid X = 1)$. The value of this a priori probability depends, however, on what other variables are present; this is the analogue of the computation of the logical form of the conditional in the logical case.

One appealing way to describe this process is by means of a Bayesian network: a graph which represents causal (in)dependencies, together with the conditional probabilities that have to be estimated. In the case of one categorical and one conditional premise, the network is of the form depicted in (figure 7.2). In this case $P(Y \mid X)$ has to be estimated, and $P(Y = 1)$ can be derived from this estimate by Bayes' rule. The processing of the second conditional is represented by the move from a Bayesian network figure 7.2, to one of the form as depicted in figure 7.3. The conditional probability that has to be estimated is now $P(Y \mid X, Z)$, and this estimate cannot be obtained from $P(Y \mid X)$ and $P(Y \mid Z)$ separately because of possible dependencies.

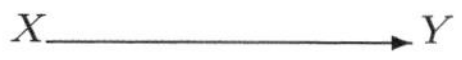

$$X\text{\textemdash}\!\!\rightarrow Y$$

Figure 7.2 Bayesian network for probabilistic modus ponens.

Indeed, the additional character of the premise is reflected in the entry in the conditional probability table associated to the network in figure 7.3 which says that $P(Y = 1 \mid X = 1, Z = 0)$ equals zero. Hence Y is dependent on Z given X, and the new $P(Y \mid X) = P(Y \mid X = 1, Z = 1)P(Z = 1)$ given by marginalization on $P(Y \mid X, Z)$ may well differ from the earlier $P(Y \mid X)$ estimated in the context of figure 7.2. As a consequence we have $P(Y = 1) = P(Y = 1 \mid X = 1) = P(Y = 1 \mid X = 1, Z = 1)P(Z = 1)$.

---

44. We are skeptical, but also think probabilistic approaches to reasoning only make sense under this assumption.

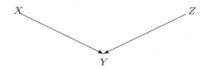

Figure 7.3 Bayesian network with second conditional premise.

Even if $P(Y \mid X = 1, Z = 1)$ is high, probabilistic MP will be suppressed in the absence of the further information that $P(Z = 1)$ is high.

Now let us see what happens in the case of an alternative premise, also represented by Z. The specific *alternative* character can now by captured by the assumption that Y is independent of Z given X: $P(Y \mid X = 1, Z) = P(Y \mid X = 1)$. In this case $P(Y = 1)$ is equal to the originally given $P(Y = 1 \mid X = 1)$, and no suppression is expected.

The upshot of this discussion of Stevenson and Over [270] is that moving to a probabilistic interpretation of the premises does not obviate the need for an interpretive process which constructs a model for the premises, here a Bayesian network, where the associated conditional probability tables are determined by the content of the conditional premises. Human reasoning may well mostly be about propositions which are less than certain, and known to be less than certain, but our processes of understanding which meaning is intended have to work initially by credulously interpreting the discourse which describes the situation, and in doing so accommodating apparent inconsistencies, repairs, and revisions. Only after we have some specification of the domain (the variables and their relations of causal dependence) can we start consistently estimating probabilities in the light of our beliefs about what we have been asked to suppose. Thus a probabilistic treatment needs the same interpretive processes as the logical treatment of section 7.3; and the alleged advantage of conditional probabilities in allowing new information to modify values can be captured easily by the enriched representation of the conditional given in section 7.2. If these observations are combined with the authors' insistence on the fact that probabilities have no cognitive reality, we see that there is no reason to prefer a probabilistic treatment over a logical one.[45]

---

45. Oaksford and Chater [203] present models of probabilistic interpretations of the suppression task and show that these models can fit substantial parts of the data from typical suppression experiments. What is particularly relevant in the current context is that these authors, like Stevenson and Over, do not present the probability calculus as a plausible processing model, but merely as a computational-level model in Marr's sense – that is, a model of what the subjects' mental processes are "designed" to perform. In contrast, the nonmonotonic logic presented here as a computational model for the suppression effect is also intended as a processing model, via the neural implementation given in chapter 8.

8 Implementing Reasoning in Neural Networks

While discussing, in chapter 5, the various "schools" in the psychology of reasoning, we adopted as an organizing principle David Marr's three levels of inquiry [183,chapter 1]

1. Identification of the information–processing task as an input–output function

2. Specification of an algorithm which computes that function

3. Neural implementation of the algorithm specified

The previous chapter can be viewed as being concerned with the first two levels: the information–processing task is credulously incorporating new information, and as an algorithm we proposed logic programming.[1] The present chapter is devoted to the third level. We show how a particular way of executing a logic program, by means of monotone operators as defined in chapter 7, section 7.2.4, corresponds to computation in a suitable recurrent neural network in the following sense: the stable state of the network is the least fixed point of the monotone operator.

In itself this observation is not new.[2] By now there exists a huge literature on "neural symbolic integration," which started from the seminal paper of Hölldobler and Kalinke [130]. Another landmark in this area is d'Avila Garcez et al. [59] which, among much else, replaced the idealized neurons (with binary thresholds) used in [130], by sigmoid activation functions, thus enhancing learning capabilities. There is much more, and the Internet fortunately excuses us from giving a complete bibliography. The reason that we devote a chapter to this topic is, first of all, that this literature is concerned with machine intelligence rather than cognitive processing, and furthermore that we propose a very different neural implementation of negation (based on three-valued logic), which does not need restrictions on the logic programs which can be made to

---

1. Strictly speaking, though, a logic program is a *specification* for an algorithm, not the algorithm itself, since control steps have to be added in the execution, for example, selection of program clauses.
2. When writing [266] we were unfortunately not aware of the results that were obtained in this direction.

correspond to a neural net.[3] In the resulting neural network a special role is
assigned to inhibition, and this may have some relevance for the study of disorders of executive function in the brain. This idea will be put to work in chapter
9, which is devoted to autism. Three-valued logic also has intrinsic cognitive
plausibility. One obvious reason is that it allows some propositions to be undecided, that is, not subject to negation as failure. An equally important reason is
that three-valued semantics treats truth and falsity as independent, unlike two-
valued semantics. One may view a proposition p as a pair (p_+, p_-), where p_+
is the "true component" of p, and likewise p_- the "false component," with the
following intuitive meaning. Evidence for p_+ and p_- can be collected independently; but of course one has to take care that as soon as enough evidence
has been gathered for one component, the other component is inhibited. Thus
computation of truth–values can proceed partially in parallel, a feature that will
become visible in the structure of the neural networks.[4]

8.1   Closed–World Reasoning and Neural Nets

There have been several attempts to model logical reasoning using neural networks, starting from McCulloch and Pitts's[188] observation that classical truth
functions can be computed using networks of idealized neurons.

Definition 14 *A computational unit,* or unit *for short, is a function with the
following input-output behavior:*

1. *Inputs are delivered to the unit via* links, *which have weights $w_j \in [0, 1]$.*

2. *The inputs can be both excitatory or inhibitory; let $x_1 \ldots x_n \in \mathbb{R}$ be excitatory, and $y_1 \ldots y_m \in \mathbb{R}$ inhibitory.*

3. *If one of the y_i fires, i.e., $y_i \neq 0$, the unit is shut off, and outputs 0.*

4. *Otherwise, the quantity $\sum_{i=1}^{i=n} x_i w_i$ is computed; if this quantity is greater
   than or equal to a threshold θ, the unit outputs 1; if not it outputs 0.*

For the time being we assume, following McCulloch and Pitts, that all links
have weight 1 or 0. The classical (binary) AND can be represented by a unit
which has only excitatory inputs and whose threshold equals 2; for OR the
threshold equals 1. NOT is represented by a unit which has one excitatory
and one inhibitory input, and whose threshold (denoted by θ) equals 1; see

---

3. These restrictions are of a technical nature and are unnatural in the course of discourse processing, one of
our aims.
4. The material presented in this chapter is a development of section 5 of [266]. Here we aim for a neural
implementation of general logic programs, whereas our concern in the paper cited was with the particular
application to the suppression task.

figure 8.1.[5] The truth–value of the proposition to be negated is fed over the

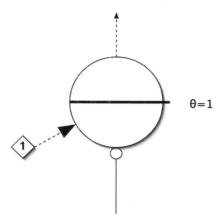

Figure 8.1   The role of inhibition in negation

inhibitory channel. The excitatory link has its origin in a bias unit **1** which fires continuously. If the truth–value is 1, the unit is shut off and outputs 0. If the truth–value is 0, the excitatory channel takes over and makes the unit output 1. By combining these units into a *feedforward neural network* every classical truth function $F(p_1, \ldots, p_n)$ can be represented in the sense that upon clamping truth–values for $p_1, \ldots, p_n$ to the corresponding input units, the output is 1 (0) if $F(p_1, \ldots, p_n)$ is true (false).

Definition 15 *A feedforward neural network is an acyclic directed graph on a set of units (cf. definition 14); the (weighted) edges will also be called links. These can be either inhibitory or excitatory. There are two distinguished sets of units, I (input) and O (output).*

With the rise of parallel distributed processing, the emphasis switched to learning: starting from a network with arbitrary distribution of weights, can one teach it, using backpropagation, to recognise classically valid argument patterns and distinguish them from fallacies? An example of this type of approach can be found in [16,chapter 5].

We mention this work here just to make clear that this is *not* what we will be doing. We have emphasized several times in the course of this book that we view planning as a precursor of logical reasoning, and therefore consider an important function of logical reasoning to be the construction of (minimal) models using closed–world reasoning. Accordingly, we look toward neural networks

---

5. In this and the following diagrams, dashed arrows represent excitatory connections and solid lines which end in a circle denote inhibitory connections.

as a way to construct models: a model corresponds to the stable state of the associated network which is reached when facts are clamped to the input units. This correspondence is motivated by the intimate connection that can be seen to exist between closed–world reasoning and the operation of neuronal units. We will first explain the main idea intuitively for a program not containing negation in the body of a clause, a case for which a two-valued semantics with values 0 (false) and 1 (true) suffices.

Suppose we have a program P consisting of the clauses $\{p_1; p_2; p_1 \wedge p_2 \to q\}$. Associate to P the (feedforward) neural network $N(P)$ whose input units are p_1, p_2, whose output unit is q, and whose structure is given in figure 8.2. The

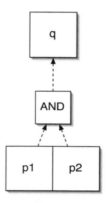

Figure 8.2 $\{p_1; p_2; p_1 \wedge p_2 \to q\}$ as a feedforward net

input units are connected by a binary AND and the link between AND and q represents the implication $\to$. We assume that all links have weight 1. In P, p_1, p_2 are both true, so that in $N(P)$ both p_1, p_2 fire, whence AND fires, and q as well. The units representing true inputs fire continuously, whence q also fires continuously. The stable state of this feedforward network thus has the units corresponding to p_1, p_2, q fire continuously, and this firing pattern codes the minimal model of P.

Now consider the subprogram P' consisting of $\{p_2; p_1 \wedge p_2 \to q\}$, i.e., P without the fact p_1. In $N(P') = N(P)$, the input unit for p_2 fires, but that for p_1 remains silent – falsity of an atom is represented by activation 0. It follows that the units for AND and q also remain silent. This stable state corresponds to the minimal model for P'.

This extremely simplified example has to be generalized in several ways in order to achieve a full correspondence between neural nets and closed–world reasoning:

1. We need output units with several incoming links.

2. We need negation in the body of a clause.

3. We need recursive programs, i.e., programs in which an atom can occur in both heads and bodies.

The first generalization is easy: output units can have arbitrarily many incoming links, and the threshold always equals 1; thus each output unit has an implicit OR built in. For negation there are various options. One solution is to add NOT units as defined above in figure 8.1. The solution adopted by Hölldobler and Kalinke [130] is to give some links negative weights and to modify AND units.[6] Suppose our program is $P'' = \{p_2; \neg p_1 \wedge p_2 \rightarrow q\}$; the associated network is $N(P'')$ (see figure 8.3), with weights indicated. The threshold of the former AND unit (denoted A in figure 8.3) is now set equal to 1. Thus, if p_1 is false and p_2 true, the weighted sum of the inputs feeding into A is 1, whence it fires. If p_1 is true, the weighted sum does not exceed 0, hence A cannot fire.

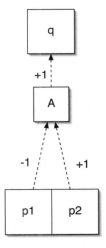

Figure 8.3   Negation via negative weights.

However, these constructions are no longer adequate if recursive programs are considered, especially those containing negation, for example, $\neg p \rightarrow p$. The type of network we need is the recurrent neural net (RNN), which differs from feedforward networks in that the graph of links may contain cycles.[7]

---

6. The earlier absolute distinction between excitatory and inhibitory links (see definition 14) is motivated by neuroscience, which has found evidence for distinct neurotransmitters involved in excitatory and inhibitory processes.

7. The definition to be given is tailored to our purposes and slightly nonstandard in that we prefer to work with absolutely inhibitory links instead of links with negative weights. It is possible, however, to give an equivalent definition in the latter format.

Definition 16 *A recurrent neural network is a set of units U_i $(1 \leq i \leq n)$ connected by links which may be inhibitory or excitatory. Activation over any inhibitory link entering U_i shuts it off completely. An excitatory link from unit U_j to U_i (where $j \neq i$) has a real-valued weight $w^i_j \in [0,1]$. There is a universal activation function $\sigma : [0,1] \longrightarrow [0,1]$ which computes the outgoing activation from the incoming excitation. In addition to the units U_i there are two bias units $\mathbf{1}$ and $\mathbf{0}$, which may be connected to some of the U_i.*[8]

We assume time ranges over the positive integers. At each instant t, the global state $\overrightarrow{U_i(t)}$ is computed as follows. At time 0, all units except bias units and possibly input units are inactive. To compute $\overrightarrow{U_i(t+1)}$, we must consider two possibilities, for each unit U_i.
If unit U_i receives an inhibitory input at time t, then $U_i(t+1) = 0$.
Otherwise U_i collects the excitatory inputs $x_j(t)$ from units U_j to which it is connected, computes $\sum_j x_j(t)w^i_j$ and outputs $U_i(t+1) = \sigma(\sum_j x_j(t)w^i_j)$.

We will mostly be interested in the case where the units obey the earlier definition 14, i.e., where the activations are 0 or 1, and σ is defined by a threshold vector $\overrightarrow{\theta_i}$ as follows: $\sigma(\sum_j x_j(t)w^i_j) = 1$ iff $\sum_j x_j(t)w^i_j \geq \theta_i$. Again, this is slightly unrealistic from a neurophysiological point of view, but it suffices for purposes of exposition. The networks can be made more realistic by exploiting the techniques of [59]. The real difference between the present construction and definition 15 is in the time lags introduced in the computation, allowing recurrence.

8.2   From Logic Programs to Recurrent Neural Networks

Now that we have defined the appropriate concept of network, we need an algorithm which transforms logic programs into suitable neural networks. We do this in two stages, corresponding to positive programs and definite programs.[9]

8.2.1   Positive Programs

Assume the proposition letters occurring in a positive program P are $p_1, \ldots, p_n$; these letters must not include $\top, \bot$. The recurrent network associated to P consists of three layers.

1. The bottom layer is formed by units corresponding to $p_1, \ldots, p_n$, viewed as inputs. Bias units are considered to be inputs.

2. The middle (or "hidden") layer is formed by AND units.

---

8. Bias units are often added for technical reasons: to make the threshold uniformly equal to 0. Here they play an essential role in coding truth and falsity.
9. Recall that the latter, but not the former, allow negation in the body of a clause.

3. The top layer is again formed by units corresponding $p_1, \ldots, p_n$, now viewed as outputs.

4. Let $\bigwedge C \to q$ be a clause in P, where C is a nonempty set of atoms.

   (a) Connect the units in the bottom layer corresponding to atoms in C to the inputs of an AND unit by means of links of weight 1.

   (b) Connect the output of this AND unit to the unit corresponding to q in the top layer.

   (c) Connect the unit corresponding to p_i in the top layer to the corresponding unit in the bottom layer.

5. If p is a fact in P, add a connection from the bias unit **1** to the *output unit p* with weight 1.

Some examples will be helpful, also for introducing our graphical conventions. The first example (see figure 8.4) is the program $P = \{p_1; p_2; p_1 \wedge p_2 \to q\}$ already discussed above, but now represented as a recurrent net. The neurons

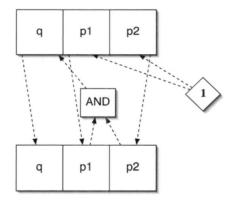

Figure 8.4 $\{p_1; p_2; p_1 \wedge p_2 \to q\}$ as a recurrent net.

are represented as squares, and in the interest of legibility inputs and outputs are only distinguished by the direction of the dashed arrows; the square does not have distinguished sides for input and output. The bias unit has been depicted separately, although strictly speaking it belongs to the input layer.

For another example consider the language $L = \{p, q, r, s, t\}$, and the following program P in L: $P = \{p, p \to q, q \wedge s \to r\}$. The network $RN(P)$ corresponding to P is depicted in figure 8.5. Units corresponding to a proposition letter q will be denoted by U_q; if we need to make a notational distinction between input and output units we shall write U_q^i and U_q^o, respectively. We show how the action of the consequence operator T_P is mirrored exactly by the flow of activation in the network; to do so we first chart the course of the computation according to T_P.

We start from the empty model $\mathcal{M}_0 = \emptyset$, i.e., the model in which all proposition letters are false. We then get the following computation:

1. $\mathcal{M}_1$ is given by $T_P(\mathcal{M}_0)(p) = 1, T_P(\mathcal{M}_0)(q) = T_P(\mathcal{M}_0)(r) = T_P(\mathcal{M}_0)(s) = T_P(\mathcal{M}_0)(t) = 0$.

2. $\mathcal{M}_2$ is given by $T_P(\mathcal{M}_1)(p) = 1, T_P(\mathcal{M}_1)(q) = 1, T_P(\mathcal{M}_1)(r) = T_P(\mathcal{M}_1)(s) = T_P(\mathcal{M}_1)(t) = 0$.

The model $\mathcal{M}_2$ is a fixed point of T_P in the sense that $T_P(\mathcal{M}_2) = \mathcal{M}_2$. It is also the least fixed point; we may consider $\mathcal{M}_2$ to be the minimal model in the sense that it makes true as few proposition letters as possible.

The time course of the computation in the network $RN(P)$ mimics the action of the monotone operator T_P. At time 0, no unit except **1** is activated. At time $t = 1$ the units compute their activation, and we get $U_p^o(1) = 1$, $U_p^i(1) = 0$, $U_q^{i,o}(1) = U_r^{i,o}(1) = U_s^{i,o}(1) = U_t^{i,o}(1) = 0$. At time 2, each unit collects its inputs as of time 1; this results in $U_p^i(1) = 1$ and the remaining units unchanged. At time $t = 3$, $U_q^o(1) = 1$, but no changes otherwise. At time 4, the output of U_q^o is fed into U_q^i, but although the network keeps cycling, there are no changes in activation. The preceding considerations are summarized in the following

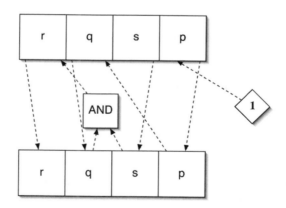

Figure 8.5   Network associated to $\{p, p \rightarrow q, q \wedge s \rightarrow r\}$.

Theorem 3 *Every positive logic program P can be associated to a three-layered recurrent neural network $RN(P)$ such that the least fixed point of T_P corresponds to the activation of the output layer in the stable state of $RN(P)$.*

Before we move on to include negation, it is worthwhile to consider the representation of closed–world reasoning in $RN(P)$. In the network depicted in figure 8.5 all units except the bias unit start inactive, representing the initial closed–world assumption that all propositions are false. The computation then propagates the activation of the bias unit **1**, but this does not affect r, s, and t, which remain inactive. In this simple case we can implement closed–world reasoning by making the following identifications: *active = true, inactive = false*. This simple picture becomes considerably more complicated when negation is included.

8.2.2 Definite Programs

To extend this correspondence to logic programs with clauses having negation in the body, one has to either restrict the class of programs one considers (as in [130] or [59]) or move to (strong Kleene) three-valued logic. Given the intrinsic cognitive plausibility of three-valued logic (the possibility to leave some propositions undecided, and the independence of truth and falsity), and since we need its functional features anyway, we choose the latter option.[10] The basis for our treatment is the following trick. Let 0 and 1 stand for "true" and "false" respectively, taken in the two-valued sense. To avoid confusion we write Kleene's three truth–values $\{u, 0, 1\}$ as $\{u, \mathbf{f}, \mathbf{t}\}$. We now represent Kleene's truth–values as pairs $(0, 0) = u$, $(0, 1) = \mathbf{f}$ and $(1, 0) = \mathbf{t}$, with the ordering inherited from that of $\{u, \mathbf{f}, \mathbf{t}\}$: $u \leq \mathbf{f}, \mathbf{t}$ and $\mathbf{f}, \mathbf{t}$ incomparable.[11] The ordering could be extended by the pair $(1, 1)$, which represents a contradiction; these four truth–values together give a diamond-shaped partial order like figure 8.6. However, in the neural networks to be constructed below we have to take special care that $(1, 1)$ does not actually occur by suitably defined consistency-checking units.

The logical operations on pairs are defined as follows.

Definition 17 *For all $i, j, k, l \in \{0, 1\}$:*

1. $\neg(i, j) = (j, i)$

2. $(i, j) \wedge (k, l) = (\min(i, k), \max(j, l))$

3. $(i, j) \vee (k, l) = (\max(i, k), \min(j, l))$

---

10. The completeness of definite programs with respect to three-valued semantics was first proved by the logician Ken Kunen using a very intricate model-theoretic argument. Subsequent treatments have simplified this somewhat (see, for example, [64]) but the proof remains one of the most difficult in the area (although the proof of soundness is fortunately much easier). In section 8.4 below we give some reasons to believe that the brain has developed the kind of neural architecture necessary for dealing with definite programs. This is not to say that the brain is capable of a complicated metaproof!

11. This trick is due to Stärk [255], who uses it in his proof of completeness with respect to three-valued semantics. Our own motivation will be given shortly.

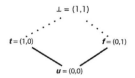

Figure 8.6   Algebra of truth–values for Kleene three-valued logic.

We leave it to the reader to check that this definition gives the same result as the truth–tables for three-valued logic given in chapter 2. We shall refer to the first component in the pair as the "plus" (or "true") component, and to the right component as the "minus" (or "false") component. We interpret a 1 neurally as "activation," and 0 as "no activation." The truth–value u therefore corresponds to no activation in the "true" and "false" components.

As a consequence of this representation of truth–values, we may now view the required neural networks *three-dimensionally* as consisting of two isomorphic coupled sheets, one sheet doing the computations for "true," the other for "false," and where the coupling is inhibitory to prevent pairs $(1, 1)$ from occurring.[12] We think of the sheets as aligned horizontally, with the plus (= 'true') sheet on top. In order to make these ideas precise, we first introduce a technical term.

Definition 18 *A node consists of two coupled competing units U_+ and U_-, that U_+ projects an inhibitory link to U_- and, conversely, U_- projects an inhibitory link to U_+. A node will be denoted by the pair (U_+, U_-).*

To see what the effect of the coupling is, consider the computational fate of the four inputs $(0,0), (1,0), (0,1), (1,1)$ to a node (U_+, U_-) corresponding to a proposition letter p (see figure 8.7).

   If $(0,0)$ is clamped to (U_+, U_-) nothing happens, and the output is $(0,0)$. If $(1,0)$ is clamped, U_+ becomes active but U_- is inhibited, so that the pair (U_+, U_-) outputs $(1,0)$; and analogously for the input $(0,1)$. If the input is $(1,1)$, both U_+ and U_- are inhibited, and the output of the pair will be $(0,0)$. Thus in our setup there is some computation going on in the input units, whereas it is usually assumed that input units do not compute anything. Although the computation is fairly trivial here, it becomes more interesting if inputs are of the more general form (a_+, a_-) with $a_+, a_- \in [0,1]$, reflecting independent degrees of activation for the "true" and "false" components of a proposition. Concretely, one may think of a situation where evidence for both the "true" and

---

12. Again this can be made more realistic by allowing both components to take values in the real interval $[0, 1]$ and defining inhibition in such a way that "winner takes all."

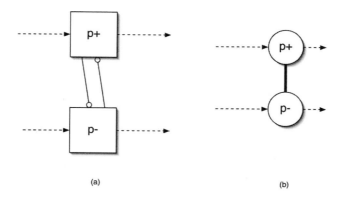

Figure 8.7   (a) Full representation of the node corresponding to p. (b) Concise representation.

"false" components is piling up independently. If in this situation "true" has collected so much evidence that the input is of the form $(1, a)$ for $a \in [0, 1)$, the node has the effect of ensuring that "winner takes all."

The nets that we will consider as implementations of definite programs have the following general form.

Definition 19 *A* coupled recurrent neural network *consists of two recurrent neural networks (cf. definition 16) such that for each unit in one layer there is a unique unit in the other layer with which it forms a node.*

We will now describe the main varieties of nodes in coupled nets necessary for computing logic programs.

Connectives AND and OR

figure 8.8 presents a simple, but fundamental, example: three-valued binary AND. What we see in figure 8.8 is two coupled neural nets, labeled $+$ (above the separating sheet) and $-$ (below the sheet). The circles indicate units, and the thick vertical lines indicate the inhibitory couplings between units in the plus and minus nets, as defined in definition 18 and depicted in figure 8.7(b). The inputs of AND are considered to lie on the left, and its output on the right. To increase perspicuity, the three-dimensional structure has been tilted, and rotated counterclockwise over 45 degrees. The horizontal arrows represent excitatory connections.

The threshold of the AND$_+$ unit is 2, and that of the AND$_-$ unit is 1. We assume all links have weight 1. As an example, suppose the two truth–values $(1, 0)$ and $(0, 0)$ are fed into the AND node. The sum of the plus components is 1, hence AND$_+$ does not fire. The sum of the minus components is 0, so AND$_-$

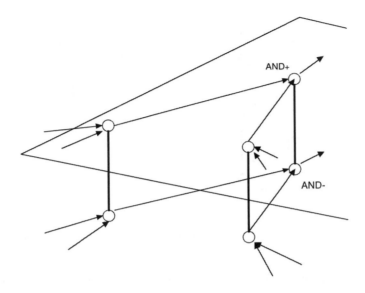

Figure 8.8   Three-valued AND

likewise does not fire. The output is therefore $(0, 0)$, as it should be.

Similarly, a binary OR gate can be constructed by setting the threshold of OR$_+$ to 1, and that of OR$_-$ to 2. The reader may check that these stipulations translate definition 17 for $\wedge$ and $\vee$ into neural terms. We obtain an AND-gate with n inputs for $n \geq 2$ (useful for representing the body of a clause) if the threshold for the plus unit is set to n, and the threshold for the minus unit is set to 1. Similarly, we obtain an n-ary OR-gate if the threshold of the plus-unit is set to 1, and that of the minus–unit to n.

Bias Units and Negation

Finally we introduce the continuously firing bias units **1** and **0**, the former for the plus sheet, where it will take care of the facts in the program as before, and the latter for the minus sheet, where it is connected to those atoms to which we wish to apply negation as failure.

Bias units also play a role in the neural representation of negation. Definition 17 shows that, strictly speaking, negation need not be represented by a unit doing a computation, as, for instance, the NOT unit defined in section 8.1, since negation can be viewed as a simple switching of the plus and minus components. In the case of a negation occurring in front of a propositional atom, this view of negation would lead to the following construction. Suppose we have a node (U_+, U_-) which has one outgoing $+$ link connected to V_+, and one outgoing — link connected to V_-, where (V_+, V_-) is a node. To negate (U_+, U_-) one must "cross the wires," so that the outgoing link from U_+ connects to V_-, and the outgoing link from U_- connects to V_+. In terms of real neural networks this crossing over does not seem to be very plausible, however, as will be discussed in section 8.4.

Because of the mutually inhibitory character of truth and falsity, it is more plausible to represent three-valued negation by means of an inhibitory process. We will elaborate on this in section 8.4. Our suggestion is given in figure 8.9. On the left side of the diagram there are two NOT nodes, one for each layer.

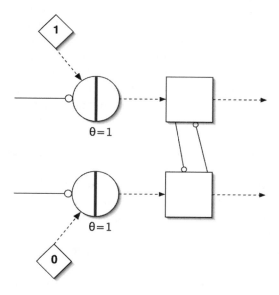

Figure 8.9   Three-valued negation through inhibition (viewed from the side).

The bias units are linked to the NOTs via excitatory links, whereas the inputs inhibit. This arrangement gives the correct outputs for $(1, 0)$ and $(0, 1)$, but not for $(0, 0)$ since it generates the output $(1, 1)$. Therefore the output also has to pass a consistency-checking node, depicted on the right. This extra complexity is the price to be paid for the parallel processing of truth and falsity.

This completes the description of the logic gates required for the construction of the coupled recurrent neural networks. Our next task is to define the network $CRN(P)$ corresponding to a definite program P. We first give a general construction, which will, however, be modified later in order to bring out the special nature of the propositional variables for an abnormality.

The network is now a three-dimensional structure consisting of a plus sheet and a minus sheet such that each sheet has at least three layers of units. We think of the input fed into the "leftmost" layer and the output read out at the "right."[13] The leftmost layer then consist of input units corresponding to the propositional variables used in P; these units are coupled into nodes. The middle or hidden layers consist of AND units (figure 8.8), and NOT units (figure 8.9) where corresponding units in the plus and minus sheets are coupled. The rightmost layers are copies of the leftmost layers, and hence also consist of units coupled into nodes.

To complete the definition we must describe the wiring of the network such that it represents the program P. Let $p_1 \wedge \ldots \wedge p_n \wedge \neg r_1 \wedge \ldots \wedge \neg r_k \to q$ be a clause in P. The network $CRN(P)$ has (at least) leftmost nodes corresponding to $p_1, \ldots, p_n, r_1, \ldots, r_k, q$, and an $n + k$–ary AND node in the middle section. The links from $p_1, \ldots, p_n$ feed directly into AND; those from $r_1, \ldots, r_k$ are first sent into NOT nodes before being linked to AND. The AND node projects to the q node. If there are more clauses with q as head, these are ORed in q, that is, to compute its output, q applies OR to its inputs. If q also occurs in a body, this rightmost node feeds back into the corresponding node on the left; inputs to the leftmost nodes are ORed. If p is a fact in P, add a link from the bias unit $\mathbf{1}$ into the plus component of p viewed as an output node. If r is a proposition letter to which negation is failure is applicable, add a link from the bias unit $\mathbf{0}$ into the minus component of r, *viewed as an output node.*

Note that this construction reflects a condition in the definition of the completion which transforms facts into conditionals: if r does not occur in the head of a clause of P, the clause $\bot \to r$ is added to P. This explains why the bias unit $\mathbf{0}$ must be connected to r as an *output* node. (Likewise for facts p, in view of the equivalence of p and $\top \to p$.) Until further notice, all links are assumed to have weight 1.

Computation in such a coupled net proceeds as follows. At time $t = 0$, all nodes are inactive in both units. At $t = 1$, the facts in P output $(1, 0)$ and the output atoms to which negation as failure is applicable (and which have no other inputs) output $(0, 1)$. All other input nodes remain inactive in both units. For larger t the computation follows the procedure given in definition 16, taking into account the definitions of the AND and OR nodes. We thus obtain

Theorem 4 *Let P be a definite program, and $CRN(P)$ the associated coupled recurrent neural network. The least fixed point of T_P^3 corresponds to the activation of the output layer in the stable state of $CRN(P)$.*

---

13. We cannot use "top" and "bottom" anymore, since this might lead to confusion with the plus and minus sheets.

8.3 Backward Reasoning and Closed–World Reasoning for Rules

We now have to consider the computations that correspond to the inferences AC (affirmation of the consequent) and MT (modus tollens). We have analysed these by means of integrity constraints, that is, statements of the form "if query $?\varphi$ `succeeds/fails`, then query $?\psi$ `succeeds/fails`." From a neural point of view, this is vaguely reminiscent of a form of backpropagation, except that in our case inputs, not weights, are being updated. However, there is a duality between weights and inputs, and this can be exploited to construct a rigorous correspondence between backward inferences and learning in neural networks. The type of learning we need is fortunately only perceptron learning, not the biologically implausible backpropagation. For expository reasons the idea will be illustrated for positive programs and recurrent neural networks only, although an extension to coupled nets is straightforward.

From now on we drop the assumption that all links have weight 1, and also allow links with weight 0. As before, if p is a fact in a program P, there is a link from the bias unit $\mathbf{1}$ to p with weight 1. What is new here is that in case p is not a fact, the link from $\mathbf{1}$ to p has weight 0.

Consider a very simple case: the AC inference of p from q and $p \rightarrow q$. The recurrent neural network corresponding to $\{p \rightarrow q\}$ is given in figure 8.10; the question mark on the link from $\mathbf{1}$ to p indicates that the weight of this link is adjustable.

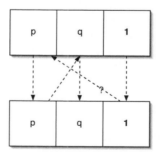

Figure 8.10 AC as perceptron learning

The learning problem can now be stated as follows. If U_p^o fires (because the link from the bias unit $\mathbf{1}$ to p has weight 1) we are done. If not, input $\mathbf{1}$ to p yields output 0 in U_q^o, although the desired output is 1. Therefore the weights in the net have to be readjusted so that the output is indeed 1. The perceptron learning algorithm (see, for example, [231,p. 84]) achieves precisely this. In this particular case it tells us that in order to approximate the right value for the weight, we have to add the initial weight (0) to the input (1). In this case the algorithm even converges in one step, because 1 is the correct value for the weight.

The same thing can be done for MT. In this case U_q^o must not be active by hypothesis. If U_p^o does not fire (because the link from **1** to p has weight 0) we are done. If it does fire, the link has weight 1, and it must learn the correct weight (i.e., 0). The perceptron learning algorithm now tells us to subtract the input (1) from the weight (1) to get weight 0, and again we have convergence in one step.

In conclusion of this discussion of how the networks compute, we may thus note that the relatively easy forward reasoning patterns such as MP and DA correspond to computations in simple recurrent networks, in which no learning occurs, whereas backward reasoning patterns such as AC and MT, which subjects typically find harder, necessitate the computational overhead of readjusting the network by perceptron learning. We propose that this difference between the processes of forward and backward reasoning can play a part in explaining various observations of the difficulty of valid backward reasoning such as MT.

8.4   Constructing the Nets

We will now briefly sketch a hypothesis on how networks as discussed above may be set up in working memory, following the highly suggestive treatment in a series of papers by von der Malsburg starting with [287] (see [286] for a recent summary), some of which were written alone [288], some in collaboration with Bienenstock [19, 289] and some with Willshaw [290, 303, 302, 291]. There are two issues to be distinguished: (1) the representation of conditionals as links, and (2) the structure of the network as coupled isomorphic graphs.

8.4.1   Fast Functional Links

For the first issue we can do no better than borrow (a lightly edited version of) von der Malsburg's own description from [287,p. 13]. The synaptic connection between brain cells i and j is characterized by a strength w_{ij}. It is a measure for the size of the postsynaptic conductance transient which is produced in the postsynaptic cell (i) upon arrival of a nerve impulse in the presynaptic fiber from cell j. It is postulated that the weight w_{ij} of an excitatory synapse depends on two variables with different time scale of behavior, a_{ij} and s_{ij}. The set $\{s_{ij}\}$ constitutes the permanent network structure. Its modification (synaptic plasticity) is slow and is the basis for long-term memory. The new dynamic variable a_{ij}, termed the *state of activation* of the synapse ij (as distinct from the activation of the cell), changes on a fast time scale (fractions of a second) in response to the correlation between the signals of cells i and j. With no

signals in i and j, a_{ij} decays toward a resting state a_0, within times typical
for short-term memory. With strong correlation between the signals the value
a_{ij} changes such that w_{ij} increases (activation). With uncorrelated signals a_{ij}
changes such that w_{ij} decreases to zero (inactivation). This behavior of the
variable a_{ij} will be referred to here as *synaptic modulation*. It can change the
value of a_{ij} significantly within a fraction of a second, thus establishing a *fast
functional link*. Not all synapses from a given cell to other cells can grow at the
same time, since an inhibitory system prevents those target cells from all firing
simultaneously; also the synapses received by a cell compete with each other,
for the same reason. The physical basis for synaptic modulation is not clear; it
might correspond to the accumulation or depletion of some chemical substance
at a strategic location in or near the synapse. The relevant postsynaptic signal
is here taken to be the cell's output spike train, but it may also be a more local
dendritic signal. As a simple example one could assume $w_{ij} = a_{ij}s_{ij}$ with
$0 \leq a_{ij} \leq 1$ and a resting state a_0 within the interval $(0, 1)$.

The variables $\{s_{ij}\}$ are controlled by what will be called *refined synaptic
plasticity*: strong correlation between the temporal fine structure in the signals
of cells i and j causes s_{ij} to grow. Absence of correlation does not directly
reduce s_{ij} . The analogy between synaptic modulation and refined plasticity
is apparent. Both are controlled by correlations in the signals of cell pairs in
a positive feedback fashion. They differ in time scale of decay (seconds for
a_{ij} , decades to permanent for s_{ij}), and of buildup; and they differ in the way
they are controlled. The a_{ij} react only to the two locally available signals and
are both increased and decreased by correlations and their absence. The s_{ij} are
only increased by local signals and are decreased in response to the growth of
other synapses.

If we apply the ideas just outlined to our representation of the suppression
task, we get something like the following. Declarative memory, usually modelled by some kind of spreading activation network, contains a unit representing the concept "library," with links to units representing concepts like "open,"
"study," "essay," and "book." These concepts may combine into propositions.
Neurally, one may view an atomic proposition ("the library is open") as a single unit (say U_p) which is activated when the units for the constitutive concepts
("library," "open") are activated; for example, because mutual reinforcement of
the units for "library" and "open" makes their combined weighted output exceed the threshold of U_p. Two propositional units p, q ("the library is open,"
"she will study late in the library") can be combined into a conditional by the
activation of a further link from p to q, possibly via an abnormality unit.[14]

All these links can be viewed at two time scales. At large time scales the links
are connections laid down in declarative memory; these links have positive (al-

---

14. We will have more to say on the neural representation of abnormalities in section 8.5.

though small) weights and correspond to the $\{s_{ij}\}$ in the above description, At small time scales, links may become temporarily reinforced by sensory input, through an increase of the $\{a_{ij}\}$. For example, upon being presented with the conditional "if she has an essay, she will study late in the library" ($p \wedge \neg ab \to q$), the link from p to q via ab becomes temporarily reinforced by synaptic modulation, and thus forms a fast functional link. As a result, the system of units and links thereby becomes part of working memory, forming a network like the ones studied above, where the $\{w_{ij}\}$ are a function of the $\{s_{ij}\}$ and the $\{a_{ij}\}$. Working memory then computes the stable state of the network, and the state of the output node is passed on to the language production system.

8.4.2 Between the Sheets

The second intriguing issue, raised at the beginning of section 8.4, is how the two layers of neurons become isomorphically wired up through inhibitory connections. What is most interesting here is von der Malsburg and Willshaw's observation [291,p. 83] that this form of coupling neural nets must actually be a fundamental operation in the brain, both at small and large time scales. In the paper cited they discuss extensively the following example. During ontogenesis, the ganglion cells of the retina send axons through the eye stalk to the brain to form connections with central structures such as the optic tectum. In order to preserve the coherence of an image, this mapping from retina to tectum must be "continuous" in the sense that neighboring retina cells project onto neighboring cells of the tectum; and indeed this is true in the adult animal – the "retinotopic" mapping. There is a clear analogy[15] with the networks described in this chapter: the map which projects units in the "true" layer via inhibitory links to units in the "false" layer has precisely this property of continuity, in the sense that neighbors in the "false" sheet are mapped to neighbours in the "true" sheet. Von der Malsburg and Willshaw mention other examples as well, now referring to "dynamic links" active at very small time scales. A good illustration is the integration of information from the left and the right eye – this can be viewed as establishing a temporary continuous map between two neural networks corresponding to the eyes. Another example at the same time scale is visual flow, where points in an image seen at consecutive moments in time must be related continuously to each other.

---

15. There is also a clear disanalogy: the retinotopic map consists of excitatory connections, whereas we need inhibitory connections. The excitatory connections are supposedly constructed via Hebb's rule which says that if two neurons fire simultaneously the excitatory connection between them is strengthened. What we need is rather the "anti-Hebbian rule," which says that if two neurons fire simultaneously, the inhibitory connection between them is strengthened. The existence of an anti-Hebbian rule has been demonstrated experimentally.

The work of von der Malsburg and his associates contains many models and simulations of how such continuous correspondences can be established by processes of synaptic growth and synaptic pruning. Translated to our context, the construction could run as follows. Initially there are two neural networks corresponding to systems of propositions, one dealing with truth, one with falsity. The results of the computations in the networks must inhibit each other, and initially a forest of inhibitory links connect the two networks. The simulations in [302] then suggest that this forest can dynamically reduce to a one-to-one projection between the isomorphically corresponding cells in the two networks. The system is able to spontaneously break the symmetry between several possible projections. We need not delve into the details here; the purpose of this section has only been to point to a striking analogy.

8.5 A Hidden Layer of Abnormalities

While the preceding constructions of neural networks are completely general, in the sense of applying to all definite logic programs, there is reason to think that abnormalities play a special role in such networks. We have seen in chapter 7, and will see again in chapter 9, that abnormalities play a special role as inhibitors in rules. They may inhibit an inference, and they may also inhibit actions. Abnormalities in rules are furthermore special in that they need not occur in the overt linguistic representation of a rule. They may, however, be activated, or suppressed, by material which is overtly represented. We therefore prefer to represent abnormalities as a hidden layer in the network and hypothesise that normally this layer is present in all networks representing the condition–action rules involved in the operation of executive function. This is a theme taken up in chapter 9, where we shall argue that the condition–action rules in motor planning can in fact be formalized as exception–tolerant conditionals like those used in the suppression task. It will be shown that, if this formalization is adopted, the resulting hidden layer of abnormalities is responsible for the possibility of flexible planning. We will furthermore see in chapter 9 that the theory that autism is a form of executive disorder can be modelled by assuming that this hidden layer is malfunctioning, thus leading to behavioral rigidity and perseverance.

Consider a conditional like $p \wedge \neg ab \rightarrow q$ together with a further determination of the abnormality as $\neg s \rightarrow ab$ and $\neg t \rightarrow ab$. We do not treat ab as an ordinary proposition letter, which would have to be included in input and output layers. Instead the effect of the abnormality is captured by a separate $ab = (ab_+, ab_-)$ node, located between the body of the clause minus $\neg ab$, which is in this case just p, and the head, here q (see figure 8.11[16]). The clauses $\neg s \rightarrow ab$ and

---

16. The diagram does not yet exhibit the symmetry of, for example, figure 8.8. This issue will be discussed at the end of the section.

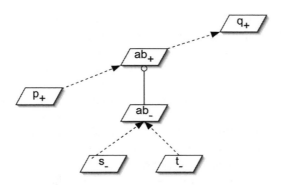

Figure 8.11   A hidden layer of abnormalities

$\neg t \rightarrow ab$ are represented by links from units labeled s_-, t_- to the unit ab_-, which contains an implicit OR. The threshold of ab_- is a small positive value. The function of the unit ab_+ in the upper sheet is only to interrupt the flow of activation from p to q if the possibility of an exception is highlighted. The connection from ab_- to ab_+ is therefore inhibitory.

One may think of the "false" sheet as gathering contextual information relevant to the inhibition of the link from p to q. This information is summarized by the unit ab_- before being relayed to ab_+ in the "true" sheet.[17] In order to visualise neural computations involving abnormalities, it is useful to allow activations strictly between 0 and 1. First suppose that s_-, t_- are not activated at all, either because the propositions s, t are known to be true, or because there is (as yet) no link from the units to ab_- in working memory. Since the threshold of ab_- is positive, ab_- does not fire, and hence the link between p and q is not interrupted. Now suppose that the possibility of an exception, say $\neg s$, is highlighted. This does not yet mean that s is known to be false, so assume this possibility is represented as a small activation in the unit s_-. If this activation is greater than or equal to the threshold of ab_-, this unit fires and thereby inhibits the link between p and q. If the proposition s is known to be false, the activation of the unit s_- is 1, and again the preceding considerations apply.

Looking at figure 8.11, it might seem that we quietly dropped a basic feature of the neural networks computing minimal models of definite logic programs: the isomorphism of the "true" and "false" sheets. The answer is yes and no: yes,

---

17. The reader may wonder why we do not represent the effect of the abnormality by means of an ANDNOT unit in the "true" sheet, since that is, after all, what is suggested by the clause $p \wedge \neg ab \rightarrow q$. One reason is that in our chosen way the role of inhibition is made more explicit, and this ties in nicely with the neurophysiological discussion of inhibition in section 9.11.1. Furthermore, the fact that ab_- is located in the "false" sheet means that new contextual information can be added on to ab_- linearly (via OR); the unit ab_- itself does not have to be modified.

because at first not all links required by the isomorphism will be present; no, because at least some of these links will be established as the result of learning. Let us be more precise.

The units labeled s_- and t_- in the diagram actually form part of a node (s_+, s_-) (and (t_+, t_-)), where the two units are connected by inhibitory links. The units s_+ and t_+ are at first *not* connected to ab_+. The unit p_+ is part of the node (p_+, p_-); here p_- need not be connected to ab_-.[18] Suppose first that s is irrelevant to ab; in this case there will not develop a link from s_- to ab_- in working memory, and there is therefore no need to have a corresponding link from s_+ to ab_+. If we now suppose that $\neg s$ is considered a possible abnormality, hence is relevant to ab, then we must assume that in working memory a link is constructed from s_- to ab_-; at first only in the "false" sheet, since we assume that it is this sheet which is responsible for the incorporation of the context, insofar as is relevant to inhibition. If one now receives the information that s is true, s_+ inhibits s_-, and hence (disregarding t) ab_- will not fire. If p is known to be true, it follows that ab_+ fires, and because s_+ and ab_+ fire simultaneously, a link will be forged between s_+ and ab_+ by Hebbian learning. One may view this process as the neural analogue of the synthesis of a new rule $p \wedge s \rightarrow q$, a synthesis that will further occupy us in chapter 9, section 9.6. The only essential difference between the network in figure 8.11 and the network consisting of two isomorphic sheets is therefore that there is no inhibitory link from ab_+ to ab_-. Indeed there cannot be such a link, otherwise activation of p_+ would by itself already inhibit ab_-, and thus discount the influence from the context.

8.6 Discussion

We showed that closed–world reasoning in its guise as logic programming has an appealing neural implementation, unlike classical logic. On our proposals the networks corresponding to logic programs become part of working memory, which then maintains a minimal preferred model of the world under description in a form in which it can be efficiently revised at any point in the light of new information. This is the kind of system required for an organism to plan, and is the kind of system which might be developed by an organism evolved for planning, as discussed in chapter 6.

We are now in a position to give some further substance to, and modify, the distinction between system 1 and system 2 processes mentioned in chapter 5. For convenience we recall Evans's view of the distinction, already quoted in

---

18. An easy calculation shows that the presence or absence of this connection does not make a difference. Suppose we add $\neg p \rightarrow ab$ to our data, which corresponds to a link from p_- to ab_-. Program completion gives $\neg p \vee \neg s \rightarrow ab$, which is equivalent to $\neg ab \leftrightarrow (p \wedge s)$. Substitution in $p \wedge \neg ab \rightarrow q$ gives $p \wedge s \rightarrow q$ as before.

chapter 5:

> System 1 is ... a form of universal cognition shared between animals and humans. It is
> actually not a single system but a set of subsystems that operate with some autonomy.
> System 1 includes instinctive behaviors that are innately programmed and would include
> any innate input modules of the kind proposed by Fodor ... The system 1 processes that
> are most often described, however, are those that are formed by associative learning of
> the kind produced by neural networks. ... System 1 processes are rapid, parallel and
> automatic in nature; only their final product is posted in consciousness[72,p. 454].

In these theories, logical reasoning is considered to belong to system 2 which
is

> slow and sequential in nature and makes use of the central working memory system [72,p.
> 454].

We believe the distinction is useful and important, but the constructions presented in this chapter challenge the idea that fast and automatic processes are
thereby not logical processes. In virtue of its mathematical properties closed
world reasoning can be modelled by fast parallel neural processes, and therefore may be taken to belong to system 1. It is not logic per se that belongs to
system 2, but some logical systems (such as classical logic) do belong there because in these systems model generation does not have a neural representation.

The reader somewhat familiar with the logical literature may have felt increasingly uneasy during our discussion of nonmonotonic logic: isn't it true
that nonmonotonic reasoning has high computational complexity and is therefore ipso facto ruled out as a formal description of actual human reasoning?
There are in fact two issues here, one pertaining to the search for possible exceptions or abnormalities in the mental database, the other to the computational
complexity of the derivability relation of a given nonmonotonic logic. The first
issue can be illustrated by a quotation from Politzer [218,p. 10]

> Nonmonotonicity is highly difficult to manage by Artificial Intelligence systems because
> of the necessity of looking for possible exceptions through an entire database. What I
> have suggested is some kind of reversal of the burden of proof for human cognition:
> at least for conditionals (but this could generalize) looking for exceptions is itself an
> exception because conditional information comes with an implicit guarantee of normality.

Translated to our formalism, the difficulty hinted at by Politzer concerns tabulating all clauses of the form $\varphi \to ab$ which are present in memory. But in
our setup we do not have a knowledge base in the sense of AI, with its huge
number of clauses which are all on an equal footing. What counts instead is the
number of links of the form $\varphi \to ab$ *which are activated in working memory*
by means of a mechanism such as von der Malsburg's "fast functional links."
This search space will then be very much smaller. There remains the issue of
how *relevant* information in long–term memory is recruited into working memory, though we assume this is achieved efficiently through the organization of

long-term memory. We do not pretend to have solved the problem, but equally we do not believe that the AI experience of the intractability of nonmonotonic logic is relevant here.

The second issue is concerned with the computational complexity of the decision problem for the relation "ψ is derivable from $\varphi_1, \ldots, \varphi_n$ in nonmonotonic logic $\mathcal{L}$," where we may restrict attention to propositional logics only. For example, one well-known nonmonotonic logic, Reiter's *default logic*, is computationally more complex than classical propositional logic, which is NP–complete, so in practice exponential (see Gottlob [104] for a sample of results in this area). By contrast, if $\mathcal{L}$ is propositional logic programming with negation as failure, the corresponding decision problem is P-complete, hence *less* complex than classical propositional logic (see Dantsin et al. [56] and references given therein for discussion).[19] This difference is mainly due to a restriction in the syntactic form of the clauses, which have to be of the form $\varphi \to A$, where φ can be arbitrary, but A must be atomic. This restriction, whose main effect is to rule out disjunctions in the consequent, is harmless in the case of the suppression task, although it may cause problems in other reasoning tasks. Again, this only serves to show that logical form determines whether a task can be solved by system 1 or just by system 2 processing.

---

19. It is true that our representation of MT goes beyond the derivability relation of logic programming. However, the fact that it can be represented using perceptron learning guarantees that it is still polynomial.

9 Coping with Nonmonotonicity in Autism

Autism is a clinical syndrome first described by Leo Kanner in the 1940s, often first diagnosed in children around 2 to 3 years of age as a deficit in their affective relations and communication. The autistic child typically refuses eye contact, is indifferent or hostile to demonstrations of affection, and exhibits delayed or abnormal communication, repetitive movements (often self-harming), and is rather indifferent to pain. Autistic children do not engage spontaneously in make-believe play and show little interest in the competitive social hierarchy, and in personal possessions. Autism comes in all severities – from complete lack of language and severe retardation, to mild forms continuous with the "normal" range of personalities and IQs. Autism is sometimes distinguished from Aspberger's syndrome – very roughly speaking, autism without language impairment – but Aspberger's is probably just the mild end of the autistic spectrum. Autistic children share many symptoms shown by deaf and by blind infants, possibly because of the social isolation imposed by these conditions. There are known biochemical abnormalities associated with autism. There is evidence of a probably complex genetic basis. As should be clear by now, we do not believe that psychological analyses of autistic functioning are inconsistent with, or exclusive of, such biochemical– or genetic–level analyses, and we will indicate something of how we think the different levels may relate to each other.

More than any other psychiatric disorder, autism has captured the imagination of the practitioners of cognitive science, because, at least according to some theories, it holds the promise of revealing the essence of what makes us human. This holds especially for the school which views autism as a deficit in "theory of mind," the ability to represent someone else's feelings and beliefs. An implication seems to be that in this respect autistic people are like our evolutionary ancestors, given that chimpanzees have much less "theory of mind" than humans. Although we believe the claims that can be made are quite different, we obviously agree that autism may well be important from the point of view of evolutionary cognitive science.

9.1   Psychological Theories of Autism

There are several current psychological theories of autism. To mention some
of the main ones: the theory of mind deficit theory (Leslie [172]), the affective
foundation theory (Hobson [127]), the weak central coherence theory (Happé
[114]), and the executive function deficit theory (Russell [237]).

9.1.1   Theory of Mind

The "theory theory" originated in Premack and Woodruff's work on chimpanzees [222], attempting to characterise the differences between human and
nonhuman primates. Alan Leslie [172] proposed that human beings have a
brain "module" that does reasoning about minds, by implementing a "theory
of mind" (often abbreviated to ToM), and that autistic development could be
seen as delayed acquisition or impairment of this module. So, the theory theory goes, in normals the module constitutes the difference between humans
and their ancestors. To paint with a broad brush, this claim gives us the two
equations:

$$\text{chimpanzee} + \text{ToM} = \text{human}$$
$$\text{and}$$
$$\text{human} - \text{ToM} = \text{autist}$$

Certainly this is a great simplification, but, we will argue, it usefully encapsulates a largely unspoken argument common in the field (although not in Happé
or in Frith [114, 88]), that autism is to be characterized by the *lack* of quali-
ties present in normals. Very little equation solving yields the consequence that
autistic people are like chimpanzees (in some relevant respects). This we find
highly counterintuitive: chimpanzees are, for example, hypersocial animals. It
may be more useful at least to entertain a different equation:

$$\text{normal human} + \text{too much "magic ingredient"} = \text{autist}$$

That is, some of whatever cognitive additions yielded humans from their ape
ancestors may be overrepresented in autistic cognition. Just for an example to
illustrate, much of autistic cognition is an obsessive attempt to extract exceptionless truth about a complicated world. This sounds to us rather more like the
scientific life than that of chimpanzees. At least this equation may allow us aca-
demics to empathize with autistic reasoners. Of course, this alternative equation has very different evolutionary implications. As we shall see, autism has
a substantial genetic component, and a high prevalence for a deleterious inherited condition, so one must ask whether there are benefits from lesser dosages
which maintain the condition in the population. Perhaps autism is the sickle cell
anaemia of behavioral traits? Sickle cell anemia is a double-recessive genetic

disease maintained in the populations of malaria–infested areas by the enhanced malaria resistance of the heterozygote. This particularly simple mechanism is too simple for autism, but there are others whereby alleles may be beneficial in one environment or one genotype, and harmful in another.

These equations raise many questions about just what nonhuman primates can and can't do in the way of reasoning about conspecifics' behavior and mental processes. Apes have considerable facility in reasoning about conspecifics' *plans* – in the sense of predicting their behavior by diagnosing their motivation – but they appear not to be able to reason about conspecifics' epistemic states. A related point is that young children seem to develop "desire" psychology before "belief" psychology, although desires are "states of mind," and so it is unclear why they do not require a theory of mind to reason about them. After all, to reason about a person's desires seems to necessitate an appropriate set of beliefs.

The theory theory can be taken as explanatory, or as an important label for a set of problems. Its authors appear to claim the former. It seems more plausible at this stage to interpret it as the latter – an important label for a problem that needs a label. So, for example, there has been a debate in philosophy contrasting "theory" vs. "simulation" accounts of reasoning about mental states (see, for example, Harris [117] and Heal [121]). This debate bears rather directly on autism, and we do not imply by our discussion of theory of mind that we are rejecting simulation-based accounts.[1]

9.1.2 Affective Foundation

Hobson's theory of autism [127] does not so much *deny* theory of mind as seek to *derive* it from more fundamental ontogenetic processes[2] – in particular from the affective foundations[3] of interpersonal communication. Humans uniquely control shared attention, especially by gaze. We diagnose where others' attention is focused from information about where they are looking. "Intersubjectivity" is established through mutual control of attention. Just as Piaget saw the child's sensorimotor activity as achieving the child's mastery of where itself left off and the world began, so Hobson sees the child's understanding of itself as a social being separated from others being achieved through joint attentional activity. The child must learn that the other can have different representations, and different wants and values. Hobson proposes that it is autistic people's *valuation* of these experiences of intersubjectivity which is abnormal. If the child does not experience the achievement of intersubjectivity as rewarding (or even experiences it as aversive), then any cognitive developments founded

---

1. In fact Stenning [258] argues that the two may not be as distinct as would at first appear.
2. But see Hobson [126].
3. The *Oxford English Dictionary* defines the relevant sense of affect as "The way in which one is affected or disposed; mental state, mood, feeling, desire, intention."

on it will not develop normally. Cognitive symptoms of autism are, on this theory, *consequences* of this valuation.

9.1.3   Weak Central Coherence

Frith and Happé's weak central coherence (WCC) theory of autism [114, 88] is built on the observation that autistic people show certain *super*normal abilities. Autistic people are good at things which can be done by attention to detail while ignoring "the big picture," particularly in some visual tasks. They show a *lack* of susceptibility to some visual illusions (e.g., Müller-Lyer[4]). Furthermore they perform very well on the Hidden Figures task, an example of which is presented in figure 9.1.

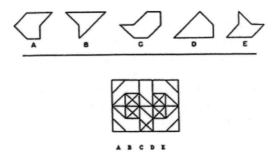

Figure 9.1   Example Hidden Figures test item. The task is to select which of the outline figures in the row above is contained in the complex pattern below.

The theoretical basis of WCC is Fodor's theory of the modularity of mind, alluded to in chapter 6. It will be recalled that Fodor postulated a central processing unit which processes the information supplied by the modules in a modality-free manner. Fodor viewed analogy and metaphor as the characteristic modus operandi of the central processor. WCC maintains that in autistic people the central processor does not fully perform its integrative function, resulting in the separate modules "pushing" their own specific information. As additional support for this account one may cite autistic people's claimed inability to understand metaphor, and also their claimed failure to exploit analogies in problem solving (see [250]). More generally, weak central coherence can be thought of as a style of cognition dominated by bottom–up information processing.

---

4. See http://www.essex.ac.uk/psychology/experiments/muller.html for an online version.

9.1.4 Executive Disorder

Russell's executive function deficit (ED) theory [237] takes yet another cluster of symptoms as basic: the observation that autistic people often exhibit severe perseveration. They go on carrying out some routine when the routine is no longer appropriate, and exhibit great difficulty in switching tasks when the context calls for this (that is, when switching is not governed by an explicit rule). This perseveration, also observed in certain kinds of patients with frontal cortex damage, is hypothesized to give rise to many of the symptoms of autism: obsessiveness, insensitivity to context, inappropriateness of behavior, literalness of carrying out instructions.[5] Task switching is the brief of *executive function*, a process (or set of processes) responsible for high-level action control such as planning, initiation, coordination, inhibition and control of action sequences. Executive function is hypothesized to be necessary for mentally maintaining a goal, and pursuing it in the real world under possibly adverse circumstances. On this view, executive dysfunction is held to be responsible for the sometimes extreme behavioral rigidity of autistic people.

The origin of the concept of "executive function" was heavily influenced by the analysis of neuropsychological patients. This has the important consequence that it is often most discussed in terms of its malfunctioning, and leaves us with little positive characterization of what executive function does when it is functioning healthily. Here AI theories of planning are perhaps helpful since they provide principled analyses of just what is involved in planning action. By contrast, the psychological study of normal undamaged planning mainly surfaces in the study of problem solving (e.g., [199]) and problem solving in turn has been most extensively studied in the guise of expertise – what is the difference between expert and novice problem solving[35]. [6]

When discussing cognitive analyses of mental malfunctioning, it is worth remembering that although much clinical literature is understandably oriented toward giving patients a unique categorization, there is an active strand of thought in contemporary psychiatry that argues that the discreteness of such categories is always to be questioned [118]. For example, autistic subjects are considerably more depressed, as measured by the relevant clinical diagnosis instruments, than are controls. Whether this is a reaction to, or rather a cause of, their condition, it becomes particularly important when considering such explanations of autism as executive dysfunction, since executive function is a component of a whole spectrum of mental disorders, including depression, but also including anxiety, schizophrenia, and attention–deficit hyperactivity disorder

---

5. Note that although autistic people may lack spontaneity, they may be able to carry out tasks involving fantasy play when instructed, as is indeed necessary if they are to engage with diagnostic tests such as the false belief task (see section 9.3 below) at all.

6. Shallice [245] provides a bridge in his studies of the Tower of London problem–solving task, which is derived from the Tower of Hanoi, a staple of the early AI literature on planning.

(ADHD). We have already noted that executive function is itself a broad category of functions. Is the executive dysfunction observed in autism the same as the executive dysfunction observed in depression, or in ADHD? If we could fractionate autistic people's problems, could the executive function subset be due to the accompanying depression? These are questions which don't currently have answers, but are nevertheless important to appreciate in thinking about cognitive accounts of such complex syndromes. They crop up again below when we survey the genetics of autism.

This quick survey of theories was intended to illustrate that there are multiple psychological characterizations of autism. Although it is the habit of the field to present these theories as alternatives, it is far from obvious that they are mutually exclusive. For example, Hobson's theory might be construed as a theory about where our theory-of-mind abilities develop from. Although there is some tension between the idea that these abilities come in a genetically determined module, and that they develop out of experiences of communication, in truth these are not really inconsistent. In any case, the theory theory does not present any evidence for the genetic basis or modularity, save for the lack of any evidence of learning and the discreteness of the diagnosing task. Similarly, executive function and central coherence are presumably *computational* capacities of systems and as such they might be components of whatever system realises theory–of–mind abilities.

9.2   Logic and Experiment in the Study of Psychiatric Disorders

Several of the proffered explanations for autism will be explored in greater depth below, but the brief synopsis given above makes plain that the relations between the theories merits greater scrutiny. It is here that a logical analysis can be helpful. More concretely, we will show that there is a common core to the theory–of–mind deficit theory and executive disorder theory, which consists in well-defined failures in nonmonotonic reasoning. Based on this analysis, one can also show in what sense theory–of–mind reasoning is more difficult (contains more components) than this common core. Furthermore, the common core leads to predictions about autistic people's behavior on our old friend the suppression task which differ from those for normals. One virtue of logical analysis is its ability to cross linguistic and nonlinguistic tasks. Another is to insist that vague distinctions between representation and processing are refined.

But the logician has another role as well. In chapter 3 we showed that dramatically different performance on superficially similar versions of the Wason task are in fact due to the different logical forms of these tasks. The same situation occurs in the "executive disorder" branch of autism research, where autistic people were shown to behave very differently on the box task (introduced in chapter 2) and the "tubes task" (to be introduced in this chapter). A careful analysis shows that in fact the logical structures of these tasks are very different, and that different behavior is therefore to be expected.

The common core has to do with autistic people's handling of nonmonotonic inference, more specifically that of closed–world reasoning. In chapter 2 we identified a number of areas to which closed–world reasoning is applicable, each time in slightly different form:

- lists: train schedules, airline databases, etc.

- diagnostic reasoning and abduction

- unknown preconditions

- causal and counterfactual reasoning

- attribution of beliefs and intentions

Autistic people have difficulties with at least the last three. They also have a special relationship with lists, in the sense that they feel lost without lists, such as timetables, to organise daily activities; they have great difficulty accommodating unexpected changes to the timetable, and try to avoid situations such as holidays in which rigid schedules are not applicable. One may view this as an extreme version of closed–world reasoning, sometimes even applied in inappropriate circumstances. But before one concludes from this that autistic people are good at closed–world reasoning to the point of overapplying it, one must carefully distinguish several components of closed–world reasoning. On the one hand, there is the inference from *given* premises which reduces to a computation of the minimal model of the premises and checking whether a given formula holds. (This is what we referred to earlier as reasoning *from* an interpretation.) As we have seen in the last chapter, this is presumably easy because automatic, as can be seen from the neural model presented there. In a wider sense, nonmonotonic reasoning also involves "preprocessing" the given situation or discourse, that is, *encoding* the law-like features of a situation in a particular type of premise (reasoning *to* an interpretation). Laws and regularities always allow exceptions, and skill at "exception handling" is required – which involves identifying and encoding the relevant exceptions, and knowing when enough is enough. The chapter heading Coping with Nonmonotonicity refers to this last aspect, at which autistic people appear to do worse than normals, although they behave normally with respect to the nonmonotonic inferences themselves. That is, autistic people appear to be worse in reasoning to an interpretation. In the remainder of the chapter we study the implicit reasoning patterns of autistic people in several well-known experimental paradigms, and show that they can be analysed as failures to engage in the difficult part of closed–world reasoning.

9.3   Theory of Mind and Reasoning

A famous experiment, the false belief task [305, 212], investigates how autistic subjects reason about other people's belief. The standard design of the experiment is as follows. A child and a doll (Maxi) are in a room together with the experimenter. Maxi and child witness a bar of chocolate being placed in a box. Then Maxi is taken out of the room. The child sees the experimenter move the chocolate from the box to a drawer. Maxi is brought back in. The experimenter asks the child: "Where does Maxi think the chocolate is?" The answers to this question reveal an interesting cutoff point, and a difference between autistic and normally developing children. Before the age of about 4 years , the normally developing child responds where the child knows the chocolate to be (i.e., the drawer); after that age, the child responds where Maxi must falsely believe the chocolate to be (i.e., the box). By contrast, autistic children go on answering "in the drawer" for a long time.

This experiment has been repeated many times, in many variations, with fairly robust results. Some versions can easily be done at home. There is, for instance, the "Smarties" or "unexpected contents" task, which goes as follows. Unbeknownst to the child, a box of Smarties is emptied and refilled with pencils. The child is asked: "What do you think is in the box?" and it happily answers: "Smarties!" It is then shown the contents of the box. The pencils are put back into the box, and the child is now asked: "What do you think your [absent] mother will say is in the box?" We may then observe the same critical age: before age 4 the child answers: "Pencils!," whereas after age 4 the child will say: "Smarties!" Even more strikingly, when asked what it believed was in the box before seeing the actual contents, the younger child will say "Pencils," even though it has just answered "Smarties!"

The outcomes of these experiments have been argued to support the theory–of–mind–deficit hypothesis on the cause of autism. Proposed by Leslie in 1987 [172], it holds that human beings have evolved a special "module" devoted specifically to reasoning about other people's minds. As such, this module would provide a cognitive underpinning for empathy. In normals the module would constitute the difference between humans and their ancestors – indeed, chimpanzees seem to be able to do much less in the way of mind-reading. In autistic children, this module would be delayed or impaired, thus explaining abnormalities in communication and also in the acquisition of language, if it is indeed true that the development of joint attention is crucial to language learning (as claimed, for instance, by Tomasello [276]).

This seems a very elegant explanation for an intractable phenomenon, and it has justly captured the public's imagination. Upon closer examination the question arises whether it is really an explanation rather than a description of one class of symptoms. For instance, as we have seen in chapter 6, the notion of a "module" is notoriously hazy. In this context it is obviously meant to be a piece of dedicated neural circuitry. In this way, it can do the double duty of differentiating us from our ancestors and being capable of being damaged in isolation. But it is precisely this isolation, or "encapsulation" as Fodor called it, that is doubtful. One reason is just our general skepticism expressed in chapter 6, section 6.4, that evolution does not generally proceed by adding new modules (rather than tweaking old ones), and another is that much of the problem of functionally characterizing human reasoning about minds is about interactions between modules. Theory of mind requires language to formulate beliefs in and it also entails a considerable involvement of working memory, as can be seen in "nested" forms of theory of mind, as in Dunbar's example

> Shakespeare intended us to realise that Othello believes that Iago knows that Desdemona is in love with Cassio [66,p. 162].

However, as soon as one realises that a module never operates in isolation, then the theory–of–mind–deficit hypothesis begins to lose its hold. We are now invited to look at the (possibly defective) interactions of the module with other cognitive functions (for example, language and working memory), which leads to the possibility that defects in these functions may play a role in autism. And there is, of course, also the problem of what the module would have to contain, given that, for instance, reasoning about other people's desires is possible for both autistic people and non-human primates.

Apart from these theoretical problems, it is experimentally controversial at what stage theory–of–mind abilities emerge. False-belief tasks were initially proposed as diagnosing a lack of these abilities in normal 3-year-olds and their presence in normal 4-year-olds (Leslie [172]). Others have proposed that irrelevant linguistic demands of these tasks deceptively depress 3–year–olds' performance. For example, in the false belief task, the child sees the doll see the sweet placed in one box, and then the child but not the doll sees the sweet moved to another. Now if the child is asked "Where will the doll look for the sweet *first*?" (instead of "Where will the doll look for the sweet?") then children as young as 2 can sometimes solve the problem (Siegal and Beattie [248]).[7] These arguments, as well as others cited earlier (see p. 164) push reasoning about intentions earlier in ontogeny.

9.4 Reasoning in the False Belief Task

In chapter 2 we made a start on analyzing attribution of belief, as it occurs in the false–belief task, as a species of closed–world reasoning. For convenience

---

7. Intriguingly, this might be read as evidence of the 3-year-olds in the original task adopting a deontic reading of the question (Where *should* the doll look? See[40]) rather than a descriptive one (Where *will* the doll look first?). Another possibility, which also echoes a problem in the selection task, is that the younger child's problem may be with sequencing contingencies in their responses.

we repeat the informal argument here, before proceeding to a rigorous logical analysis.

An agent solving the task correctly first of all needs to have an awareness of the causal relation between perception and belief, which can be stated in the form: "if φ is true in scene S, and agent a sees S, then a comes to believe φ." Applied to the situation at hand, this means that Maxi comes to believe that the chocolate is in the box. An application of the principle of inertia now yields that Maxi's belief concerning the location of the chocolate persists unless an event occurs which causes him to have a new belief, incompatible with the former one. The story does not mention such an event, whence it is reasonable to assume – using closed–world reasoning – that Maxi still believes that the chocolate is in the box when he returns to the experimenter's room. An explanation for performance in the false belief task also needs to account for the incorrect answers given by children younger than 4 and autistic children. These subjects almost always answer "in the drawer," when asked where Maxi believes the chocolate to be. To model this, we borrow a notion from executive dysfunction theory, and hypothesise that the "prepotent response" is always for the child to answer where it knows the chocolate to be. In some children, this response can be inhibited; in other children it cannot, for various reasons which we shall explore below.

The formal analysis we are about to present has to combine reasoning about beliefs and about the world, as well as to link a subject's beliefs with her responses (verbal as well as nonverbal). This last component, usually omitted in discussions of a theory–of–mind "module," but which we consider an integral part of the task, is the brief of executive function. We therefore preface our analysis with a brief discussion of some logical features of executive function. This will pay dividends in later parts of this chapter, when we treat the explanation of autism as a form of executive dysfunction. In fact, it will be seen that the executive components in false-belief tasks make them formally very similar to tasks not involving beliefs about other people at all.

Recall from section 9.1.4 that executive function can be decomposed in planning, initiation, inhibition, coordination, and control of action sequences leading toward a goal held in working memory. In the following we abstract from the coordination and control component, and concentrate on goal maintenance, planning, and (contextually determined) inhibition. We have seen in chapter 7 that at the level of competence, planning can be described as a form of closed–world reasoning, which is applied in particular to implicit preconditions for actions. Viewed in terms of executive function, the suppression effect is a special case of inhibition of a response. In the logical model of executive function proposed here, inhibition is represented through the special logical form of causal properties of actions, as a conditional in which the link from say action to effect is mediated by the slot labeled $\neg ab$:

$$A \wedge \neg ab \rightarrow E \tag{9.1}$$

To recapitulate the discussion in chapters 7 and 8: the conditional (9.1) is read as "if A and *nothing abnormal is the case*, then E," where the expression *nothing abnormal is the case* is governed by closed–world reasoning. For instance, if there is nothing known about a possible abnormality, i.e., if the causal system is closed, one concludes $\neg ab$, hence from A it follows that E. If, however, there is information of the form $C \rightarrow ab$, i.e., if there is a context C which constitutes an abnormality, and C is the case, then the link from A to E is inhibited. In the neural model of closed–world reasoning proposed in chapter 8, ab corresponds to a neuron situated between the neurons for A and E, such that C is connected to ab via an inhibitory link; and this is the general way of incorporating contextual influences. The theories describing task competence will all consist of sets of such conditionals. We begin by formulating languages in which these theories can be expressed.

9.4.1 Formal Language and Principles

The languages we need comprise at least the following predicates[8]:
$R_a(p)$: agent a reports her belief that p
$see_a(p)$: agent a sees that p
$told_a(p)$: agent a is told that p
$ded_a(p)$: agent a deduces that p
$B_a(p)$: agent a has the belief that p
$l(i, t)$: the chocolate is at location i at time t
ab_a: an exception which obstructs agent a's inferences
$clipped(s, i, t)$: at some time between s and t, the chocolate ceases to be at location i. The agent's information state $B_a(\varphi)$ satisfies properties such as the following[9]:

$$
\begin{aligned}
see_a(\varphi) &\rightarrow B_a(\varphi) & (9.2) \\
told_a(\varphi) &\rightarrow B_a(\varphi) & (9.3) \\
ded_a(\varphi) &\rightarrow B_a(\varphi) & (9.4) \\
B_a(\varphi \rightarrow \psi) &\rightarrow (B_a(\varphi) \rightarrow B_a(\psi)) & (9.5)
\end{aligned}
$$

---

8. The formalism introduces just what is necessary to model the various tasks. A fully general formalism would have to use the "event calculus," for which see [282]. Our formulation uses predicates which can take formulas as arguments. Strictly speaking this is not allowed in first–order logic, but there are a number of technical tricks to deal with this issue. A general approach is given in [282,chapter 6].
9. The properties of $B_a(\varphi)$ assumed in the analysis of the standard false–belief task are very minimal. We shall have occasion to use deeper principles concerning $B_a(\varphi)$ in section 9.4.5.

Suppose b is an agent thinking about the behavior of agent a. We model b's responses as the result of a competition between two rules, both of which are instantiations of the general response rule schema

$$B_b(\varphi) \wedge \neg ab_b \rightarrow R_b(\varphi) \qquad (9.6)$$

where ab_b indicates a possible circumstance which prevents b from reporting his belief.[10] This response schema says that if b believes φ, his prepotent response is to report that φ; but the rule is *inhibitable* in that the occurrence of ab_b may prevent the report. Obviously this response is itself an instance of the more general schema (9.1).

The first substitution instance of rule (9.6) says that if b knows what the location of the chocolate is, he will report that location, barring exceptional circumstances:

$$B_b(l(i,t)) \wedge \neg ab_b \rightarrow R_b(l(i,t)), \qquad (9.7)$$

which arises from rule (9.6) by the substitution $\varphi := l(i,t)$.

The second rule, which reflects partial comprehension of the task instructions, says that b will report a's information state:

$$B_b(B_a(l(i,t))) \wedge \neg ab_b \rightarrow R_b(B_a(l(i,t))) \qquad (9.8)$$

It arises from rule 9.6 by the substitution $\varphi := B_a(l(i,t))$.

In the case of a false belief, these rules are in competition, and we have to ensure that only one is operative; i.e., the rules must inhibit each other mutually. This is achieved by means of the abnormalities. The inhibitory effect of (9.7) on (9.8) is modelled by the clause

$$R_b(l(j,t)) \rightarrow ab_b \qquad (9.9)$$

which expresses that b's own response interferes with 9.8 if $j \neq i$.

The inhibitory effect of 9.8 on 9.7 is modelled by a clause which expresses another part of task comprehension: b should report a's beliefs, even if he knows them to be wrong:

$$B_b(B_a(l(i,t))) \rightarrow ab_b \qquad (9.10)$$

This formula expresses that b's prepotent response 9.7 is inhibited if agent b has information that agent a has (possibly incorrect) information about the location of the chocolate.

It is essential to note that the false–belief task not only involves fairly modest reasoning about beliefs, but more importantly also reasoning about the world.

---

10. The abnormality ab_b may be different for each concrete φ, but in order not to overload notation we will not indicate this explicitly.

The interaction between the inertial properties of the world and the information of an agent a is given by

$$B_a(l(i, s)) \wedge s < t \wedge \neg B_a(clipped(s, i, t)) \rightarrow ded_a(l(i, t)) \qquad (9.11)$$

with *clipped* governed by clauses such as

$$l(i, s) \wedge chocolate\text{-}moved(r) \wedge s < r < t \rightarrow clipped(s, i, t); \qquad (9.12)$$

$$l(i, s) \wedge chocolate\text{-}melted(r) \wedge s < r < t \rightarrow clipped(s, i, t). \qquad (9.13)$$

9.4.2 Closed–World Reasoning in the Normal Child Older Than 4 Years

Let the location variable i range over $\{1, 2\}$, where $1 = $ box, $2 = $ drawer. Also let a be Maxi, b the child, t_0 the time at which Maxi leaves the room, and $t > t_0$ the time at which b must answer the experimenter's question, i.e., report Maxi's belief state. We will represent b's report as a statement of the form $R_b(B_a(p))$. We assume that b believes that $l(2, t)$, and we omit the derivation of this fact. We must explain why the normal child responds with $R_b(B_a(l(1, t)))$, and not with $R_b(l(2, t))$. As mentioned above, the explanation assumes that of the competing conditionals (9.7) and (9.8) the first is inhibited by the second through a condition on ab_b reflecting the child's understanding of the task:

$$B_b(B_a(l(i, t))) \rightarrow ab_b \qquad (9.14)$$

We first show that in these conditions b will not respond with his own knowledge of the whereabouts of the chocolate. The response $R_b(l(2, t))$ would require $\neg ab_b$, i.e., that ab_b cannot be derived. Now ab_b reduces to $B_b(B_a(l(i, t)))$ by equation (9.10): if the latter can be proved, so can the former. But as we will prove next, one has $B_b(B_a(l(i, t)))$, whence also ab_b. Thus the prepotent response (9.7) is inhibited and $R_b(l(2, t))$ is not a possible response for b. This will help in showing that the antecedent of rule (9.8) is satisfied.

The second part of the proof shows that b will report a's beliefs. We know $l(1, s) \wedge see_a(l(1, s))$ for some $s < t_0 < t$. It follows that $B_a(l(1, s))$ by equation (9.2). Intuitively, because nothing happens between s and t_0, and Maxi leaves after t_0, one may conclude $\neg B_a(clipped(s, i, t))$, i.e.,

$$?B_a(clipped(s, i, t)) \; \texttt{fails}.$$

Formally, one can show a query like

$$?B_a(chocolate\text{-}moved(r) \wedge s < r < t)$$

fails, even though the chocolate is actually moved. Indeed, applying equation (9.2)

$$?B_a(chocolate\text{-}moved(r) \wedge s < r < t)$$

reduces to queries such as the following, which all fail:

$$?see_a(\textit{chocolate-moved}(r) \wedge s < r < t)$$

It thus follows that
$$?B_a(\textit{clipped}(s,i,t)) \texttt{ fails.}$$

By inertia (i.e., equation (9.11)), we then have $ded_a(l(1,t))$, whence $B_a(l(1,t))$ by (9.4). Since b can perform the preceding deduction, it follows again by (9.4) that $B_b(B_a(l(1,t)))$. We have already seen in the first part of the argument that therefore $\neg R_b(l(2,t))$, and it follows by clause (9.9) that $\neg ab_b$. We must therefore have $R_b(B_a(l(1,t)))$ by rule (9.8).

9.4.3   Attribution of Beliefs and Closed–World Reasoning in the Younger or Autistic Child

As mentioned in the introduction to this section, in this case b's response rule is effectively of the form

$$B_b(l(i,t)) \rightarrow R_b(l(i,t)), \tag{9.15}$$

i.e., rule (9.7) without the inhibiting condition. In the Maxi task we thus get the response $R_b(l(2,t))$. This response cannot be inhibited: the form of the rule does not even allow b to consider a's information sources. But the effect of the response $R_b(l(2,t))$ is that rule (9.8) is inhibited, whence $R_b(B_a(l(1,t)))$ is not a possible response.

The rule (9.15) may be primitive, or a consequence of failed task comprehension. In the latter case, the child has not yet incorporated rule (9.10), so that closed–world reasoning leads to $\neg ab$. In this case cognitive development may be viewed as relating the variable for an exception in (9.7) to internal theories about mental processing and about the world. The child may also substitute the rule (9.10) with the following theory relating world and information

$$l(i,t) \rightarrow B_a(l(i,t)) \tag{9.16}$$

introducing a short circuit which bypasses the set of principles (9.2) – (9.4), (9.11), and (9.12) and its analogues for other events affecting the chocolate. The rules (9.15) and (9.8) are then no longer in competition, but yield the same answer.

It is also possible that (9.15) arises as a failed neural encoding of a rule of the form (9.7). As in chapter 8, section (8.5), consider what is the neural analogue of having a node $\neg ab$ in a rule like (9.7) (see figure 8.11, repeated here for convenience as figure 9.2). The inhibitory effect of the node $ab = (ab_+, ab_-)$ is captured by the link from ab_- to ab_+: if ab_- fires because it is activated by contextual material, it inhibits the unit ab_+, whence the linked from p to q is blocked. If this inhibitory channel is defective (e.g., because of insufficient inhibitory neurotransmitters such as GABA, see [235]), chances are that the link from p to q is not interrupted, even if the input ab_- is active. In case there is such a deficit, cognitive development may not make much of a difference. The same argument applies to the $\neg B_a(clipped(s, i, t))$ node in the inertial rule (9.11), which is an ab node with more structure built in.

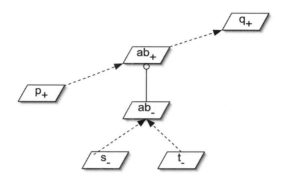

Figure 9.2 The relation between inhibition and abnormalities.

9.4.4   Reasoning in an Unexpected Contents Task

It is of some interest to inquire whether the above analysis extends to the entire family of false–belief tasks. A full treatment would exceed the bounds of this chapter, but as an illustration we sketch the reasoning in the Smarties task, when viewed as a species of closed world reasoning.

We first recapitulate the task at issue. A box of Smarties is emptied, refilled with pencils, and then shown to a child who is ignorant of the change. The child is asked: "What do you think is in the box?" and it answers: "Smarties!" The child is then shown the contents of the box. The pencils are put back into the box, and the child is now asked: "What do you think your [absent] mother will say is in the box?" We may then observe the same critical age: before age 4 the child answers: "Pencils!," whereas after age 4 the child will say: "Smarties!" Also, when asked what she believed was in the box before seeing the actual contents, the younger child will say "Pencils," even though she has just answered "Smarties." Here we are interested in the responses to the second question.

This type of answer seems to be related to the development of episodic memory in children. Young children have no "source memory" for when they have learned a particular piece of information. Parents of 3–year–olds will recognise the calm self-confidence with which the child claims to have "always known" a particular fact she recently learned. In our formalization, source memory is encapsulated in principles such as (9.2), together with closed–world reasoning; if $B_a(p)$, then one of $see_a(p)$, $told_a(p)$, ... must be the case.

We need the following primitive propositions, in addition to the language introduced for the false–belief task:

p: Smarties inside

q: pencils inside

Again we start from an instance of the general response rule (9.1), now indexed to time (compare (9.6)):

$$B_a(\varphi, t) \wedge \neg ab_a(t) \rightarrow R_a(\varphi, t) \tag{9.17}$$

where $B_a(\varphi, t)$ means that agent a has information that φ at time t. Let t_0 be the time of the first question, $t_1 > t_0$ that of the second question. A particular instance of (9.17) is what can be called the prepotent response in this task

$$B_a(q, t_1) \wedge \neg ab_a(t_1) \rightarrow R_a(q, t_1) \tag{9.18}$$

Proper task comprehension requires that the response rule (9.18) is inhibited when the task is to report the subject's belief at time t_0; this is achieved via the inhibitory condition

$$B_a(B_a(p, t_0), t_1) \rightarrow ab_a(t_1). \tag{9.19}$$

As in the false–belief task, the competence response is governed by another instance of rule (9.17), namely

$$B_a(B_a(p, t_0), t_1) \wedge \neg ab'_a(t_1) \rightarrow R_a(B_a(p, t_0), t_1)) \tag{9.20}$$

with the associated inhibitory condition

$$R_a(q, t_1) \rightarrow ab'_{(a)}(t_1). \tag{9.21}$$

The reasoning now proceeds as in the false–belief task. The older child invokes the principle (9.4), relativized to time:

$$ded_a(p, t_0) \rightarrow B_a(p, t_0) \tag{9.22}$$

The child deduces at t_0 that there are Smarties inside the box from the fact that it is a Smarties box. As a consequence she comes to believe that there are Smarties inside: $B_a(p, t_0)$. At the time the second question is asked (t_1), source memory comes into play: the child remembers what she deduced at t_0, so that we get $B_a(ded_a(p, t_0), t_1)$; by monotonicity of B_a (principle (9.5)) it follows that $B_a(B_a(p, t_0), t_1)$. The prepotent response (9.18) is inhibited because of (9.19), whence we get (by closed–world reasoning), $\neg R_a(q, t_1)$ and $\neg ab'(a)(t_1)$. The rule (9.20) now produces the right response.

The younger child may experience several problems. If she has no source memory, i.e., if she does not infer $B_a(ded_a(p, t_0), t_1)$, task-understanding (rule (9.19)) cannot be applied, and the child will give the prepotent response (9.18). The same would happen if the child experiences the difficulties with inhibition outlined in section 9.4.3. Notice that these difficulties are very different. It might well be that the normal child younger than 4 fails the task because of underdeveloped source memory, whereas the autistic child fails it due to problems with inhibition.

9.4.5 What This Analysis of the Child's Reasoning Tells Us

Let us first explain some of our design decisions. The reader might wonder why a task called the "false–belief task" is not analysed logically in terms of one of the several available logics of belief. And indeed the predicate B_a, applied to propositions, acts somewhat like a modal belief operator as used in multiagent epistemic logics (since we need iterated belief operators, for instance, in the clause reflecting task understanding (9.10), and in rule 9.8). The trouble with such an analysis is that, on the one hand, standard axioms for belief such as positive and negative introspection appear to play no role in the derivation of the responses of the two categories of subjects, and on the other hand, the real work in the derivation is done by assumptions concerning the relation of belief and sensory information, concerning persistence of belief over time, and concerning belief reports. In other words, the reasoning is mostly about belief formation, not so much about belief manipulation. For the same reason it does not appear to be very useful to analyse the false–belief task in terms of a possible world semantics for epistemic logic, since such a semantics is concerned with how to get from one belief state to another, which is not the main issue in the false–belief task.

This said, there remain intuitive considerations on the false–belief task which suggest that some sort of modal principle of positive introspection is operative after all. An experiment by Clements and Perner [41] shows that normal 3–year–olds may give the wrong answer in the false–belief task, while simultaneously looking at the right place. Hauser's interesting paper 'Knowing about knowing' [120] glosses this result by saying that these 3–year–olds have (implicit) knowledge about the right response, but no knowledge of their knowledge, i.e., no explicit knowledge. This distinction can be represented by a slight change in the setup. We keep the predicate $R_a(p)$ for "agent a (verbally) reports her belief that p," but introduce a new predicate $A_a(p)$ with the intended meaning "agent a *acts out* her belief that p," for example by looking. We then get two general response schemata instead of the one given as (9.6), namely

$$B_b(\varphi) \wedge \neg ab_b \to A_b(\varphi) \tag{9.23}$$

and

$$B_b(B_b(\varphi)) \wedge \neg ab_b \to R_b(\varphi). \tag{9.24}$$

Only positive introspection leads to congruent answers here. That is, the argument given above for the normal child older than 4 now applies to "acting out" only, i.e., with R_b replaced by A_b everywhere; positive introspection is needed to give the corresponding verbal response.[11]

On the assumption that the analysis captures the processing that is going on in the child's mind, we can isolate the executive and "theory" components in the false–belief task. To start with the latter, the theory component for the normally developing child consists of the rules (9.2), ..., (9.11), (9.12) and its analogues, and the response rule (9.7). If we define executive control generally as concerned with maintaining a goal, and planning, coordination, inhibition, and control of action sequences leading toward that goal, then in this particular task executive control has to maintain the goal "Find out what Maxi's belief state is, and report truthfully," and to set up a sequence of steps leading to this goal. This first involves keeping the linking rule (9.10) active in working memory, and also the goal $?B_a(l(i, t))$. Second, a computation has to be started, regressing from the activated goal; this is essentially the closed–world argument given above. Given the connection between closed–world reasoning and planning, one can see from this analysis that executive function is essentially involved in solving the false–belief task. Inhibiting the prepotent response (9.7) is only one, relatively minor, facet of this involvement.

These two components together explain competent verbal performance in the false–belief task. If one of these is lacking, one may expect wrong answers. If the child does not answer that Maxi believes the chocolate to be in the box, this may thus be due to a failure to maintain the goal, or rule (9.10), in working memory, a failure to apply closed–world reasoning, for instance due to rule (9.16), a failure to grasp inertia (principle (9.11) plus closed–world reasoning),

---

11. The reader may well wonder why we identified B and BB with implicit and explicit belief, respectively. The reason is mainly that matters may be arranged such that $BB\varphi$ implies $B\varphi$, but not conversely, so that, at least formally, BB represents a stronger form of belief. It is possible to give more refined analyses, e.g., in terms of graded modalities, or of Halpern's awareness operator. (See, e.g., [191] for notions not explained here.) Investigations of the neural correlate of the distinction between implicit and explicit belief may well need such a more refined analysis. The reader may think of the neural implementation of the belief operator in the following way. So far we have assumed that outgoing signals always have activation strength 1 (cf. definition 14); this roughly corresponds to the assumption that one is always fully aware of the truth. With a model of the neuron which is less simplified than that of definition 14 one can relax this assumption, and allow output strength to correlate with the number of iterated B's in front of a proposition, or with the strength of the graded modality. Technically, one can do this by making bias nodes amplify the signal emanating from a neuron representing a proposition φ; the meaning of $B\varphi$ is that the bias node is switched on. The principle of positive introspection then says that one type of bias node suffices.

a failure to grasp the connection between sensory input and information state (principles like (9.2) together with closed–world reasoning), or simply having a different primitive response rule replacing (9.7), one which cannot be inhibited, as in (9.15). We know that children below the cut-off age overwhelmingly answer that Maxi believes the chocolate to be in the drawer, whereas a possible answer could also be "anywhere." This reduces the possible causes of the failure to those which generate a response rule which is essentially of the form (9.15). As shown in section 9.4.3 this still leaves several possibilities, from deficient neural encoding of rules to a failure in closed–world reasoning about information sources. That is, the defect could be located at the level of neurotransmitters, at the level of executive function, or at the level of theory of mind; at the moment one cannot say which.

What the analysis also shows is the implausibility of a theory–of–mind *module*, in the sense of an encapsulated piece of neural tissue dedicated exclusively to theory of mind. The force of the set of rules (9.10), (9.2), . . . , (9.11), (9.12) and its analogues comes from combining notions which have to do with mental representation, and notions useful in understanding (and acting in) the natural world, by means of a powerful inference engine operated by executive function. Theory of mind must be viewed as a superstructure built on top of a theory of causality in the world, powered by a theorem prover in executive function.

Although this superstructure is a quite considerable extension, and so could be differentially affected, some researchers have claimed that in autism the foundation itself, the theory of causality, is compromised. This will be discussed next, in section 9.5. We then turn to a more detailed discussion of executive dysfunction in section 9.6, and will provide a formalization of one of its important experimental paradigms, the box task. The formalization of the false belief task reveals formal similarities with the suppression task, a reasoning paradigm much studied in the adult reasoning literature. The box task exhibits even stronger similarities to the suppression task, and this has led us to try the latter task on a population of autistic subjects. The results (see section 9.7) are highly suggestive of a very specific deficit in autism.

9.5   Counterfactual Reasoning

The 'theory of mind deficit' hypothesis lays great stress on normal children's supposed discovery that the mind forms representations of the world and reasons on the basis of these representations. By thus distinguishing between world and representation, there arises the possibility of a mismatch between the two. Some researchers claim that it is in fact this last step, appreciation of the possibility of a mismatch, that is most important:

> . . . the important step taken between 3 and 5 years . . . is not the discovery that the mind is
> a representational device, but rather the appreciation that mental states . . . can be directed

> at situations that the child rules out as part of reality as it stands. This discovery is part
> of a more wide-ranging ability to think about and describe counterfactual substitutes for
> current reality (Harris [117,p. 131]).

In other words, between ages 3 and 5 the child learns to appreciate what philosophers call the *intentional* character of mental states: they are always about something, but that something need not be there.

At first blush, there still is a difference between false–belief reasoning and counterfactual reasoning: the former is more specific in that the child must also appreciate that the intentional character of mental states holds for others as well, whereas this is not necessary for counterfactual reasoning. This suggests that one should fractionate false–belief reasoning into different components, and try to determine experimentally which component is responsible for the observed behavior.

A purely counterfactual version of the false–belief task due to Riggs and Peterson [227] was designed with the purpose of showing that (in normally developing children) indeed failures in counterfactual reasoning lie at the root of unsuccessful performance in the false belief task, as Harris proposed. Briefly, the setup is as follows. In each condition, a false–belief task and a corresponding physical state task based on the same ingredients were constructed. For instance, the analogue of the Maxi task was the following. A child, a mother doll and an experimenter are in a kitchen. The child sees that there is a chocolate in the fridge. The mother doll now bakes a chocolate cake, in the process of which the chocolate moves from fridge to cupboard. The experimenter now asks the child: (*) Where would the chocolate be if mother hadn't baked a cake?

In two of the three experiments, the pattern of answers is highly correlated with that on the false–belief task. Below the cutoff age of 4, the child answers: "in the cupboard"; afterwards, it answers "in the fridge." Apparently there is no theory of mind involved in answering this question correctly; instead one needs insight into the "inertia" of the world: "things only change places when there is an explicit cause." It is interesting to inquire what prompts the younger child to answer "in the cupboard"; a simple failure to apply inertial reasoning might as well lead to the answer "it could be anywhere," say, because of the events that could have happened in this alternative world. Answers such as this would be a consequence of applying causal reasoning without closed–world reasoning for occurrences of events. The answer "in the cupboard" more likely reflects a failure to apply causal reasoning altogether, reverting instead to the prepotent response. It must be noted here that in one of Riggs and Peterson's three experiments, the false–belief task was considerably more difficult for the children than the counterfactual task, which is what one would expect given the analysis of section 9.4. We will return to this issue below, in connection with autistic children's behavior on this task.

We will now restate the previous considerations in terms of the formal machinery introduced for the false–belief task; this will allow a more precise comparison. The main difference with the argument in section 9.4 is that the child now compares two belief states of herself: what she knows to be true and what she is asked to assume. To economize on notation we will not introduce a separate operator for knowledge, and will continue to use B to mark beliefs which are not necessarily true.

The general form of the response rule is now

$$\varphi \wedge \neg ab_{ch} \rightarrow R_{ch}(\varphi) \tag{9.25}$$

where the subscript ch indicates that the rule is applied by the child herself. The substitution instance of interest to us is

$$l(i,t) \wedge \neg ab_{ch} \rightarrow R_{ch}(l(i,t)). \tag{9.26}$$

The analogue of the substitution instance (9.8) is now the simpler

$$B_{ch}(l(i,t)) \wedge \neg ab_{ch} \rightarrow R_{ch}(l(i,t)), \tag{9.27}$$

which comes together with a clause inhibiting (9.26), where $j \neq i$:

$$R_{ch}(l(j,t)) \rightarrow ab_{ch} \tag{9.28}$$

Let $t = 0$ denote the time of the initial situation, $t = 1$ the time of moving the chocolate, $t = 2$ the time of asking question (*). The child is asked to imagine that $chocolate\text{-}moved(1)$ did not occur. Understanding this task amounts to the adoption of the rule

$$\varphi \wedge B_{ch}(\neg \varphi) \rightarrow ab_{ch}, \tag{9.29}$$

which inhibits the child's report of the true situation φ if she pretends to believe $\neg \varphi$. The child may derive by closed–world reasoning that $\neg clipped(0, fridge, 2)$, whence by equation (9.11) $ded_{ch}(l(fridge, 2))$. It follows that $B_{ch}(l(fridge, 2))$, whence the child will report $l(fridge, 2)$ by rule (9.27), if in addition $\neg ab_{ch}$. To establish this latter formula, we have to show (using (9.28)) that $\neg R_{ch}(l(cupboard, 2))$. That the response $R_{ch}(l(cupboard, 2))$, triggered by the rule (9.25), is indeed inhibited, follows from the fact that $l(fridge, 2)$ and $l(cupboard, 2)$ are incompatible, so that $B_{ch}(\neg l(cupboard, 2))$, whence ab_{ch} by 9.29, which inhibits the rule (9.25).

The younger child is again hypothesized not to use (9.25), but to use the uninhibitable prepotent response ((9.25) stripped of $\neg ab_{ch}$) instead, for any of the reasons outlined in section 9.4 (failed task understanding, deficient neural encoding etc.).

If we now compare the two tasks, we see that the reasoning involved is very similar, but that the false–belief task requires a more extensive set of principles. Thus, *failure* on the counterfactual task may be expected to lead to failure on the false–belief task, because in both cases it is the prepotent response that is assumed to be operative, perhaps as a derivative effect. Success on the counterfactual task by itself does not imply success on the false–belief task, because the calculations for the latter involve combining reasoning about information sources, inertial properties, and closed–world reasoning. In this sense false–belief reports are a proper subspecies of counterfactuals, and it would be interesting if they could be shown to be harder for some populations.

There is some experimental evidence which bears on this issue. Peterson and Bowler [215] have compared performance on false–belief tasks and counterfactual tasks in populations of typically developing children, children with severe learning problems, and autistic children. The normal children showed high correlation on these tasks, but a dissociation became apparent in the other two groups. In all groups, those who failed the counterfactual task overwhelmingly failed the false–belief task, suggesting that the kind of reasoning going on in the former is a necessary ingredient of the latter. Seventy-five percent of the typically developing children who pass the counterfactual task also pass the false–belief task, but these percentages get lower in the other groups: 60% in children with learning difficulties, 44% in autistic children. The authors speculate on the additional factors going into a false–belief computation, and suggest that one factor is the necessity to "generate" Maxi's false–belief, whereas in the counterfactual task the false statement is given. They then go on to relate this feature to other supposed failures of generativity in autism, such as the difficulty of spontaneous recall compared to cued recall. While we would not put it in precisely this way, there is something to this distinction, in that in the false–belief task the child has to see the relevance of Maxi's not witnessing the crucial event, for the ensuing computation. In the counterfactual task all the ingredients are given, and only an inertial computation is necessary.

In the next section we shall provide an analysis of the theory which views autism as *executive dysfunction*, that is, as a failure of executive function. We will take one of the experiments illustrating the theory, the box task, and provide a logical analysis to exhibit similarities and differences with the other tasks discussed. This includes the suppression task, whose formal structure will be seen to be very similar to the false–belief task, counterfactual task and box task.

9.6 Executive Dysfunction and the Box Task

As noted above when introducing the concept of executive function, Russell [237] takes as basic the observation that autistic children often exhibit severe perseveration. Executive function is called upon when a plan has to be re-designed by the occurrence of unexpected events which make the original plan unfeasible. Autistic people indeed tend to suffer from rather inflexible planning. Here are two examples, furnished by a single (Aspberger's) patient, to illustrate the phenomenon.

(1) If she wants to go to the supermarket, she must make a shopping list. If she finds items in the supermarket that she needs, but which do not figure on her list, she has to go home, append the needed item to the list, and return to the supermarket. Occasionally she has to go through this loop several times.

(2) She has a fixed route from home to work. If a detour is necessary because of construction work on the road, she does not know what to do, because she has only one plan, whose execution is now thwarted [131,p. 503].

The second example is an instance of the inability to inhibit the prepotent response to a stimulus, even when it is known that the response is inappropriate. This phenomenon is illustrated in an experiment designed by Hughes and Russell [131], the box task, which we have already encountered in chapter 2 (see figure 9.3).

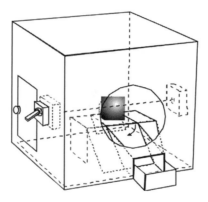

Figure 9.3   Russell's box task

The task is to get the marble which is lying on the platform (the truncated pyramid) inside the box. However, when the subject puts her hand through the opening, a trapdoor in the platform opens and the marble drops out of reach. This is because there is an infrared light beam behind the opening, which, when interrupted, activates the trapdoor mechanism. The switch on the left side of the box deactivates the whole mechanism, so that to get the marble you have to flip the switch first. In the standard setup, the subject is shown how manipulating the switch allows one to retrieve the marble after she has first been tricked by the trapdoor mechanism.

The pattern of results is strikingly similar to that exhibited in the false–belief task: normally developing children master this task by about age 4, and before this age they keep reaching for the marble, even when the marble drops out of reach all the time. Autistic children go on failing this task for a long time. The performance on this task is conceptualized as follows. The natural, "prepotent," plan is to reach directly for the marble, but this plan fails. The child then has to replan, taking into account the information about the switch. After age 4 the normally developing child can indeed integrate this information, that is, inhibit the prepotent response and come up with a new plan. It is hypothesized that autistic people cannot inhibit this prepotent response because of a failure in executive function. But to add precision to this diagnosis we have to dig deeper.

It is important to note here, repeating a point made in chapter 6, that the ability to plan and re-plan when the need arises due to changed context, is fundamental to human cognition, no less fundamental than theory–of–mind abilities. Human beings (and other animals too) act not on the basis of stimulus-response chains, but on the basis of a (possibly distant) goal which they have set themselves. That goal, together with a world model leads to a plan which suffices to reach the goal in the assumed circumstances. But it is impossible to enumerate a priori all events which might possibly form an obstacle in reaching the goal. It is therefore generally wise to keep open the possibility that one has overlooked a precondition, while at the same time not allowing this uncertainty to inhibit one's actions. It is perhaps this flexibility that autistic people are lacking. This point can be reformulated in logical terms. The autistic person's concept of a rule is one in which the consequent invariably follows the antecedent. By contrast, a normal subject's rule is more likely to be of the exception–tolerant variety. Indeed, Russell writes (following a suggestion by Donald Peterson)

> [T]aking what one might call a "defeasibility stance" towards rules is an innate human endowment – and thus one that might be innately lacking . . . . [H]umans appear to possess a capacity – whatever that is – for abandoning one relatively entrenched rule for some novel ad hoc procedure. The claim can be made, therefore, that this capacity is lacking in autism, and it is this that gives rise to failures on "frontal" tasks – not to mention the behavioral rigidity that individuals with the disorder show outside the laboratory [236,p. 318].

Russell goes on to say that one way this theory might be tested is through the implication that children with autism will fail to perform on tasks which require an appreciation of the defeasibility of rules such as "sparrows can fly." This is what we shall do; but to get started we first need a logical description of what goes on in the box task, refining the description given in chapter 2.

9.6.1   Closed–World Reasoning in the Box Task

For the formalization we borrow some self-explanatory notation from the situation calculus.[12] Let c be a variable over contexts, then the primitives are
the predicate $do(a, c)$, meaning "perform action a in context c";
the function $result(a, c)$, which gives the new context after a has been performed in c.

---

12. The situation calculus is a standard formalism in AI. A good reference is Russell and Norvig [238,chapter 10]. Note that these authors use the variable s (for "situation") where we use c (for "context").

The actions we need are g ("grab"), u ("switch up"), d ("switch down"). We furthermore need the following context-dependent properties:
$possess(c)$: the child possesses the marble in c,
$up(c)$: the switch is up in c (= correct position),
$down(c)$: the switch is down in c (= wrong position).

The following equations give the rules appropriate for the box task

$$down(c) \wedge do(u, c) \wedge \neg ab'(c) \rightarrow up(result(u, c)) \qquad (9.30)$$

$$do(g, c) \wedge \neg ab(c) \rightarrow possess(result(g, c)) \qquad (9.31)$$

We first model the reasoning of the normal child older than 4 years. Initially, closed–world reasoning for $ab(c)$ gives $\neg ab(c)$, reducing the rule (9.31) to

$$do(g, c) \rightarrow possess(result(g, c)), \qquad (9.32)$$

which prompts the child to reach for the marble without further ado. After repeated failure, she reverts to the initial rule 9.31, and concludes that after all $ab(c)$. After the demonstration of the role of the switch, she forms the condition

$$down(c) \rightarrow ab(c) \qquad (9.33)$$

. She then applies closed–world reasoning for ab to 9.33, to get

$$down(c) \leftrightarrow ab(c), \qquad (9.34)$$

which transforms rule (9.31) to

$$do(g, c) \wedge up(c) \rightarrow possess(result(g, c)). \qquad (9.35)$$

Define context c_0 by putting $c = result(u, c_0)$ and apply closed–world reasoning to rule (9.30), in the sense that $ab'(c)$ is set to $\perp$ due to lack of further information, and $\rightarrow$ is replaced by $\leftrightarrow$. Finally, we obtain the updated rule, which constitutes a new plan for action

$$down(c_0) \wedge do(u, c_0) \wedge c = result(u, c_0) \wedge do(g, c) \rightarrow possess(result(g, c)) \qquad (9.36)$$

As in the previous tasks, both the normal child younger than 4, and the autistic child are assumed to operate effectively with a rule of the form

$$do(g, c) \rightarrow possess(result(g, c)) \qquad (9.37)$$

which cannot be updated, only replaced in toto by a new rule such as (9.36).

It is tempting to speculate on the computational complexities of both these procedures. Russell wrote that "humans appear to possess a capacity – whatever that is – for abandoning one relatively entrenched rule for some novel ad hoc procedure [236,p. 318]." The preceding considerations suggest that "abandoning one relatively entrenched rule" may indeed be costly, but that normal humans get around this by representing the rule in such a way that it can be easily updated. It is instructive to look at the computation that the normal child older than 4 is hypothesized to be performing. The only costly step appears to be the synthesis of the rule (9.33); the rest is straightforward logic programming which, as we have seen in chapter 8, can proceed automatically. The rule (9.31) is never abandoned; a new rule is derived without having to ditch (9.31) first.

To close this discussion, we compare the false–belief task to the box task from the point of view of the formal analysis. The tasks are similar in that for a successful solution one must start from rules of the form $p \wedge \neg ab \rightarrow q$, identify conditions which constitute an abnormality, and apply closed–world reasoning; and also that in both cases a failure of ab to exercise its inhibitory function leads to the inability to inhibit the prepotent response. A difference is that in the false–belief task, one needs a "theory" relating ab to sensory, or inferred, information via clauses such as $see_a(l(i,t)) \rightarrow B_a(l(i,t))$, $\neg B_a(l(i,t)) \rightarrow ab_a(i,t)$, etc., whereas it suffices to operate with rules for actions in the box task.

9.6.2   The Suppression Task as a Formal Analogue of the Box Task

The reader who has followed the above computation will have noticed its striking similarity to the essential step in our derivation of the suppression effect as a form of closed–world reasoning. Given the formal analogy between the box task and the suppression task, we were led to expect that autistic people have a very specific difficulty with closed world reasoning about exceptions. This should show up in a refusal to suppress the inferences MP and MT, in case the second conditional premise is of the additional type. To show that the problem is really specific to exceptions, and not a problem about integrating new information, or with closed–world reasoning generally, one may compare autistic people's reasoning with AC and DA,. In these cases, suppression of the inference by addition of an alternative motivation, for example, is independent of exception handling. Here one would expect behavior which is comparable to normals. One must thus distinguish two forms of closed–world reasoning that play a role here. On the one hand there is closed–world reasoning applied to abnormalities or exceptions, which takes the form: "assume only those exceptions occur which are explicitly listed." On the other hand there is closed–world reasoning applied to rules which takes the form of diagnostic reasoning: "if B has occurred and the only known rules with B as consequent are $A_1 \rightarrow B, \ldots, A_n \rightarrow B$, then assume one of $A_1, \ldots, A_n$ has occurred." These forms of closed–world reasoning are in principle independent, and in our autistic population we indeed observed a dissociation between the two.

9.7 Autists' Performance in the Suppression Task

In order to test these hypotheses, formulated generally as

(1)   Autistic people can apply closed–world reasoning, but have a decreased ability in handling exceptions to rules.

Smid [250] conducted an experiment on a population of six autistic subjects (young adults) with normal intelligence (IQ > 85) and language abilities from a psychiatric hospital in Vught (Netherlands). The tests administered to the subjects involved a false belief task (the Smarties task[13]) propositional reasoning with two premises (MP, MT, etc.), the Wason selection task, the suppression task, reasoning with prototypes, and analogical reasoning. The method consisted in engaging in tutorial dialogues with the subjects.

The data strongly suggested that in autistic people there is indeed a dissociation between the two forms of closed–world reasoning. As predicted, suppression of fallacies (DA and AC) with an alternative premise did occur and the percentages we found are roughly the same as those found in research with normal subjects. Suppression of MP, by contrast, was much rarer in our subjects than in normals. In the dialogues, subjects often ignored the additional premise completely in their overt reasoning. With regard to suppression of MT the results were less dramatic, and harder to interpret, in particular because the rate of endorsement for MT with an alternative premise is somewhat higher than that for the base case. Nevertheless, the percentage of MT conclusions drawn in problems with an additional premise is higher than for the normal subjects – autistic subjects are not suppressing. What is of especial relevance is that the experimenter's interventions, pointing to the possible relevance of the additional conditional premise, had no effect. Another finding in the dialogues that deserves to be noticed is the diverse and sometimes unusual interpretation of the conditional. Particularly the hypothetical character of the antecedent appears to be hard to represent; for instance, subjects sometimes take the antecedent as stating something which is the case.

While suggestive, the data from this experiment were obtained in a small population and so lacked statistical significance. The experiment was redone on a much larger scale at the F.C. Donders Centre for Cognitive Neuroimaging (Nijmegen, Netherlands).[14] The experimental group consisted of twenty-eight autistic individuals, who were tested also on a standard battery of neuropsychological tests. The control group consisted of twenty-eight subjects, each matched to a unique autistic subject with respect to intelligence and verbal mental age. The reasoning problems were presented as a list of two or three premises, followed by the question: "is [conclusion] true?" where the allowed

---

13. Five out of six subjects performed normally on this task.
14. The experimenter is Judith Pijnacker, who kindly gave permission to include some of her data here.

answers were yes, no or maybe. Table 9.1 gives the percentages, the prefixes a-indicating the autistic population, and c- the controls. We discuss some salient features of this table.

With regard to the two-premise inference patterns MP, MT, AC, and DA, this study found an unexpected difference between the groups: in all four inference patterns the autistic subjects volunteered significantly more maybe answers.[15] Given this result, it is somewhat surprising that there is no significant difference between the groups in rate of endorsement of MP, of MT, and of AC.[16] In the case of DA, inspection of the table shows there is a difference in rate of endorsement between the groups; in fact this difference approaches significance ($p = .054$).

Turning to the three premise arguments, results are almost as expected. In MP$_{add}$, autistic subjects answer yes significantly more often than controls ($p = .011$), while in MT$_{add}$ the autistic subjects answered no more often, although the difference only approaches significance ($p = .066$). For MP$_{alt}$ and MT$_{alt}$ there are no significant differences between the two groups, nor are there among AC$_{alt}$, AC$_{add}$, DA$_{add}$, and DA$_{alt}$.[17]

These observations lend some support to the hypothesis (1), that it is specifically processing exceptions that creates difficulties for autistic subjects.[18] DA and AC showed the pattern familiar from normals, suggesting that this type of closed–world reasoning, where exceptions do not figure, presents no atypical difficulties. The behavior in MP and MT conditions (especially the former), where implicit exceptions need to be acknowledged to achieve suppression, was different from normals, showing much less suppression. Moreover, the tutorial dialogues show that nonsuppression in MP$_{add}$ and MT$_{add}$ is caused by a total disregard of the additional premise, even though these same subjects had no trouble incorporating the alternative premise in AC$_{alt}$ and DA$_{alt}$. We have seen in chapter 7 that nonsuppression may be due as well to a form of nonmonotonic reasoning: introducing, for example, "the library is closed" as a presupposition. The dialogues with the autistic subjects do not show this pattern; here nonsuppression is due to rigid rule following, and the experimenter's attempts

---

15. The full results are as follows – MP: $p = .031$; MT: $p = .011$; AC: $p = .040$; DA: $p = .059$. (Strictly speaking, of course, the result for DA only approaches significance.) The fact that there are more "maybes" in all four conditions suggests that the increased frequency is not related to the logical properties of these argument patterns.

16. MP: $p = .156$; MT: $p = .091$; AC: $p = .078$.

17. In this experiment also reaction times were measured. One interesting finding is that in both groups the 'fallacial' responses of the type AC and DA were given significantly faster than the answers dictated by the classical logic. Perhaps there is a relation here with the straightforward neural implementability of closed–world reasoning discussed in chapter 8.

18. The behavioral task whose outcome is given in table 9.1 is actually a prelude to an ERP experiment involving the suppression task. Very roughly speaking, the prediction is that upon presentation of the additional premise in MP$_{add}$, controls show the characteristic 'surprise response' called the N400 (see Kutas and Hillyard [166] for definition and discussion), whereas this response will be much less in evidence in autistic subjects.

Table 9.1   Results on suppression task in autists (n=28) and matched controls (n=28)

argument	a-yes	a-no	a-maybe	c-yes	c-no	c-maybe
MP	89.0	0.0	10.4	96.1	2.5	1.4
MP_{add}	71.0	1.1	28.9	51.1	0.7	48.2
MP_{alt}	92.9	0.4	6.7	97.5	0.7	1.8
MT	1.4	79.6	19.0	2.5	92.8	4.7
MT_{add}	0.7	62.1	37.2	0.7	45.0	54.3
MT_{alt}	0.4	90.3	9.3	1.1	95.0	3.9
AC	45.0	1.1	53.9	67.1	2.1	30.8
AC_{add}	28.1	1.1	70.9	35.7	0.0	64.3
AC_{alt}	12.2	2.2	85.6	9.6	0.0	90.4
DA	1.1	48.0	50.9	0.4	69.1	30.5
DA_{add}	2.9	28.9	68.2	2.5	33.6	63.9
DA_{alt}	3.2	15.7	81.1	1.1	10.4	88.5

to induce some flexibility were to no avail. [19]

9.8   Dialogue Data

We now present some conversations with subjects from the experiment conducted by Smid [250] while they were engaged in the suppression task. The subjects were presented with either two or three premises, and were asked whether another sentence was true, false, or undecided. We then proceeded to ask them for a justification of their answer.

The first example gives something of the flavor of the dialogues. We see subject A engaged in MT with three premises, having refused to endorse MT in the two-premise case. The excerpt is interesting because the subject explicitly engages with the possibility of exceptions.

If Marian has an essay to write she will study late in the library.
(*) If the library stays open then Marian will study late in the library.
Marian will not study late in the library.
Does Marian have an essay?

A: It says here that if she has an essay, she studies late in the library.... But she doesn't study late in the library ... which suggests that she doesn't have an essay ... But it could be that she has to leave early, or that something else came up ... *if you only look at the given data*, she will not write an essay ... but when you realise that something unexpected has come up, then it is very well possible that she does have to write an essay ... [our italics] [250,p. 88ff]

---

19. For an analogous use of the logical framework to predict discourse processing style in children with ADHD , see [267].

The sentence beginning "But it could be that ... " suggests considerations of possible exceptions; the italicized phrase looks like closed–world reasoning applied to these exceptions. The interesting point is that the information in (*) is nowhere integrated; the step *library-closed* $\rightarrow$ *ab* is not made.

9.8.1 Excerpts from Dialogues: MP

We recall the argument:

> If Marian has an essay to write she will study late in the library.
> (*) If the library stays open then Marian will study late in the library.
> Marian has an essay to write.
> Does Marian study late in the library?

Here is subject C, first engaged in the two-premise case, i.e., without (*):

> C: But that's what it says!
> E: What?
> C: If she has an essay then she studies.
> E: So your answer is "yes"?
> C: Yes.

The same subject engaged in the three-premise argument:

> C. *Yes*, she studies late in the library.
> E. Eh, why?
> C. Because she *has to write* an essay.

Clearly the possible exception highlighted by the second conditional is not integrated; the emphasis shows that the first conditional completely overrides the second.

9.8.2 Excerpts from Dialogues: MT

In this case the argument pattern is

> If Marian has an essay to write she will study late in the library.
> (*) If the library stays open then Marian will study late in the library.
> Marian will not study late in the library.
> Does Marian have an essay?

Here is again subject C:

> C. No, she has ... oh no, wait a minute ... this is a bit strange isn't it?
> E. Why?
> C. Well, it says here: if she *has to write* an essay ... And I'm asked whether she has to write an essay?
> E. Mmm.
> C. I don't think so.

This is probably evidence of the general difficulty of MT, but note that the second conditional does not enter into the deliberations. In the dialogue, E then prompts C to look at second conditional, but this has no effect: C sticks to his choice.

Here is a good example of the way in which a subject (in this case B) can be impervious to the suggestions of the experimenter. The dialogue refers to the argument with three premises; we give a rather long abstract to show the flavor of the conversations.

B: No. Because if she had to make an essay, she would study in the library.
E: Hmm.
B: And she doesn't do this, so she doesn't have an essay.
E: Yes.
B: And this means ... [inaudible]
E: [laughs] But suppose she has an essay, but the library is closed?
B: Ah, that's also possible.
E: Well, I'm only asking.
B: Well, according to these two sentences that's not possible, I think.
E: How do you mean?
B: Ehm, yes she just studies late in the library if she has an essay.
E: Hmm.
B: And it does not say "if it's open, or closed ..."
E: OK.
B: So according to these sentences, I know it sounds weird, but ....
E: Yes, I ...
B: I know it sounds rather autistic what I'm saying now [laughs].
E: [laughs]
B: Eh yes.
E: So it is like you said? Or perhaps that she ...
B: Yes, perhaps the library closes earlier?
E: You may say what you want! You don't have to try to think of what should be the correct answer!
B: OK, no, then I'll stick to my first answer.
E: OK, yes.
B: [laughs] I know it's not like this, but [laughs].
E: Well, that's not clear. It's possible to say different things about reasoning here, and what you say is certainly not incorrect.

In the above we have seen examples of how our autistic subjects refuse to integrate the information about exceptions provided by (*). The next extracts show that this need not be because they are incapable of integrating a second conditional premise, or of applying closed–world reasoning. We here consider the "fallacies" DA and AC, which can be valid if seen as a consequence of closed–world reasoning, and which can be suppressed by supplying a suitable second conditional premise, e.g., (†) below.

9.8.3   Excerpts from Dialogues: AC

The argument is

> If Marian has an essay to write she will study late in the library.
> (†) If Marian has an exam, she will study late in the library.
> Marian studies late in the library.
> Does Marian have an essay?

Here is subject C, in the two-premise argument without (†).

> C: Yes.
> E: Why?
> C: It says in the first sentence "if she has an essay then she does that [study late etc.]"
> … But Marian is just a name, it might as well be Fred.

Now consider the three-premise case.

> C: Mmm. Again "if," isn't it?
> E: Yes.
> C: If Marian has an essay, she studies late in the library…
> E: Yes.
> C: If Marian has an exam, she studies late in the library …
> E: Hmm.
> C: Marian studies late in the library. Does Marian have an essay?
> E: Hmm.
> C: No.
> E: Hmm.
> C: It does not say she has to make an essay.
> E: Hmm. But she studies late in the library, can you conclude from this that she has to make an essay?
> C: No you can't, because she could also have an exam.

We see in this example that C correctly judges the import of (†): after having applied closed–world reasoning to the two-premise case, he notices that it is powerless in this case.

9.9   A Similar Task with very Different Outcomes

After having explained the importance of defeasible reasoning for the study of autism, Russell was forced to add a caveat. The box task is superficially similar to another task devised by Russell, the tubes task (depicted in figure 9.4), but performance on the latter task is very different from that on the former.

What one sees in the schematic drawing in figure 9.4 is a series of six holes into which a ball can be dropped, to land in a small container below. A ball dropped through the leftmost opening will end up in the catch tray directly underneath, but a ball dropped through the opening which is second from left travels through an opaque tube to end up in the catch tray which is third from

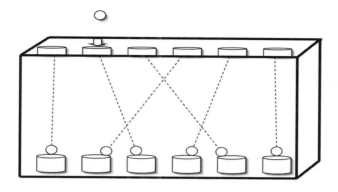

Figure 9.4 Schematic drawing of the tubes task.

left. The child sees the ball being dropped through an opening, and has to retrieve it from one of the catch trays below. When the ball is dropped in the second from left opening, children of age 3 or younger tend to look in the catch tray directly underneath the opening, probably applying the (defeasible) rule that things fall vertically. Older children, *including also autistic children*, manage to inhibit the "prepotent" response and search in the correct catch tray, adequately representing the trajectory of the ball as guided by the tube.

The apparent puzzle posed by performance on this task is that in this case also autistic children older than 3 are able to switch rules effortlessly. Russell originally explained this by a distinction between "arbitrary" rules imposed by the experimenter (as in the box task), and rules based on fairly transparent physical principles (as in the tubes task). Autistic children would be impaired on the former but not the latter, incidentally showing that autism, viewed as executive dysfunction, must be a rather specific executive deficit. If both kinds of defeasible rules require the same kind of closed–world reasoning about abnormalities, the hypothesis that it is this form of reasoning that is difficult for autistic subjects is defeated.

The first thing to observe here is that the rules involved in the two tasks have different logical forms, and so require different reasoning. In the box task, correct performance hinges on the ability to amend the *antecedent* of the rule, whereas in the case of the tubes task it is the consequent (i.e., the catch tray) that has to be changed. In the box task, the original plan has to be changed by incorporating another action, whereas in the case of the tubes task one action has to be replaced by another. This suggests that what happens in the tubes task need not be viewed as rule switching, but can also been seen as the application of a *single* IF-THEN-ELSE rule, where the action to be taken depends on the satisfaction or not of an explicit precondition: unimpeded fall of the ball. On this analysis, the difference between box and tubes task would be that the former forces synthesizing a new rule on the spot by exception handling, whereas in the latter case the switch is between components of a single rule.

The experimental literature shows that autistic subjects have less difficulty with synthesizing an IF-THEN-ELSE rule from instructions shown to them, than with rule construction by exception handling. Indeed, a standard Go/No Go task is of the IF-THEN-ELSE form. For instance, in one such task, subjects were shown different letters of the alphabet that flashed one at a time on a computer screen. They were asked to respond by pressing a key in every case except when they saw the letter X. The first task was a Go task, in which the letter X never appeared and in this way subjects were allowed to build up a tendency to respond. Immediately afterward, subjects performed a Go/No Go task in which the letter X did appear in the lineup, at which point the subject had to control the previously built-up response tendency. Autistic subjects are not particularly impaired at such a task,[20] although they do become confused when they have to shift rapidly between one target stimulus and another (Ozonoff et al. [208]). At a more abstract level, what the analysis of the empirical difference between the box and tubes tasks just given highlights is that, before one can discuss whether autistic subjects have difficulties with rule switching, the proper definition of "rule" in this context has to be clarified. If the preceding considerations are correct, then autistic subjects can be successful with rules more general than the "condition–action" format.

9.9.1   The 'A not B' Task

The above method of analysis is actually a general scheme for the analysis of executive tasks,[21] as we will illustrate here using Piaget's famous 'A not B' task, for which see Baillargeon [10] and the references given therein. Suppose one shows a child between ages 1 and 2 two opaque screens, A and B, and suppose furthermore one hides a toy behind A. The child is asked to retrieve the toy. Once she successfully and repeatedly retrieves the toy behind A, the experimenter switches sides, hiding it behind screen B. Surprisingly, the child searches behind A, not behind B, and keeps doing so over many trials. This looks like the building up of a prepotent response, but as Hauser [120] observes, it is a response tendency built up by the actual reaching, not by the bare fact that the toy was observed to go behind A.

> If an experimenter repeatedly hides and then reveals the object behind A, but doesn't allow the child to search until the switch trial to B, the child shows no deficit, searching

---

20. In contrast, for example, to ADHD kids.
21. See [267] for an elaboration of this point.

right away at B. This shows that actively searching is crucial; simply observing passively, is not.[120,p. 4]

In a further twist reminiscent of Clements and Perner's observation of the dissociation between verbal and nonverbal responses in the false–belief task (see section 9.4.5), it was observed that sometimes a child will *look* at the B screen even when reaching for the A screen. However, in this case there is clearly a dissociation within the nonverbal domain, one between looking and reaching. We will now formalise this task, again using exception-tolerant rules allowing inhibition, as we did above.

We refer to the screens as s_1 and s_2, and use B for "belief." As in the Smarties task, a single B will stand for implicit knowledge, whereas the iterated BB represents explicit knowledge. We assume the child knows implicitly that the toy is either behind s_1 or behind s_2: $B(toy\text{-}at(s_1) \vee toy\text{-}at(s_2))$, and that she either (implicitly) knows that the toy is behind s_i or (implicitly) knows that it isn't: $B(toy\text{-}at(s_i)) \vee \neg B(toy\text{-}at(s_i))$. From these assumptions it follows that $\neg B(toy\text{-}at(s_i)) \rightarrow B(toy\text{-}at(s_j))$ for $i \neq j$. The following rules then describe the task, incorporating the distinction between looking (9.38,9.39) and reaching (9.40,9.42). We use $intention(toy)$ to express that the child has the intention to get the toy.

The first set describes the looking response, in which the child looks at the correct screen even when reaching for the wrong screen; this response is supposed to be driven by implicit knowledge.

$$intention(toy) \wedge \neg ab_i \rightarrow look(s_i) \qquad (9.38)$$

$$\neg B(toy\text{-}at(s_i)) \rightarrow ab_i \qquad (9.39)$$

If the child has implicit knowledge that the toy is at s_2, i.e., $B(toy\text{-}at(s_2))$, it follows that $\neg B(toy\text{-}at(s_1))$, whence ab_1, so that closed–world reasoning shows she does not look at s_1. That she must look at s_2 follows because $B(toy\text{-}at(s_2))$ implies $\neg ab_2$, whence $look(s_2)$.

The second set describes the grasp response, where the difference with the previous set is that now explicit knowledge, i.e., iteration of the belief operator, is needed to generate the correct response. The observation that it is the reaching system that builds up the prepotent response is reflected in the abnormality conditions, which are asymmetric, in contrast to the previous case.

$$intention(toy) \wedge \neg ab_i' \rightarrow reach(s_i) \qquad (9.40)$$

$$reach(s_2) \rightarrow ab_1' \qquad (9.41)$$

$$\neg BB(toy\text{-}at(s_2)) \rightarrow ab_2' \qquad (9.42)$$

In this case, if positive introspection fails, it may happen that $B(toy\text{-}at(s_2))$ but not $BB(toy\text{-}at(s_2))$. It follows that ab_2', whence $\neg reach(s_2)$ and by closed–

world reasoning $\neg ab'_1$, so that we must have $reach(s_1)$. If the child has positive introspection, $B(toy\text{-}at(s_2))$ implies $BB(toy\text{-}at(s_2))$, whence by closed–world reasoning $\neg ab'_2$ and $reach(s_2)$.

The analyses just given hinge on the difference between implicit and explicit knowledge, i.e., between $B(toy\text{-}at(s_2))$ and $BB(toy\text{-}at(s_2))$. A neural interpretation of this difference was given in footnote 11 (this chapter). Applied to this case, that interpretation implies that the signals governing the looking response can be of weaker strength than that governing the reaching response. Indeed, the A not B task shows differentiation of an attentional system (looking) from an action system (pointing). There is evidence of a different time scale for registration of learning episodes in the two systems – the pointing system lagging behind the looking system at least in this context. The degree of organization required for information to control the attentional system is clearly less than for the action system. To put this in slightly different terms, the young child "knows" it can get things done by acting, not just by looking, and therefore the responses built up by the reaching system are at first stronger than that built up by the attentional system. An equilibrium between the two systems is reached only later.

9.10   Summing up the Cognitive Analyses

We can now briefly discuss what can be said about the various explanations for autism, based on experimental data and logical analysis.

At first sight, the analyses presented here appear to have little relevance for the assessment of Hobson's "affective foundation" theory, although they do raise important general questions about the relation between cognition and affect, which are relevant to assessing the relation between Hobson's theories and cognitive accounts. Most specifically, planning logics incorporate reasoning goals within their accounts of reasoning in a way which classical logic does not. Goals are part of motivation, and motivation is intimately related to affect.[22] There has, for example, been much discussion recently of defects of reasoning which can be understood as abnormalities of motivation (see, for example, Damasio [55]). Inasmuch as reasoning and motivation for reasoning can be separated, these patients (also with frontal lobe damage and executive function deficits) have intact reasoning but defective motivation for reasoning. They seem to "discount the future" in assessing the relevance of lines of reasoning. Damasio cites a patient who is trying to decide whether or not to enter into a business relationship with the arch enemy of his best friend. The patient

---

22. Less specifically, there are issues about how we are to conceptualise the implementations of logical systems in the mind. Stenning [258,p. 266ff.] has argued that affective reactions are as much implementations of aspects of logical reasoning systems as is cold calculative machinery. The particular case of the affective element of "cheating detection" is taken as an example.

enters into an elaborate calculation of costs and benefits which would normally be pruned from the reasoning space by emotional rejection. This sounds not a million miles from some aspects of autistic people's failure to empathise.

There are somewhat more specific things to say about Frith and Happé's weak central coherence theory. The computations involved in the false–belief task seem to call for some kind of central processor, because they combine ingredients from different "domains," in particular reasoning about information and mental states, and reasoning about inertial properties of the world.[23] We have seen that decoupling these domains, for whatever reason, leads to anomalous behavior on the false–belief task. Perhaps, then, weak central coherence fosters this decoupling. The weak central coherence theory is all about attention and its distribution. Attention is controlled by motivation even if attention may be interrupted bottom–up by environmental events whose motivational significance then has to be assessed. Autistic motivation and attention appear to be gripped by detail, and difficult to shift.

One of the contributions of affect to cognition is its capacity for abstraction (Stenning [258,p. 217ff.]). Although we often think of emotion as being a concrete reaction (for example, experienced in the gut), affect is peculiarly abstract in that the same affective state can be a response to almost any object, state, or event, given the right circumstances. Stenning [258,p. 203ff.] argues that affective mappings are the wellspring of our earliest analogical recognition. Perhaps the decoupling highlighted by weak central coherence theory is related to the affective abnormalities which are the basis of Hobson's theory.

The most specific comparisons are between the theories which propose theory–of–mind failure and executive dysfunction. In making this comparison, we draw on a survey paper by Perner and Lang [211], who suggest five possible relationships between these theories:

1. Executive control depends upon theory of mind.

2. Theory–of–mind development depends upon executive control.

3. The relevant theory of mind tasks require executive control.

4. Both kinds of tasks require the same kind of conditional reasoning.

5. Theory of mind and executive control involve the same brain region.

We discuss each of these except the last (since so little is known), and evaluate them in the light of the foregoing considerations.

---

23. One should not take "central processor" too literally. The importance of the neural implementation of default reasoning is precisely that it shows how reasoning can be "distributed" across a network, though the network itself may be operating as a central processor relative to some peripheral systems.

Executive Control Derives from Theory of Mind

Perner and Lang suggested that both theory–of–mind and executive inhibition tasks require the child to appreciate the causal power of mental states to initiate action. This is clear in the false–belief task. In the case of executive inhibition, such as found in the box task, the child would need to see that the mental picture of the apparently fully accessible marble causes her to make the unsuccessful reaching movement. Thus there would be a common mental factor underlying both types of tasks.

This conceptualization suffers from an unduly narrow view of executive control as concerned only with inhibition. Even if Perner and Lang's invocation of mental causation would apply to inhibition, it is not clear at all how it could explain the closed–world reasoning, in other words the planning, that takes place during the computations.

Theory of Mind Essentially Requires Executive Control

Under this heading we will discuss both 2 and 3 from our list above. Russell suggested that self monitoring (as part of executive control) is a prerequisite of self awareness, which is in turn necessary for the development of ToM. Less strongly, false belief tasks would all involve an executive component in that a prepotent response has to be inhibited. Perner and Lang claim that there are versions of the false–belief task which do not involve inhibiting a prepotent response. One example is the "explanation task," which (translated to the language of our running example) runs like this: when Maxi returns to the room, he looks for his chocolate in the (empty) box. The child is then asked why he is doing this. Children above the cutoff age give the correct explanation, whereas younger children appear to guess. The authors claim that this is in marked contrast to the standard task, where these children consistently answer "in the drawer," thus showing that no (failed inhibition of the) prepotent response is operative in the explanation task.

Here one may well wonder what the younger children can do except guessing, given that Maxi is looking in what is (according to the child) evidently the wrong place. It is precisely because the prepotent response is not inhibited that the child must guess.

Defective Conditional Reasoning as a Root Failure in Autism

In their survey, Perner and Lang here refer to work by Frye, Zelazo, and Palfai [89], who claim that all the relevant tasks can be formalized as reasoning with *embedded* conditionals of the form

$$\texttt{if } p \texttt{ then (if } q \texttt{ then } r \texttt{ else } r') \texttt{ else} \ldots$$

The difficulty with embedded conditionals is then presumably that they put heavy computational demands on working memory.

Unfortunately there are two serious problems with the proposed explanation. The first is that conditionals such as the above do not involve embedding essentially, since they can be rephrased as

$$(\text{if } p \text{ and } q \text{ then } r) \text{ and } (\text{if } p \text{ and not-}q \text{ then } r') \text{ and } (\text{if not-}p\ldots)$$

Thus the embedded conditionals can be replaced by a conjunction of noniterated conditionals, where the antecedents enumerate the various possibilities: $p \wedge q, p \wedge \neg q, \neg p \wedge q, \ldots$ Indeed, avoidance of iterated conditionals that cannot be eliminated by such conjunctive paraphrase seems to be a general tendency in natural languages. The description in terms of a conjunction of conditionals is more systematic and probably quite easy to code into working memory; although perhaps some people never re-represent the embedded conditional into this simpler form.

Furthermore, while it is readily apparent that the logical form of card–sorting tasks can be given in this way, the application to false–belief tasks, via rules such as

if the question is from Maxi's perspective then (if he is looking for his chocolate then predict that he goes to the cupboard) ...

is much more dubious. In the case of a card–sorting task, or a Go/No Go task, the embedded conditional is provided by the experimenter, and autistic subjects have no difficulty with this as long as the nesting (i.e., the number of different antecedents) is not too deep. But the whole problem with the other tasks is that the subject has to synthesise the relevant rules herself, for instance by means of the closed–world reasoning illustrated here.

It will be clear, however, from the analyses presented in this chapter that we fully endorse the view that all these tasks are ultimately about conditional reasoning, once a more reasonable concept of conditional is adopted. Thus, our considered view of the relation between theory of mind and executive function is a combination of (3) and (4): theory of mind is built on top of executive function, and all tasks ultimately reduce to applying closed–world reasoning to suitable sets of conditionals.

9.11   The Biological Setting of Autism

We will end this chapter with some biological background to autism and with a discussion of its possible significance in evolutionary analyses. We do this for two reasons. First, in discussing logical accounts of reasoning tasks which diagnose autism, it would be easy to leave the reader with the picture that autism is the result of a few implementations of logical rules going awry – that is certainly not our position. We present this biological background to give some idea of what may be involved in understanding the relation between our "neural" model and its brain implementation. Second, autism offers an opportunity to elaborate our conjectural account of the part played by altriciality in cognitive evolution given in chapter 6, section 6.5. Remember, the main purpose of that conjecture was to offer an alternative way of thinking about cognitive evolution from the approaches which dominate evolutionary psychology. We emphasized the importance of changes in timing of developmental processes. Whether our conjectures about autism turn out to be true or wild, they can serve to illustrate what we claim is a more reasonable general biological approach.

In chapter 6, we introduced altriciality as an important example of a biological innovation, which is a good candidate for playing an organizing role in many of the changes responsible for the emergence of humans and their minds. *Homo sapiens* is an altricial species – it is born at an immature stage with regard to a whole host of features. The changed pattern of timing of maturation persists long after birth. Biological adolescence as a delay of sexual maturity is a related human innovation. The growth of neural tissue in the frontal cortex is now understood to continue until about the age of 20. These are uncontested biological innovations of humans relative to their immediate ancestors.

We believe that autism can insightfully be considered as a disturbance of the timings of developmental processes. Autism is therefore particularly relevant to our more general effort to interpret human cognitive evolution in the light of changes in the temporal patterning of development. To take one example, it has often been reported that autistic children have rather large heads, typically about 15% to 40% having macrocephaly, defined as a head circumference greater than two standard deviations above the mean [193]. Although many conflicting reports of data have appeared, macrocephaly is one of the most often reported gross correlates of autism spectrum disorders. Even more interesting for our concerns with changes in timing is that the conflicts appear to arise because autistic children have a changed temporal profile of head growth (see figure 9.5).

The difficulty of getting data on early head circumference growth is that autistic children are often not diagnosed until about the age of 2 years. But retrospective studies indicate that the head growth profile of those subsequently diagnosed as autistic is even more surprising [225]. As can be seen in the figure, at birth they have *smaller* heads than average, but by 1 year their heads are substantially larger than average, and by 2 years this growth spurt is leveling off. By adulthood, the normal population has caught up (not shown). Several studies [62, 271] have reported that it is particularly *accelerated brain growth* rather than absolute size that correlates with autistic symptoms. However, their results show *better* cognitive function (relative to autistic peers) with growth

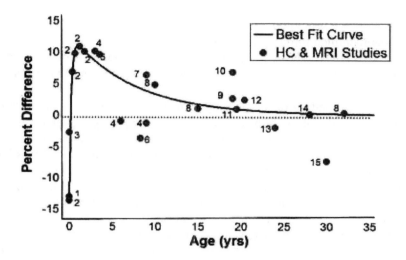

Figure 9.5   Head circumference (HC) and magnetic resonance imaging (MRI) percent difference (%Diff) by age. %Diff values from all HC and MRI studies are plotted by the mean age of the study. The best fitted curve shows the most rapid rates of increased deviation from normal brain size in autism within first year of life and the greatest rates of decrease in deviation from normal during middle and late childhood. Study number is given next to each percent difference value. HC, head circumference; MRI, magnetic resonance imaging. (Reprinted from [225,Figure 1, p. 5] by permission of the Society of Biological Psychiatry.)

spurts, whereas the analysis of Courchesne et al. indicates *worse* behavioral deficits. It is as well to note that macrocephaly is common in other related psychiatric categories such as ADHD [97, 94]. Since macrocephaly is normally given an extreme definition, and since temporal profile data from longitudinal studies are not available, it is hard to say how many autistic spectrum children exhibit brain growth spurts, but from the figures available it *could* be a very considerable proportion.

Some possible genetic determinants or concommitants of this pattern of head growth are surfacing. [197] following up work by [45] and [138] have shown that the gene HOXA1 appears to be both related to autism, and a controller for head growth rates in some normal populations as well as autistic ones. Children with at least one g allele of this gene show more rapid head growth than those without, whereas the a allele is associated with an increased suceptibility to autism. The head growth rate is not associated with larger heads in adults—it is a growth rate difference. HOXA1 is a member of the homeobox family of highly conserved genes responsible for laying down the 'body plan' of organisms. Its particular influence is on the differentiation of head from body, and its main known effects are seen in innervation of posterior portions of the head. It is therefore related to another well-known homeobox gene, FOXP2. which was identified through the disruption of articulation in a family with a mutated form [181]. These are genes close to the foundations of the modern "evo devo" understanding of relations between development and evolution (see section 6.2.4).

This disturbed pattern of the phasing of head growth prompts the possibly wild speculation that it might be an adaptation to the problems of human birth as discussed in chapter 6, and argued there to be the focus of major evolutionary changes in the period of emergence of modern human cognition. Perhaps having a slightly smaller head at birth and compensatnig with accelerated gowth thereafter is one contribution to safer birth. Perhaps some autistic children have overdone such an adaptation. Regardless of how this speculation fares, here is clear evidence of changed temporal patterning of a developmental process with pervasive effects on brain development and consequent behavior [123]. At the very least we can organise our enquiries into the autistic brain around the question of how this grossly changed pattern of head growth relates to neural developmental processes.

We will now explore two avenues that lead from viewing autism as a change in the temporal pattern of development. First we seek to link these observations of the timing of brain development, through executive function interpretations of autism, to our neural implementations of closed–world reasoning in chapter 8. Second, we will review some of what is known about the genetics of autism, which will serve to further link autism, through the phenomenon of genetic imprinting, to our organizing theme of altriciality in human evolution. What follows is rather dense neuroscience and we do not claim more than amateur status here. Nor could we reasonably expect readers to be or become experts. Until rather recently we too were skeptical ourselves whether neuroscience or genetics was sufficiently developed to bring to bear on computation models of functional characterizations of reasoning. However, things are moving fast, and our purpose here is to find some areas where the gap may be closing.

9.11.1 Brain Development and Implementations of Closed–World Reasoning

Understanding autistic brain function as it implements autistic cognition requires a demanding integration of data from different time scales: developmental, learning, and online computation. This is true of many developmental disorders, to say nothing of "neurotypical" cognition, as is eloquently argued by Scerif and Karmiloff-Smith [241]. What is so intriguing coming from a perspective dominated by the shortest of these time scales (in discourse processing) is both that the developmental processes which construct the brain are themselves computational processes not unrelated to those of learning and reasoning, and conversely, that with what we already know about the brain, online adult discourse interpretation and reasoning processes could plausibly involve construction of bits of brain. As an example of brain development as computation, neurons migrate from one place to another, and their axons and dendrites grow to make their connections by following chemical gradients – a kind of hill climbing. Neurons and synapses survive or are pruned according to their activity levels as defined by algorithms closely related to Hebb's law. Examples of on-line brain construction are recent demonstrations that adult neurogenesis plays a functional role in some kinds of learning, as described above (p. 151). Our own models of neural implementation of discourse understanding require some combination of construction and activation of new networks on the time course of online discourse comprehension. Large parts of our working memory networks may be the reactivated parts of long–term memory, but to the extent that they have to incorporate modifications based on episodic information, and this information subsequently gets consolidated and can be reactivated, there is network construction going on at this time scale too. There is a fine line between the adjustment of synaptic weights to extremes, and the making or severing of connections, but as we shall see, the evidence grows that "weight-adjustment" and "activation level" are not the only structural changes wrought on the brain by experience. Modelers need to think more broadly.

Needless to say, these considerations make any idea that "the DNA determines brain structure" thoroughly obsolete, just as obsolete as the idea that "learning registers experience on a tabula rasa." We begin with attempts to provide higher functional level models of autistic "neural computation," proceed through what is known about autistic brain development, and finally discuss the genetics of the condition.

Functional Level Considerations

Levy [174] reviews functional properties of autistic neural computation through several neural network models of aspects of autistic cognition. Cohen [43] uses over- and underprovision of hidden units in multilayer networks to explain "overfitting" and failure to generalize respectively. These hidden-unit layers of cells would presumably be interneurons, which might be of some significance when we come presently to discuss neurogenesis. Gustafsson [111] sees abnormalities of self-organizing map networks explaining autistic perceptual functioning. Maps that are smaller than normal lead to perceptual discrimination that is greater than normal, but also to problems with abstraction. Interestingly, narrow selectivity is claimed to be due to "excessive lateral feedback inhibitory synaptic strengths." McClelland [187] emphasizes the tension between generalization and interference in the storage of memories, with reference to his work on memory and the interaction between cortex and hippocampus. McClelland's suggestion is that the parts of autistic brains devoted to semantics and conceptual representations rely on conjunctive encoding too much and are thus unable to take advantage of generalizations but are good at learning specific associations. The idea is related to weak central coherence and might be the consequence of mechanisms such as those suggested by Cohen and Gustafsson.

Levy's review [174] points to the importance of numbers of units and the balance of excitation/inhibition as modeling factors in understanding autism. It turns out that these two factors are intimately related in brain development. Our earlier discussion of neurogenesis in chapter 5 reviewed the phases of brain neuron generation and their mapping onto the phases of brain growth. We alluded to the process of overproduction of neurons and synaptic connections, followed by a combination of pruning of connections and cell death. Pruning differentially affects excitatory and inhibitory synapses, reducing the number of the former far more than of the latter (see Luciana [176,p. 161]). Chris Frith [87] has proposed that some aspects of autistic functioning may be explicable in terms of abnormalities in pruning – underpruning leading to their overspecific, bottom-up style of cognition. If pruning is mainly of excitatory synapses and less pruning goes on in autistic people's brains, then the result will be more excitatory synapses relative to inhibitory ones.[24]

It is a fascinating question how to map microscopic brain development processes onto macroscopic models of brain growth, as [292] shown in figure 6.4 in chapter 9, both in normal and abnormal development. On Frith's account, underpruning might well be a direct explanation of the course of autistic head growth. It is interesting that Vrba labels the phase of her model corresponding to this period as the "cerebellar period" and the cerebellum is one brain area which develops abnormally in autism, but the cerebellum is relatively small (compared, say, to the frontal lobes) and unlikely to account for gross head-size differences. Then there is the further difficulty in thinking about the timing of these developmental processes, since there may be delayed effects. Just as a hypothetical example, although the *number* of a class of cells may be determined early, perhaps in utero, it is possible that the resulting contribution to brain volume might only show up later due to maturational effects such as myelination. Finally, before we leave the issue of mapping Vrba's model to the detailed subprocesses of development, we have to ask how does human brain

---

24. Frith relies on Huttenlocher [137] for his data: "In visual cortex, the total number of synapses at birth is less than 10% of the maximum. It reaches a maximum number at about age 6 months, and decreases to about half the maximum between ages 1 and 5 years. Synapse number remains stable after age 5. In medial frontal gyrus, synaptic density reaches a maximum between ages 24 and 36 months, synaptic density begins to decrease at about age 7 years, and adult synaptic density, about 60% of the maximum, is reached by early adolescence. Preliminary data from left angular gyrus and left Broca's speech area show curves that fall between those for visual cortex and medial frontal gyrus [137,p. 348]." If these data are correct, pruning also differentially affects different areas of the brain.

development change the timings of subprocesses relative to our primate ancestors. Is everything merely slowed down? Or is there shear between processes? If conditions such as autism can be interpreted as distortions of timing, then they may provide valuable evidence about normal development and evolution.

Despite the gross differences in head size growth patterns, at a structural level autistic brains were, until relatively recently, chiefly characterized by their structural similarity to normal brains. Postmortem examination, and imaging with increasingly sophisticated technology, revealed only small differences, often inconsistent from study to study. Certainly the frontal lobes and the cerebellum were often mentioned in dispatches, but sometimes as too large, sometimes as too small, sometimes as more and sometimes as less interconnected. It is only in the last few years that that more stable characterizations of these differences, so hard to detect at a gross level, have begun to emerge.

For example, Courchesne and Pierce [51] review what is known about frontal lobe abnormalities in autism. Despite the multiply conflicting data about gross structural abnormalities there is a growing body of evidence for microscopic maldevelopment. Minicolumns, a basic unit of neocortical organization, are narrower and more numerous in autistic brains, and there are differences in gray/white matter balance. These authors particularly stress recent evidence from [285] that autistic children suffer from an immunological inflammatory response in their temporal lobes and cerebella. The response is primarily by the glia and astrocytes rather than neurons themselves. Inflammation might account for some of the head size observations. One might be tempted to dismiss the behavioral significance of inflamed astrocytes and glia as these are not neurons. But it turns out that whereas astrocytes and glia have long been thought of as passive maintenance agents supporting neurons, it now seems that they play critical roles in controlling the architecture of the developing brain [198]. These immune responses are not reactions to infectious agents but are "innate immune reactions." They may be related to the differences in cell death patterns discussed presently under "pruning." They are interpreted as persistence of a "pre-natal" state or process – all the more surprising since they showed up postmortem in a sample of fifteen autistic people ranging from 5 to 40 years old – and adding further encouragement that autism may be understood as a disturbance of the timing of developmental processes. The upshot of Courchesne and Pierce's discussion [51] is that autist people show overdevelopment of local, and underdevelopment of longrange, connections, together with some abnormalities of inhibitory processes (Rubinstein and Merzenich [235]). The authors encapsulate their conclusions in the memorable claim that the autistic temporal lobe is cut off from the rest of the brain, "talking to itself".

Three further aspects of autistic brain development deserve brief mention as possibly relevant to our earlier modeling proposals. One is differences in the timing of development of feedforward and feedback connections in the neocortex. The second is the phenomenon of adult neurogenesis mentioned earlier in connection with brain growth. The third is the balance between excitation and inhibition.

Feedforward and Feedback Connections   The phasing of the development of feedback and feedforward connections may be functionally relevant because of the earlier mentioned differences in ease of reasoning forward and backward. It is a very striking feature of adult neocortical microstructure that nearly as many projections go in the direction from brain to retina as from retina to brain, reflecting the role of expectation in perception, at a functional level. Most of what is known about the development of feedforward and feedback projections comes from study of the topographically mapped visual system in which the two are easier to distinguish, though it is assumed that the observations may be more generally applicable in areas of less convenient microanatomy. These studies show that feedforward connections develop earlier than feedback connections (Burkhalter [27]). Friston [86] proposes a mapping from brain to computational models which places the issue of directionality and the role of forward models of expectations at centerstage. These forward models are continuous control theory models, but they are functionally closely related to our logical models for closed–world reasoning.

Neurogenesis and Brain Growth   With respect to adult neurogenesis, we described in chapter 6 how it is now known that neurons continue to be added to various areas of the mammalian brain throughout adult life, and these neurons can be shown to function in certain kinds of learning and memory tasks, especially in the hippocampus, an area known to be involved in working memory tasks. This fact is especially relevant to our neural models of default discourse interpretation. A central proposal of these models is that networks are actually constructed in working memory on the time course of discourse processing. This is functionally necessary since it is implausible that preexisting networks can provide the range of structures which are required. The anatomical and functional relation between working and long–term memory is contentious. The activated portion of existing default rules in long–term memory plays some role in constituting these networks, yet the networks must also be capable of incorporating new connections to represent episodically new information, which may later be consolidated into long–term memory.[25] In the light of the role of

---

25. We have been careful to emphasize that the relation between the units and links in our models and the neurons and axons in the brain is at this point open. Our units and links may represent a considerable abstraction over groups of neurons, rather than single neurons [304, 1]. But plausible cognitive models need to be able to create structure, and furthermore the adult brain does literally continue to create structure in performing working memory tasks (and possibly in consolidating the results). Our models may well describe this process of creating structure.

inhibitory disturbance in autism, it is intriguing that the particular class of neurons claimed to be created in the adult neocortex are GABA-ergic inhibitory interneurons (Dayer et al. [60]). Levitt et al. [173] propose that it is exactly this subclass of neurons which are undersupplied in autism, and that a mouse model of this deficiency yields related behavioral deficits in social interaction.

Autism and the Ratio of Excitation to Inhibition   Inhibition brings us to the third issue of the balance between excitation and inhibition. Rubinstein and Merzenich [235] propose a model of autism as a family of brain disorders whose common factor is too high a ratio of excitation to inhibition, especially in frontal areas of the brain.[26] This work is primarily focused on neurotransmitters, and so is complementary to issues of pruning at the structural level. Glutamate is the prime excitatory and GABA the prime inhibitory neurotransmitter – a pair that operate over a wide area of the brain. Their model discusses many factors and other neurotransmitters, but GABA insufficiency plays a large role in increasing the ratio of excitation over inhibition. Just to complicate matters, it has recently been discovered that whereas GABA is inhibitory in the adult brain, it actually has an *excitatory* function during early neuron development. GABA's switch from excitatory to inhibitory function appears to play an important role in neurons' switching from early embryonic modes, in which activity is driven by gross factors such as giant polarizing potentials giving rise to synchronized waves of activity, to later modes in which neurons modulate each other's activity through synaptic connnections in more complex patterns [18]. On the face of it, this switch by GABA is occurring at a much earlier stage than the appearance of autism, but nevertheless may be significant for the later balance between inhibition and excitation. Rubinstein and Merzenich [235] describe the close relation between GABA and the brain growth factors which play important roles in ending critical developmental periods. This is particularly intriguing for an interpretation of autism as arising from disturbances of the timing of developmental processes. We return to GABA in our discussion of the genetics of autism.

Neural Underpinning of Closed–World Reasoning   The neural implementation of our model of closed–world reasoning offers many points of contact with this biological background. The central role of abnormalities in closed–world reasoning couches the whole process as the spread of excitation and its inhibitory control. As we discussed above and illustrated in figure 9.2, insufficient inhibitory resources (either at the transmitter level or through pruning),

---

26. Needless to say, these proposals about inhibitory deficiency do not sit well with the idea that excessive lateral inhibition lies behind the narrowness of autistic perceptual maps, though there are many factors, not least timing discrepancies, that might or might not account for the apparent contradiction.

would have specific effects on the processing of conditionals' abnormality conditions.[27] The two-tiered architecture of our net with its truth and falsity sheets bound by corresponding inhibitory connections also gives a prominent role to inhibition, although it seems unlikely that the symmetry of the net's sheets as presented can be the whole story. On the biological side, there is no shortage of evidence implicating the relevance of the balance of excitation and inhibition, but much of it is speculative. We make no apology for this: we intend to give some feel for how much is settled and just how much is not.

9.11.2 The Genetics of Autism and Parental Resource Allocation

The power of modern genetic analysis offers great opportunities for understanding the processes of cognitive change involved in human speciation. While human speciation as a process presents immense difficulties of investigation – neither brains nor behavior fossilise, the nearest extant species are 5 million years diverged, etc. – genetics represents one of the main sources of evolutionary information. It really is possible to get information about which genes have been under selection pressure and something about when. Genetics has barely entered into cognitive science yet, but it will be worth a detour here in making our example of altriciality more vivid.

The Importance of Epigenesis

In chapter 6 we contrasted the concept of innateness, still much discussed in psychology, with the genetic concept of heritability which has replaced it in biology. The realization that heritability could only be studied relativized to an environment crystallized the contrast between genetic and epigenetic factors controlling development. The known role of epigenetic factors in development is growing by the day. The brain growth processes we have been describing are ones in which the chemical soup in which neurons develop has all sorts of environmental effects on the resulting brain structures. Of course the composition of the soup is partly genetically controlled, but at each stage close analysis shows interaction between gene and environment, always remembering that the other genes and their products are environment in these calculations.

Our understanding of the genetic control of autism is rudimentary, but developing fast. There is good evidence that genes are involved. In fact autism highly genetically influenced: observations of the concordance of autism in monozygotic (identical) twins run as high as 90%. In dizygotic twins it is about 3%, similar to nontwin siblings. This concordance *rises* to 90% for monozygotic

---

27. It must be noted though that at present our treatment of abnormalities is rudimentary in the sense that insufficient analysis is given of how propositions are identified as abnormalities in configuring a network, and how relevant abnormalities are differentiated from irrelevant ones within a context.

twins if the criteria for autism are *relaxed* [141]. That is, there is a somewhat higher concordance if a broader definition of autism spectrum disorders is adopted. This strongly suggests that the inheritance mechanism involved applies to a wider spectrum of characteristics than full-blown autism, raising the possibility that the benefits of autistic spectrum characteristics may play a part in the maintenance of autism in the population. The pattern whereby monozygotic twins show more than double the concordance of dizygotic twins suggests that multiple interacting genes play a role [232]. In fact, a specific gene-gene interaction which affects the GABA metabolism has recently been identified in some autistic cases [178]. Such gene interaction is a common situation, but needless to say, it hugely complicates the business of analysis.

While this is strong evidence that genes are involved, the patterns do not fit simple patterns of inheritance (many genetic conditions do not, so this in itself is unsurprising). These high concordances in monozygotic twins, coupled with concordances for dizygotic twins similar to nonsiblings, suggests at least some epigenetic influence and/or some de novo factors (e.g., mutation). The sex ratio, variously estimated at between three and ten to one times as many males affected as females, is not easy to explain by a sex-linked trait on the Y chromosome. Again, one possibility is that there are many genes involved, possibly with varying degrees of expression, possibly interacting with each other to determine the phenotype. Another, not exclusive possibility, is that epigenetic factors are involved.

Imprinting: Generalities

One class of epigenetic factors, recently discovered, and especially pertinent to analyses of altriciality, is genetic *imprinting*, whereby alleles of maternal origin have different effects than the same alleles of paternal origin [139]. Alleles of genes with normal Mendelian characteristics have the same effect whether they are paternal or maternal genes. Imprinting is an epigenetic process which applies to relatively few, and only mammalian, genes which overwhelmingly control aspects of resource allocation in development. An increase in parental investment in offspring is one defining characteristic of mammals, carried to extremes in altricial *Homo sapiens*. With an imprinted gene, one parent, most often the mother, suppresses the effects of the other parent's allele, often by a process known as methylation which takes place at conception. So, although the offspring has, say, two dominant alleles (DD), one of those alleles is suppressed and is not expressed in the phenotype.

The dominant theory of imprinting is that it is part of a competition between mother's and father's interests in reproductive resource allocation. Whenever females mate with more than one male, there is a divergence of genetic interests of the two parents. This conflict theory of imprinting has more recently been joined by a "dose dependence" theory of imprinting, specifically for genes on the X chromosome [140]. One can make a good case for a noncompetitive explanation for imprinting on the X sexchromosome.[28]

Whether or not there is parental conflict under conditions of polyandrous mating, mothers and fathers also share interests in having advantageous sexual dimorphism in their offspring. Since females have a double dose of the X chromosome, it seems that they have evolved imprinting to switch off the X chromosome they contribute *for genes on X for which too great a dose (i.e., a double dose) would disrupt other genes which must contribute to the phenotypes of both sexes.* This is called "dosage compensation." So *if* it is advantageous, for example, for females to have greater social skills, then this must be represented on the X chromosomes that fathers contribute to their daughters, because mothers have to turn this off on their Xs which they contribute to both sons and daughters. So the crucial issue is whether a gene benefits males more than females (size perhaps), females more than males (social skills perhaps), or both equally (brain development perhaps) [209].[29] Note that this analysis presupposes that having greater social skills has to actually be *deleterious* for males, to explain why imprinting in the form of dosage compensation by the female would take place. Ramsay et al. [196] in a recent review of imprinting, considers the status of several theories of its evolutionary origin, as well as its extent, and the considerable divergence in imprinting between mouse and man which may suggest the importance of imprinting in our evolution. The authors also argue that a high proportion of imprinted "transcriptional units" are noncoding RNAs (not DNA at all). Imprinted genes are important as "controllers" of genetic cascades as we emphasized in our discussion of the importance of control elements in explaining macroevolution (chapter 6, section 6.2.4), and in discussing altriciality as an example.

Imprinting and Brain Growth

Whatever the status of these particular examples it has been shown that imprinting is rife among the genes which control brain growth, and that there are distinctive spatial and temporal patterns to the maternal/paternal imprint-

---

28. The XX (female) and XY (male) sex chromosomes in mammals exercise genetic control of the organism's sex, but this is *not* imprinting. Imprinting can happen on non-sex chromosomes (autosomes), or on the X chromosome. It cannot happen on the Y chromosome since all Y chromosomes are contributed by fathers. But autosomal imprinting generally affects both sons and daughters.

29. These particular example characteristics are taken from claims in the literature, but should be treated with a healthy skepticism – their purpose here is illustrative only.

ing. Interestingly, the X chromosome appears to disproportionately influence the development of the brain and cognitive traits [309]. For example, the genes contributing to mental deficiency are overrepresented on the X chromosome. There are some very basic biological reasons why speciation genes (those under particular selection pressure as two varieties of a species drift toward reproductive isolation and full specieshood) are particularly likely to be related to sexual behavior, and expressed in brain, testes, and placenta. An old observation of Haldane was that when hybrids between two subspecies are sterile, it is usually the heterogamous sex (i.e., XY males in mammals) which is sterile.

Many imprinted genes do not control the synthesis of any protein but are the elements controlling other clusters of genes which were mentioned in chapter 6 as being particularly important in tweaking old modules in macroevolutionary change. Imprinted genes are independently identifiable, and are evidently prime candidates for controlling the changed pattern of fetal maturation in altricial *Homo sapiens*, and especially of brain development – big brains are supremely metabolically expensive as well as being difficult to give birth to.

Neuroscientists now have sophisticated techniques for mapping both spatially and temporally the patterns of expression of genes. The molecular signatures of imprinting have enabled researchers to track down genes controlling brain growth during maturation (the techniques have currently been applied mostly in mice – 70 million years diverged from our ancestral line). Maternally imprinted genes are responsible for controlling the growth of the frontal lobes (one of the areas of greatest human innovation in development, and a prime seat of the planning functions we are focused on in our cognitive analysis of executive function). Paternally imprinted genes control growth of the hypothalamus [103]. To put it facetiously, mom controls the development of civilization and dad the animal urges. Slightly more intricately, the unique degree to which human brains, and especially the planning frontal lobes, continue growing after birth may prove to be an innovation controlled by the mother's interest in reproductive resource allocation – specifically her interests in her offsprings' capacities for inducing their father and his relatives to provide resources.

If such accounts hold up, then they provide evidence about the originating selection pressures for the explosive growth of human planning, reasoning, and communication capabilities. Just so stories about evolution get grounded in selection pressures, as evidenced by molecular genetics. These capabilities may have proved useful for mammoth hunting or for mate attraction, but to the extent they are controlled by imprinted genes, their evolution is more likely to have been driven by changes in maternal reproductive resource allocation, or pressures for sexual dimorphism of particular characteristics involved in these processes.

Imprinting and Lifestyle in Primates

This distribution of imprinting in the brain suggests a return to reconsider Foley's paradox (p. 140). Keverne et al. [156] present a table of forty-five primate species, with data on their brain part sizes and such lifestyle factors as whether they are diurnal or nocturnal, herbivore or fructivore, their living group size, the sexual composition of groups, and the timing of mating. They divide the brain into "executive brain" and "emotional brain" on the basis of the maternal vs. paternal imprinting of genes expressed, and show that there is a positive correlation between sizes of parts within the executive and the emotional brain, but negative correlations between parts across these two areas. They then study the relation between lifestyle variables and brain part size for each of the two divisions of brain. For the executive brain there were significant correlations between its size and living group size (+), number of females in the group (+), but not number of males, or arboreal/terrestrial (-), nocturnal/diurnal (-) lifestyles, or restricted/confined mating times (+). Imprinted genes have reciprocal effects on body and brain size: maternally imprinted genes suppress body size (to decrease maternal investment) but paradoxically increase brain size; paternally imprinted genes increase body size (to increase maternal investment) but decrease brain size. There is something inverse about investment in brain, the hypothesis being that a bigger brain (at least some parts) leads to better social skills at extracting resources from others. These authors interpret the decrease in the emotional brain and increase in executive brain in the course of primate evolution as resulting from appetitive behaviors becoming less under neuroendocrine control, and more under the control of strategic behaviors, controlled by the frontal cortex and social skill. As an example, they remark that dominant males in higher primates are often not particularly aggressive, achieving their ends by more cerebral methods of clique formation or what–have–you.

Keverne et al.[156], like their colleague Foley, note the female bonded groups of many Old World monkeys, although they don't mention his observation of how male-bonding plays such a distinctive role in the great apes. Much of the genetic experimentation involves the mouse, so it is far from clear exactly how these patterns changed and affected human evolution. It seems likely that the shift from female– to male–bonded group living, combined with the huge increase in reproductive resource requirements, must have had a large impact on the balance between maternal and paternal control of brain development. Although the details of the last phase of human evolution are not settled, we can be sure that they will need interpretation against this long–run backdrop of primate evolution.

Imprinting and Autism

Claims have also been made that imprinting plays a role in determining the sex-ratio of cases of autism (Skuse [249], Jiang et al. [141]). It does in mouse models of autism, where a particular gene can be shown to affect analogues of executive function tasks [58]. Skuse's model proposes a paternally imprinted gene on X suppressing the effects of multiple autosomal (non-sex chromosome) genes which are responsible for the actual phenotype when expressed. Fathers would normally pass this suppressor factor to their daughters, which would ensure they were free of the kinds of social skills deficits associated with autism.

Already a number of human behavioral syndromes are known to be related to abnormalities of imprinting (e.g., Prader–Willi, Angelman's , Silver-Russell, and Beckwith-Wiedemann syndromes [80]). There is evidence that Angelman's syndrome particularly is associated in at least a subgroup of cases with autism. In one study, nine of nineteen Angelman's subjects fulfilled the diagnostic criteria for autism [214]. Badcock and Crespi [8] make the proposal that autism is a syndrome of generally imbalanced imprinting. Their paper contains an extensive review of the current state of knowledge of the involvement of imprinted genes, and links this aspect of autism to evolution through the parental competition for investment in the offspring theory of imprinting and the "male brain" theory of autism.

Of course, imprinting is not the whole story in the genetics of autism. There are plenty of unimprinted genes which show evidence of affecting the development of autism. Rubinstein and Merzenich [235], already discussed with respect to inhibition, provide a useful review of some of the candidate genes, oriented toward neurotransmitter effects. Another useful review is [213]. As mentioned above, the complex pattern of inheritance makes it likely that many genes are involved – estimates vary between ten and a hundred. And it should not be forgotten that the expression of nonimprinted genes may be controlled by imprinted ones, and vice versa. Even more recent advances in the unravelling of what is called *copy number variation* in genetics has opened up the alternative possibility that hundreds of different genetic anomalies may individually cause autistic symptoms—the "rare-alleles" model of common genetically influenced diseases [69, 186].

On a concluding note, both positive and cautionary, an important contribution of genetic population studies is that they study random samples more or less representative of whole populations rather than populations of subjects filtered through clinical diagnostic criteria which constitute almost all other data on autism. Here is a source of evidence which avoids the distorting selection of data (see Harvey et al. [118] for discussion). Intriguing examples are two papers by Happé and colleagues [232, 115] which ask the question whether the social and nonsocial deficits in autism are correlated and/or genetically related in the general population. Since the clinical criteria guarantee an association in clinical populations, this is a first preliminary indication (using a not yet fully normed scale for autistic tendencies in the normal population) that in fact these symptoms may not be highly correlated, and although both are under substantial genetic influence, they appear to be under *independent* genetic (or epigenetic) influence. We agree about the probable phenotypic heterogeneity of autism as stated above, but these authors believe that individual genes will map onto phenotypic characteristics of the varied disorders. This seems to us most unlikely for the reasons stated here. Interaction between genes in determining phenotypic characteristics is to be expected as the default case however difficult it is to identify specific interactions with current methods. This is a powerful reason for thinking in terms of changes in timing of developmental processes, since changes in timing are inherently likely to produce interactions.

To the extent that imprinting is involved in the epigenetic control of autism, then that is evidence that the condition has something to do with the selection pressures on parental investment in the rearing of offspring, and/or the requirements of sexual dimorphism and its (epi)genetic control. Against this background of evolution of the species, the fact that autistic people exhibit such a marked temporal profile of head growth is a striking observation.

In normal human development, altriciality means that the human infant's brain is dumped out into the external environment at a very much earlier stage of development than that of our ancestors, and that it goes on developing for very much longer. The particularly "hyperdeveloped" part of the human brain, the frontal lobes are the most extreme part of this pattern, even to the degree that it has been suggested that mothers essentially function as their infants' frontal lobes in the early months of development. This closeness of coupling of two individuals has long been understood as playing an organizing role in human learning and development. In the next few years we are likely to learn a great deal more about the genetic and epigenetic control of this process and thence about its evolutionary significance.

Focusing on altriciality as a biologically recognisable human innovation, offers the possibility of connecting cognition to the burgeoning information sources offered by genomics. Perhaps genetic imprinting can offer a methodology to identify some candidate genes for involvement in human speciation.

Another Source of Genetic Information on Brain Growth   Certainly another recent genetic method has already yielded dividends – the identification of "human accelerated regions" in the genome. Now that the sequencing of the chimpanzee's genome has largely been completed, it is possible, though by no means straightforward, to compare it to the human genome and to identify sites of divergence. The basic problem is that most divergence is random, and it is only functional divergence which is of interest. Previously, the only way of circumventing this problem was to study only protein–coding genes which can be screened for selection pressure, as noted above (page 150). But we believe, for the reasons explained in chapter 6, that control genetic elements which are typically non-protein–coding are likely to be of most interest in our speciation.

Pollard et al. [220] present a study of an "RNA gene" called *HAR1F* and its twin *HAR1R*, whose identification is the first fruit of a new direct approach. HAR stands for "human accelerated region." The genomes of chimpanzee and human are compared (along with several other more distantly related species), first to find highly *conserved* regions which are assumed to be functionally important because preserved by selection pressure *against* genetic change. The resulting collection of what we can think of as *mammalian decelerated regions* is then screened for regions showing evidence of high rates of genetic change between chimpanzee and human. Thus the argument is that although the resulting HARs are functionally important (because of having been preserved by selection pressure *against* change in a long line of mammals), their *rapid change* between chimpanzee and human is indicative of a significant evolutionary role in the speciation and evolution of *Homo sapiens*. Random variation of highly conserved regions would not be tolerated because of their functional significance.

This technique identified forty-nine HARs ranked for the rapidity of their recent evolutionary change. The first-ranked *HAR1* is a 118 base-pair region of human chromosome 20 which is mostly the overlap between two previously unknown RNA genes:[30] HAR1F and HAR1R. This region is the top-ranked HAR out of the 49, and the only one yet functionally analysed. A high proportion of HARs (96% of the 49) are non-protein-coding elements. A high proportion of adjacent genes are related to DNA binding or transcriptional regulation, and 24% are adjacent to neurodevelopmental genes. *HAR1F* and *HAR1R* are RNA genes expressed in cortical development in Cajal-Retzius cells, a class of cells which are probably involved in producing some of the cytoarchitecural peculiarities of human cortex.

HAR1F is strongly and specifically expressed in developing brain, starting between 7 and 9 gestational weeks, in the dorsal telencephalon (the cortex primordium). These Cajal-Retzius cells are transient cells which do not survive into adulthood, and are known to be involved in leading the migration and development of other neocortical neurons. They form distinctive horizontal networks, chiefly in layer 1. Their function and differentiation from other cell classes is currently under review [190]. We noted in our discussion of brain growth (page 149) that layer 1 is the cortical layer most differentiated in humans. The gene expression patterns suggest that *HAR1F* and *HAR1R* may reg-

---

30. RNA genes are also a novel concept, arising from recent discoveries of "RNA interference," the subject of a Nobel Prize in 2006. RNAi is the phenomenon whereby RNA controls the expression of DNA genes, thus leading to the notion of an RNA gene.

ulate each other through a sense-antisense relation,[31] and it may be a shift in the balance of control which is the human innovation. Diffuse expression of the *HAR1* genes in the adult brain is also observed, especially in forebrain, hippocampus, cerebellum, thalamus, and hypothalamus. One speculation is that *HAR1R* suppresses much adult expression of *HAR1F*. Outside the brain, expression of *HAR1F* and *HAR1R* also show up in testes, ovary, and placenta – one classic pattern for speciation genes (page 291).

Just to give an idea of the disparities in evolutionary "speed" picked up by this technique, in *HAR1* only two base pairs are changed between chicken and chimpanzee (diverged 310 million years ago), but eighteen are changed between chimpanzee and human (diverged about 6 million years). The *HAR1* region has no orthologues in fish or invertebrates, so probably originates less than 400 million years ago.

We describe this technique here to give further indication of how rich genetic information can be and how rapidly techniques are developing, but also because the very first information yielded by the technique supports Waddington's long–standing functional contention that control elements are all–important in explaining macroevolution.

Conclusion

Embedding the example of autism inside the framework of altriciality as an organizing force in human cognitive evolution provides a good illustration of how rich and complex a phenomenon autism is, and how many levels of analysis are required for a full understanding. The details of our speculations are undoubtedly wrong, but nevertheless this is an infinitely better biological model for understanding at least one important aspect of human evolution than the adaptationism typical of evolutionary psychology. If the temporal profile of human head growth and its implications for obstetrics is one organizing selection pressure of human evolution, then altriciality is at least partly an adaptation to this pressure. This must have led to the exaptation of existing learning mechanisms to the new environment in which the immature brain dealt with an external environment, an environment organized overwhelmingly by the mother. Of course there would also be myriad secondary adaptations (all the way from cognitive and affective changes to social organizational ones) produced by the pressures of surviving altriciality. Stenning [257] describes some of these, paying special attention to the resulting shift in the balance of intentional and causal analysis of the newborn's environment.

---

31. DNA's double helix unwinds into a sense and an antisense strand – the latter a "negative" of the former. The former may code for a protein, but the antisense strand (transcribed into RNA) can inhibit such coding by combining with the messenger RNA, in what is called RNA interference.

10 Syllogisms and Beyond

10.1 Putting It All Back Together

The "psychology of reasoning" as a field coalesced from studies of syllogistic reasoning, but we have deliberately stood history on its head in leaving syllogisms to the end.[1] This choice reflects the fact that the syllogism requires just about enough derivation to provide a microcosm for studying the integration of several strands of our argument so far. The selection task and the suppression task present interpretation problems to subjects, but once an interpretation is settled, barely any derivation is required. At least for some subjects, syllogisms evoke both interpretation processes of reasoning to an interpretation *and* derivational processes of reasoning from the interpretation imposed. Indeed, syllogisms are one area where substantial interpretational theories from linguistics and philosophy have been applied by psychologists and, as we shall see, have met with self-proclaimed failure.

This slightly greater role of derivation is sufficient to introduce representational issues which do not play a large role in the selection task. In chapter 5, we expressed skepticism that the models vs. rules debate about *mental* representations had been given any empirical substance, and we will revisit that debate here on its home territory. But we are not at all skeptical that contrasting external representations (for example, rule systems or diagrams) have real impact on subjects' reasoning, and especially on their conceptual learning, and we review evidence to that effect here. Along with the variety of representation strategies come individual differences in reasoning styles. Individual differ-

---

1. From a purely logical point of view, syllogisms are only special in being the first logical system to be presented formally. Apart from this, they just form a fragment of predicate logic; moreover, a fragment in which the quantifiers $\forall$ and $\exists$ do not come into their own, because iteration is not allowed. It is therefore not clear to what extent results of experiments on syllogistic reasoning extend to reasoning with quantifiers generally. We have some anecdotal data on children's reasoning which may be relevant in this respect. It has been known since Piaget that children have nonstandard truth conditions for "all circles are blue," judging this sentence to be false if there are blue things which are not circles. Our data show that if one gives the same child a sentence in which quantifiers are iterated ("All boxes contain a key which fits the lock on all boxes"), it has no trouble processing this according to the standard truth conditions.

ences in interpretation were seen to underlie subjects' decisions in the selection task, but the range of available responses allowed to the subject was insufficient to tease them apart without resorting to Socratic dialogue, and there was barely enough derivation from interpretations to approach issues of derivational strategy. In the syllogism, with its requirement to integrate two propositions, the differences in interpretation continue, but now there are also potential differences in reasoning from interpretations. The problem set is now sufficiently rich that data analysis becomes a more substantial task. For the reader coming from a chiefly logical background, this is the first encounter with the analysis problems that occupy psychologists. For the psychologically based reader, this material provides methodological issues for the standard hypothesis testing approach, and some resolutions offered by a background of logical theory.

And finally, because the syllogism is blatantly intended to require classical logical reasoning from a skeptical stance, it is a microcosm for examining the "information–packaging" structures which are designed to assist the credulous processing of natural language, and their effects on subjects' reasoning. We will argue that these structures are inherently part of credulous reasoning, but produce interesting conflicts with the skeptical stance.

The chapter begins with a logical specification of the syllogism, and the presentation of some alternative representations and methods of solution. Then some studies of the interpretation of single syllogistic premises are described which have been used to claim that premise interpretation cannot predict syllogistic reasoning. With a view to establishing just such a relation, we describe an exploratory analysis of interpretation data, and its use to build a syllogistic reasoning model which incorporates interpretation differences. The results give clear evidence of qualitative individual differences in subjects' reasoning as a function of their interpretations, and a simple process account, the source–founding model, is presented. Finally, the chapter ends with a logical reappraisal of mental models theory, and an assessment of the appropriateness of its goals given the evidence available for qualitative individual differences.

10.2   What is the Syllogistic Task?

One of the focal points for empirical studies of deductive reasoning is the syllogism. This is probably mainly because of the tractability for the experimenter afforded by this domain – a finite number of problems, a wide range of difficulty for naive subjects, etc. But there is also the possibility that this is a psychologically interesting fragment of logic for the empirical study of human reasoning precisely because of its tractability for the reasoner – more on this below. Another reason for the possible psychological importance of syllogisms is that there is some evidence that monadic reasoning (reasoning about one-place predicates) may have an important status due to its relation to discourse processing which will become clear in what follows. Since the syllogism deals with monadic predicates only, it is perhaps helpful to think of the syllogism as the logic of taxonomy whereby individuals are sorted into types defined by the possession (or not) of properties.

10.2.1   Syntax

A syllogism consists of two premises which relate three terms (a, b, and c), one of which (the *middle* term, b) occurs in both premises, while the other two (the *end* terms, a and c) each occur in only one premise – a is the end term in the first premise, and c is the end term in the second premise.

There are four *moods* or premise types, distinguished by the quantifiers "all," "some," "none," and "some... not." The quantifiers *all* and *none* are *universal*. The quantifiers *some* and *some... not* are *existential*. There are four possible arrangements of terms in the two premises, known as *figures*, as shown in table 10.1.[2] We use the term *diagonal figures* to refer to the first pair of figures (ab/bc and ba/cb) and *symmetric figures* to refer to the second pair (ab/cb and ba/bc). Since each premise can be in one of four moods, and each premise pair can have one of four figures, there are $4 \times 4 \times 4 = 64$ different syllogisms.

Table 10.1   The four figures of the syllogism

	diagonal		symmetric	
Figure Number	1	2	3	4
1st premise	$a - b$	$b - a$	$a - b$	$b - a$
2nd premise	$b - c$	$c - b$	$c - b$	$b - c$

10.2.2   Semantics

The semantics of the syllogism concerns *types* of individuals defined by combinations of properties. Because there is no identity relation, it is never of logical significance how many of a type of individual exist – hence the talk of *types*. Properties are denoted by the terms of the syllogism – given the term a, any individual is either an a or not an a ($\neg a$). Fully specified types are specified with respect to all three properties, and there are eight such types: abc, $ab\neg c$, $a\neg bc$, $a\neg b\neg c$, $\neg abc$, $\neg ab\neg c$, $\neg a\neg bc$, and $\neg a\neg b\neg c$.

Due to the restriction to monadic predicates, we can express the semantics of syllogisms in terms of sets of types. This can be seen as follows. If we think of predicates as denoting sets of individuals, then a model of a syllogism is an interpretation of the predicates which makes both predicates true. In principle

---

2. Care is needed in reading the literature because different numbering schemes are used.

there are a great many such models for a given syllogism, since the cardinality of the domain can be varied. However, because the language contains monadic predicates only and does not have the identity relation, individuals can only be distinguished by the types which define them, and differences in cardinality therefore do not play any role. Thus, a model of the premise "some A are B" can be given as any of the following sets of types: $\{ab\}$, $\{ab, \neg ab\}$, $\{ab, a \neg b\}$, ..., $\{ab, \neg ab, a \neg b, \neg a \neg b\}$. A model of a syllogism is a set of fully specified types whose existence is consistent with the truth of both premises. Thus suppose the second premise of the syllogism is "all B are C." To compute the models of both the premises, first the set of models of "some A are B" is expanded so as to incorporate all the possibilities for the predicate C. This yields as sets of types $\{ab \neg c\}$, $\{abc\}$, ..., $\{abc, \neg abc, a \neg bc, \neg a \neg bc\}$. These sets are then pruned to take into account that all B are C, and we get $\{abc\}$, ..., $\{abc, a \neg bc\}$, ..., $\{abc, \neg abc, a \neg bc, \neg a \neg bc\}$. Each set can be thought of as a possible syllogistic world described at the level of abstraction with which the syllogism deals; that is, with predicates rather than individuals. Erasing the bs from the fully specified types then yields types which satisfy the conclusion "some A are C."

In the psychological literature, but not generally the modern logical literature, the syllogism is conventionally interpreted under the assumption that none of the three sets of things with the properties a, b, and c are empty.[3] Sometimes this assumption is explicitly included in the instructions to subjects, although as we shall see, it is an open question whether they take this instruction on board. It is a pity that there does not appear to be any empirical studies of this issue. The no empty sets axiom reduces the number of possible models somewhat. A modern logical treatment would make these existential assumptions explicit, separately from its definition of the quantifiers.

Given this semantics, of the sixty-four syllogisms, twenty-seven have valid conclusions which can be formulated by applying one of the four quantifiers to the two end terms. The remaining thirty seven syllogisms do not allow any valid conclusions of this form. As we shall see, an extension of the set of quantifiers slightly extends the set of problems with valid conclusions (see figure 10.5).

---

3. This strong "no-empty-sets" assumption appears to stem from Strawson [274,p. 174] although even he describes it as one that logicians have "hesitated to adopt." For Aristotle, positive quantifiers carried existential assumptions, but negative ones didn't. There are interesting historical reasons for the adoption of existential assumptions: the distinction between the domain of interpretation of an argument and the universal domain (cf. the discussion in chapter 2) wasn't clarified until the twentieth century. See section 10.3.2 for further discussion.

10.3   Euler Circles

We choose to introduce this logical fragment diagrammatically, drawing on Stenning and Oberlander [263], for two reasons. First, such a presentation further dispels any illusion that logic is concerned only with reasoning about sentences. Second, it helps us to explore some of the semantic properties of diagrams which are particularly closely associated with models, to which, as we mentioned above, we will return.

Most diagrammatic methods for solving syllogisms are based on the same spatial analogy – the analogy between an item's membership in a set and the geometrical inclusion of a point within a closed curve in a plane. Euler took this analogy, represented the first premise as a pair of circles, represented the second premise by adding a third circle; and finally read off the conclusion from this construction. So, for example, figure 10.1 shows how one might solve the syllogism *All A are B. All C are B.*

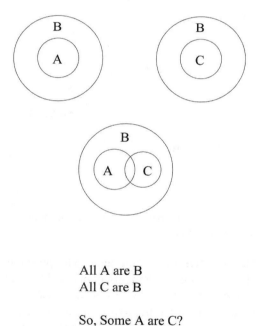

All A are B
All C are B

So, Some A are C?

Figure 10.1   A syllogism and potential conclusion represented by Euler circles.

This is an interesting example illustrating the *in*expressiveness of diagrams. While we may feel that figure 10.1 is helpful in clarifying the reasoning, as a method of reasoning it is obviously fallible. Even setting aside the several different diagrams we could have chosen to exemplify the premises individually, there are several ways of combining the two premise diagrams that we could have chosen. The conclusion drawn here is true in the combination we chose, but if we had only tried a different combination, we might have found that the conclusion did not hold. Diagrams exhibit specificity. How are generalizations to be extracted from them? Figure 10.2 shows the mapping of the

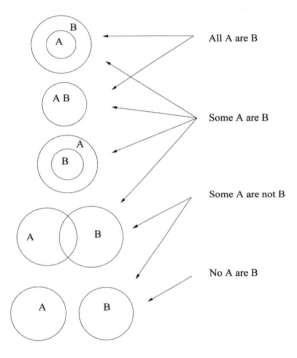

Figure 10.2   The five spatial relations between two circles mapped onto the quantified sentences they model – the Gergonne relations.

sentence forms onto primitive Euler diagrams. The problem of the explosion of combinations of diagrammatic elements is particularly acute in the case of *some* where four of the five spatial relations between two circles exemplify the sentence. Imagine having to solve the syllogism *Some A are B. Some B are C* by this method. There are four diagrams of the first premise, four of the second, and several ways of making each combination to derive a composite diagram. There are about fifty diagram combinations we should consider. In many of these diagrams, it is true that some *A* are *C* (or, diagrammatically, that circle *A* intersects circle *C*), but not in all. If we chanced to construct a diagram where some *A* were *C*, we might make this conclusion without realizing that it does not follow because there are other situations which made the premises both true, but in which this conclusion was nevertheless false.

This problem with diagrammatic methods of reasoning stems exactly from the lack of abstraction inherent in diagrams. This problem has been used by Johnson-Laird to argue for the hopelessness of diagrammatic methods. How could a brilliant mathematician like Euler make such a fundamental mistake? How did the poor German princess who was his original pupil gain anything from this flawed system?

10.3.1   Strategies for Combining Diagrams

The answers, of course, are to be found in what Euler taught about the *strategy* for choosing which diagrams to use when. Euler taught that one should select what we might think of as the "weakest" case. If we want to represent *Some A are B* we do not choose a diagram where all *A* are *B*. If we want to add a third circle to a diagram, we do so in the way that represents the most possibilities – graphically we include the most circle intersections that are consistent with the premises. Although Euler diagrams are usually presented without an explicit notation for these strategies, it is rather simple to do so. Figure 10.3 shows four diagrams for representing the four premises. The crosses (intro-

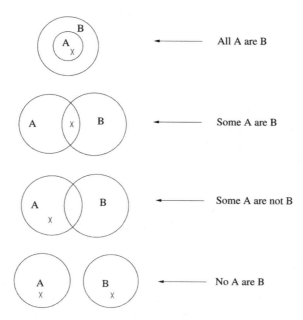

Figure 10.3   The four quantifiers mapped onto their characteristic diagrams using the cross notation for their smallest models.

duced in Stenning and Oberlander [263]) mark smallest models.[4] If there is a cross in a minimal subregion of the diagram, then there *must* be something in the world represented with the properties corresponding to that subregion. One thing corresponding to a cross is the absolute minimal "furniture" there must be in a world for the sentence to be true in that world. There may be more, but this much there must be. If there is more than one cross, there is more than one smallest model. It is an important property of the syllogism, that smallest models are always single-element models.

The crosses help capture the right strategy for combining diagrams. Figure 10.4 shows the process of solving the syllogism *All A are B. Some C are not B.* exploiting the cross notation. The two–premise representations are combined by superposing the *B* circles (which are, after all, the same circle). There is then a choice about the relation between the *A* and *C* circles. They could be placed in one of three arrangements consistent with the premises. The rule is that the arrangement which creates most subregions is chosen. A simple rule determines whether the crosses persist or are eliminated during this combination process. If a subregion containing a cross is bisected in combining the diagrams, then its cross is eliminated. If not, then the cross persists.

Finally, we need to determine what if any conclusion follows from the represented syllogism. It turns out, as the reader might want to verify, that every valid conclusion is based on the three-property description of a subregion containing a cross. For example, in the case of figure 10.4, the subregion with a cross in the final three-circle diagram corresponds to *C*s that are not *A* and not *B*. No cross, no valid conclusion. Conversely, if there is a cross remaining in the final diagram, then, with a couple of interesting exceptions which we shall come to directly, there is a valid conclusion. To generate a conclusion, first describe the type of individual corresponding to the cross's region and eliminate the *B* term. In the case of figure 10.4 this yields "things that are *C* and not *A*." Now, if the subregion containing the cross is circular, its label becomes the subject of a universal conclusion. Otherwise the conclusion is existential (with *some* or *some not*). If the cross is outside one of the *A* and *C* circles, then the conclusion will be negative; otherwise it will be positive. This algorithm will generate all the valid conclusions of the sixty-four syllogisms. Try some!

The attentive reader will be asking why this graphical rigamarole leads to the right answer. How is it any more insightful than the medieval logician's mnemonics about Barbara and her friends? Stenning [258] presents studies which show that subjects differ greatly in their facility for learning from diagrams, but that at least for some subjects diagrammatic presentation makes real differences in their learning. Be that as it may, a few hints might be helpful.

---

4. We use "smallest" to avoid confusion with the different sense of "minimal" which is important in chapter 7.

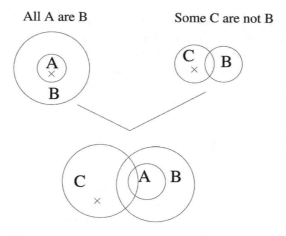

Figure 10.4   An example syllogism solved by Euler's method augmented by the cross notation.

Combining the circles to give the maximum number of subregions consistent with the premises guarantees the exhaustiveness of the search for kinds of things there may be in a world in which the premises are true. A cross's subregion is guaranteed to have something in it. If the region is bisected during the addition of the third circle, then it is no longer clear which subregion the cross should go in, and so neither of the new sub–subregions is guaranteed to have anything in it. And so on for the rules about drawing conclusions. If there is no cross left in the diagram there is no type of individual defined for all three properties which must exist. It turns out that the syllogism has the rather special metalogical property that all its valid conclusions follow in respect of such maximally defined individuals. If there is such a cross, then its subregion defines the type of thing that must exist. At least an existential conclusion is therefore justified. The rules about when universal and negative conclusions are warranted are left as homework.

The cross notation abruptly turns Euler's method from one mired in up to more than fifty diagrams for a syllogism, to one which provides a one-pass algorithm constructing a single diagram for solving any problem. The cross notation is an abstraction trick. It allows exactly the abstractions required, but little more. The result is a kind of mechanical calculating device. Imagine the circles as wire hoops of variable size, and the crosses as thumbtacks. This mechanical device models the logical constraints of the premises. If a thumbtack prevents the A and C wire hoops from being pulled horizontally apart, then a positive conclusion follows about the fact they must intersect. If the thumbtack prevents the A and C hoops from being pushed into complete correspondence, then a negative conclusion is justified by their non-correspondence. No thumbtack – no conclusion. Euler's genius here was to appreciate this correspondence between logical and mechanical constraints.

10.3.2   Metalogical Considerations

Euler's method exposes metalogical properties of the syllogism which are important to their implementation in representation systems. As we just noted, conclusions require there to be a cross in the final diagram, and the cross corresponds to a completely described type of individual. The diagrammatic representations make this especially easy to see. The geometrical properties of closed connected areas (such as those of circles) mean that every point in a plane is either inside or outside any closed area. Therefore any cross defines its corresponding type of individual with regard to all three properties. Every valid argument can be made in virtue of a cross in a final diagram. We shall call this property of the syllogism revealed by the diagrammatic system *case identifiability*, there being always a single "case" that founds a valid argument. Most logical systems do not have this property. A further obvious question is whether the converse of this "no cross ⇔ no conclusion' generalization is also true. Does every cross give us a valid conclusion?

For Aristotle's system the answer is no. There are syllogisms which give rise to final diagrams containing crosses which do not allow any Aristotelian conclusion. Figure 10.5 shows two such syllogisms and their diagrams. If we think for a moment about whether there *should* be a conclusion to these problems, we can see that in all cases it is true that *Some not-A is not C*. However, this would have failed to qualify as an Aristotelian syllogism because it contains a fourth term not-A and extra reasoning is required to accommodate it, and also because Aristotle would not have accepted 'not-A' as a subject term.

Since the conventional abbreviations for *all, some, none, some_not* are respectively **a, e, i, o** (from the Latin mnemonics), we shall abbreviate this new quantifier by the one remaining vowel, **u**.

The Deeper Meaning of u-Conclusions

Aristotle's rejection of these arguments as syllogisms is on the one hand a superficial matter of form: extra reasoning is required to eliminate their fourth term, and so they fail the syntactic definition of syllogism. But the reason why this superficial rejection was perhaps felt reasonable takes us near the heart of one of the critical developments of twentieth–century logic.

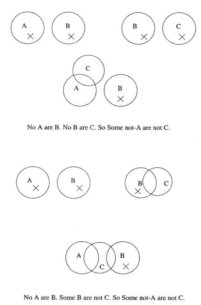

No A are B. No B are C. So Some not-A are not C.

No A are B. Some B are not C. So Some not-A are not C.

Figure 10.5   Syllogisms with valid conclusions *Some not-A are not C* – the "**u**-conclusions."

For Aristotle, and indeed logicians up to the 19th century when mathematical influence began to be felt, the concept of domain was not much discussed, and a quantifier's domain was taken to be determined by the sentence in which it occured. Logicians were quite comfortable with discussions of empty properties (such as square circle). From the modern point of view one might ask, whether they would have been equally comfortable with primitive properties which were empty—perhaps square circle can be accommodated because square and circle both have instances? But it is not clear whether this discussion could or did take place within the conceptualisation of the day.

The development of twentieth-century semantics occured when Frege generalized the notion of domain to what we now mean by the universal domain – all individuals, classes, functions, . . . – and it was rapidly noticed that this notion is incoherent. Russell's paradoxes thus brought it home that languages must be interpreted on local domains and cleared away Frege's objections to a formal approach to semantics. This twentieth-century insight into the distinction between local and universal domain is the logical motivation for our cognitive focus on the importance of reasoning externally about logics, and choosing between them in the process of interpretation.

Quite apart from his formal or syntactic reasons, Aristotle might have had some discomfort about admitting these **u**-conclusion syllogisms as valid because they violated one of his two major metalogical generalizations about validity, namely:

1. for a syllogism to have a valid conclusion, at least one of the premises must have a universal quantifier;

2. for a syllogism to have a valid conclusion, at least one of the premises must have a positive quantifier.

The syllogisms with only valid **u**-conclusions (figure 10.5) violate this second dictum. These logical observations are not merely historical curiosities. They raise interesting psychological questions about whether logically untrained students have any metalogical, if implicit, grasp of these principles. And does their grasp agree with Aristotle, or with these more recent insights? We return to these questions when some data on how students reason allow logical insights to be put to good psychological effect (section 10.4).

Consistency

A final metalogical property of the syllogism that is emphasized by Euler's system is what we might call its self-consistency. Euler's system is self-consistent in that no single diagram can represent an inconsistent set of propositions – the diagrams are models. Strictly speaking, we need to make some assumptions explicit before this statement is true. We have been assuming that Euler's system represents properties by *continuous* closed curves (those curves which are not composed of separated regions); and that distinct closed curves in the same diagram represent different properties. For an example of a discontinuous closed curve, imagine the two B circles in figure 10.4 interpreted as a single closed curve labeled B. The possibility of discontinuous curves would be incompatible with the reasoning algorithms. Similarly, in the same figure, if the two circles C and B denoted the same property, then the diagram would express a contradiction. Self-consistency is a consequence of the style of interpretation of Euler diagrams – a mode of interpretation we have called *direct* (see Stenning [258]).

The above observations of the concreteness of primitive diagrammatic systems, and the fact that in this little domain there are strategies for always selecting a single diagram which can be an appropriate basis for reasoning, are interestingly reminiscent of the contrast between credulous and skeptical reasoning that has been an important strand in this book. Constructing a single diagram is like credulously seeking an intended model of a discourse. But this domain has the very special property that if we choose our intended model wisely, then it can suffice to serve as the basis of reasoning which will fulfill the more demanding skeptical goal of only producing *classically* valid conclusions – ones true in *all* models of the premises. So here, the two stances of reasoning *can* collapse, though, as we shall see, they do not have to. So another interest of the syllogism is that in this peculiar domain, the relation between credulous and skeptical processing becomes very close.

10.4   Individual Differences in Interpretation

Nothing is apparently easier than to ask subjects to engage in syllogistic reasoning. One simply asks them to assume that the two premises are true, and then asks whether it follows that the conclusion is true, or asks them to generate a conclusion that follows from the assumptions. However, as we shall see presently, subjects do not universally construe these instructions as instructions to reason with a classical concept of "follows." Lest there be any doubt at this stage that this is a real possibility with subjects, there is evidence in the literature that experimenters also sometimes adopt a different notion of validity. For example, in a pioneering study into the interpretation of syllogistic premises which is our experimental setting–off point in this section, Newstead [200] instructed subjects to assume single premises, and then used the following instruction: "Now judge whether (1) the following candidate conclusion must be true, or (2) whether it must be false." Subjects were not given the chance to respond (3) "the conclusion might be true or might be false" – the necessary response to reflect any grasp they have of the concept of logical independence between premise and conclusion. The construal of the task reflected in Newstead's response set is nearer to a credulous one than a classical skeptical one. Later Newstead added the necessary third response option as what he called a "more sensitive measure," seemingly without realizing that this was a measure of a different concept of validity. If experimenters can have nonclassical interpretations, it is hardly surprising that subjects turn out to have them too.

Although syllogistic premises are simple sentences which may appear stony ground for growing multiple interpretations, our earlier discussions of the selection and suppression tasks are sufficient to make it likely that multiple interpretations will be possible simply because universal quantifiers invoke conditional logical form. *All A are B* is analysed as *If it's an A then it's a B*.[5] Here, then, is another illustration that logical form is as much a function of the inferential task we engage in, as of the sentences in the materials presented. Adopting a credulous goal may lead to different interpretations than a skeptical one.

Newstead's interest in syllogistic interpretation was sparked not by considerations of credulous and skeptical processing, but by the very closely related philosophical and linguistic literature on the theory of cooperative communication (Grice [108]; see also chapter 5). Just to remind the reader, in *cooperative*

---

5. As an historical aside, we note here that the representation of the universal sentence *All A are B* via a bound variable (here "it") seems to have originated with Kant. Longuenesse [175,p. 86ff] discusses why this representation is important in Kant's philosophy.

communication, the hearer assumes that the speaker is being helpful, and will tell the hearer exactly what he needs to know to construct the intended model of the discourse. By contrast, in *adversarial* communication, the participants adopt a skeptical stance of seeking countermodels.

As Grice pointed out, cooperative communication gives rise to *implicatures*, inferences that can be made on the assumption that the speaker is helpful, although not from their classical logical entailments. Thus, if the speaker says "Some *A* are *B*," the hearer generates the implicature "Some *A* are not *B*": for if the speaker actually knew that *all A* are *B*, he would have said so.[6] Questions about the exact relation between Grice's account, and the distinction between credulous and skeptical reasoning will arise in what follows.

We now summarise an experiment (Stenning and Cox [262]) which investigated just what naive subjects' interpretations of syllogistic quantifiers are like, alongside Newstead's analysis of his experiments.

10.4.1 Immediate Inferences and the Understanding of Deductive Tasks

Newstead dubbed his one-premise task, the "immediate inference task" to distinguish it from the "extended" inferences across the two premises of syllogisms. Newstead presented his subjects with all thirty-two combinations of assumptions (the four quantified forms) with candidate conclusions (the four quantified forms, plus their four "conversions"). In his later experiments and our subsequent ones, for each of the thirty-two items, subjects were asked whether the conclusion was true, false, or could be either (see figure 10.6).

Thus there are 3^{32} possible patterns of responses which subjects could make – a large number. Newstead pursued the hypothesis that subjects' reasoning in the two-premise syllogistic task was influenced by their interpretations as evidenced in the one-premise immediate inference task. This seems a highly reasonable hypothesis. Indeed, if it were to turn out to be false, one might question how that could be. Reasoning just has to be influenced by interpretation, though clearly there might be more to the two-sentence task than merely multiplying sentences, and the range of possible influences is broad.

Newstead's hypothesis testing approach was the conventional one. The concept of Gricean implicature was operationalized in terms of particular responses to four of the thirty-two questions in the immediate inference questionnaire. These four questions include the *some A are B* and *some A are not-B* premises (which would implicate each other, even if they do not logically entail each other), but also *all A are B* (possibly "inconsistent" with *some A are B*) and

---

6. Note that to conclude some *A* are not *B*, the hearer also has to assume that the speaker knows what the relations between *A* and *B* are. This goes beyond being helpful. The speaker may be helpful and not know that all *A* are *B*, without knowing that some *A* are not *B*. In this case, the implicature generated is only "the speaker does not know that all *A* are *B*." These knowledge requirements are much neglected in discussions of Grice.

This is a study of the way people draw conclusions from information. On each of the following pages there is a statement at the top of the page. An example is 'All A's are B's'. Assume that these statements at the top of the page are true and that there are both A's and B's.

Below each statement is a line. Below the line are some more statements. For each of the statements below the line, decide whether you believe it is true, false or one can't tell (because either is possible), given the truth of the sentence at the top of the page. Indicate your belief by circling ONE of either 'T' (true) , 'F' (false) or 'CE' (could be either). \\
Examples:

  if you believe that 'No As are Bs' must be true given the true statement 'All A's are B's' then circle T
  if you believe that 'Some As are not Bs' must be false given the true statement 'No As are Bs' then circle F
  if you believe that 'No As are Bs' could be true and could be false given the true statement 'No As are Bs', then circle CE

Again, please note that you should interpret 'some' to mean 'at least one and possibly all'.

Figure 10.6   The instructions with example material from the immediate inference question-naire.

no A are B (possibly "inconsistent" with *some A are not-B*). This measure of "Gricean interpretation" was examined for internal correlations between the drawing of implicatures to different questions in the immediate inference task, and later correlated with conclusions drawn from syllogisms where different conclusions would become valid if the Gricean implicature were added to the premises.

Newtead's results did produce high rates of Gricean interpretation in the immediate inference task. About 80% of subjects produced Gricean implicatures from at least some assumptions, but there was little correlation between drawing one expected implicature and drawing the others. Newstead then turned to the question whether these implicatures could predict subsequent reasoning. He interpreted his results as resoundingly negative. Syllogistic conclusions were not predicted by premise implicatures. Newstead concluded that there was no relation between what subjects did in the two tasks – presented with one premise they applied Grice, but presented with two premises they threw a switch and applied mental models.

We applaud Newstead for adopting an extremely interesting large-scale question informed by philosophical, logical, and linguistic literatures – can Grice's theory of cooperative communication contribute to an explanation why subjects do not conform to classical logic when solving syllogisms? Since credulous reasoning is so closely related to Grice's theory, the authors of this book would have to hope the answer is positive. Our argument is that the answer is positive, but Newstead's project was derailed by conventional experimental psychology hypothesis testing methodology. Instead of first asking exploratory questions such as "What are undergraduate subjects' interpretations of syllogistic quantifiers like?" the standard psychological approach is to operationalise on a narrow base of specific stimuli and responses, and then to test the operationalization's ability to make predictions of another narrow range of responses identified by another operationalization. Of course, in order to explore, one needs some guidance as to how to condense the 3^{32} response patterns into a description of "what naive logical intuitions are like," but there is plenty of guidance available from elementary logical concerns.

10.4.2   A New Experiment on Immediate Inference

We will pay rather more attention to the sequence by which our findings were arrived at than is normal in reporting experimental results. Exploration is not much taught as a psychological method, but it is an important one for progress in this area.

The first principle employed in our fishing expedition into the interpretation data was: pay close attention to the "could be either" responses. These responses are judgments to the effect that assumption and conclusion sentences are logically independent. Logical independence is transformed in going from credulous to skeptical reasoning. Many premise-conclusion pairs that are valid credulously become logically independent once viewed classically. Of course, exploration is aided by a rough guide, and it is very useful to bear in mind what one's guide is, because it certainly will affect what is found. But rough guides are not hard to come by, and if one doesn't find much with one guide, then one can resort to another.

Rashness and Hesitancy

There are therefore two classes of cases of particular interest – cases where classical logic tells us that assumption and conclusion are logically independent, but significant numbers of subjects respond that either the conclusion or its negation does follow. We will call this general kind of response "rash" – subjects are rashly overinferring (by a classical logical criterion). The second kind of case is where classical logic tells us that something does validly follow, but subjects respond that the conclusion could be either true or false. We will call these responses "hesitant" – subjects hesitate to draw a valid conclusion. The rash case is generally to be expected if the interpretation is credulous. The hesitant case is more puzzling, since classically valid conclusions tend to be valid under at least some credulous interpretations. Many cases of the former (rash) kind are already well known to logic teachers down the ages as fallacies, and observed in the history of experimental investigation of syllogistic reasoning. The most prominent example is the fallacy known as "illicit conversion" [34]: from *All A are B* it follows that *All B are A*. The second kind of response, as far as we are aware, has not been reported, but asking whether it occurs is an obvious initial exploratory question which is at the very least an important backdrop to interpreting rash responses.

As an aside to be picked up later, it is important to realise that conversion, at least of conditionals, can be related to closed-world reasoning and is therefore another case of credulous reasoning. It isn't hard to see informally that closed–world reasoning in discourse can lead to "conversion." The rough principle is: "only add to the model what is necessary to understand what has been said." So, if a discourse begins "All *A* are *B*," then at this stage we get a model in which the only way that something can get to be *B* is because it is *A*, and in such a model it will be true that "All *B* are *A*."

Examination of the data quickly revealed some striking cases of rashness and hesitancy. For example, there was a substantial minority (about 20%) of subjects who refused to draw the conclusion *Some B are A* from the assumption that *Some A are B* where subject and predicate of the premise are inverted in the conclusion. Our logically sophisticated colleagues, even those who teach logic, often react to these responses by saying they must just be random noise – how could anyone possibly refuse this inference? A little further eyeballing of the data demonstrates that it is not random noise. When all the questions that are cases of classical logical dependence are tabulated ($N=12$), it turns out that there are quite a few of them that produce similarly large proportions of hesitant responses. The next observation is that this is *only* the case when the conclusion has subject and predicate "inverted" from their positions in the assumption ($N=8$), as in our example.

The third observation is that subjects who make these hesitant responses on one inverted question tend to make them on other inverted questions. In fact when a histogram is drawn up tabulating the number of subjects who make 0, 1, 2, ... 8 hesitant responses, the distribution is bimodal. Most subjects make none or few, but there is a substantial tail of subjects who make every, or nearly every, possible hesitant response (figure 10.7). Without any statistical testing, or better, with only the simplest of intuitive models of what might be expected, this is pretty strongly flavored stuff.

The fourth observation is that subjects who make several of these hesitant re-sponses to inverted conclusions, are disjoint from the subjects who make several rash responses to inverted conclusions. There are about a quarter of subjects in each category, but there is no overlap. Random this is not. Wonderful thing following one's nose, especially when kept pointing forward. These obviously

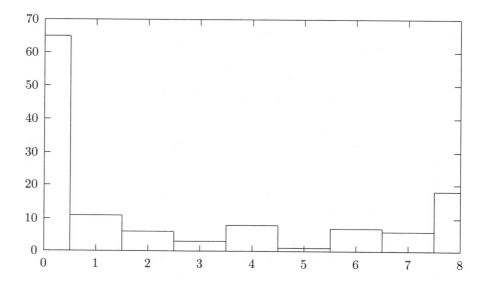

Figure 10.7   The number of subjects responding to N out of eight questions that invert subject and predicate with the answer "Neither conclusion follows," when this is incorrect.

intriguing observations suggest a scheme for classifying subjects' answer pat-terns on a small number of dimensions. Let "T," "F," "CE" abbreviate the responses "true," "false" and "could be either." Above we dubbed subjects who tend to answer T or F when the answer should be CE: *rash*, and subjects who tend to answer CE when the answer should be T or F, *hesitant*. As mentioned above, the rash subjects are the ones who tend to apply a cooperative model of communication.

Immediate Inference and Information Packaging

Now consider a specific structural feature of an immediate inference, namely whether it conserves the structure of subject and predicate (henceforth an *in-place* inference), or whether that structure is reversed (an *inverted* inference). Both rashness and hesitancy can be further evaluated along the in-place/inverted dimension. Thus, a subject who is rash on in-place inferences is one who tends to answer T or F instead of the correct CE on immediate inferences which preserve subject/predicate structure; cf. the classical examples of Grice's implicatures. It turns out that no subjects were hesitant on in-place questions, which leaves three combinations of properties: hesitant on inverted inferences, rash on in-place inferences, and rash on inverted inferences. Interestingly, 94% of subjects fall into one of the following four groups: neither rash nor hesitant on any inference (17%); rash on in-place questions but neither rash nor hesitant on inverted inferences (22%); rash on both kind of inferences, but not hesitant (35%); and hesitant on inverted inferences plus rash on in-place inferences (20%). It is also striking how many subjects are rash on in-place inferences: 80%! Thus there is, as Newstead already remarked, good evidence for the prevalence of a Gricean model of communication (or credulous interpretation) in this task.

What intuitions are available to explain what hesitancy might reflect? "Some A are B" is different from "Some B are A": about a quarter of subjects deny that the latter sentence follows from the former.[7] Linguists employ the metaphor of "information packaging": the same information is realized (packaged) linguistically in different ways, and this because each packaging serves a different communicative function.[8] For example, the two sentences are natural answers to different questions. While linguists would not normally use this term for describing the subject/predicate structural difference between these two sentences, in the very restricted class of abstract syllogistic materials this metaphor applies. If a logically naive subject is asked whether "Some B are A" follows from "Some A are B," he may not realise that he should strip the sentences of their information packaging, nor that that is what the graphical representation using Euler circles does. Information–packaging is related to credulous interpretation because speakers use appropriate packagings to help hearers arrive at the intended model. To take a skeptical attitude one often needs to strip off the packaging to find possible counterexamples. Syllogisms can be divided into those whose information packaging points toward valid conclusions, and those where it obscures them. The latter are sometimes called "counterfigural," and they produce a lot of "no valid conclusion" responses.

Subjects who are rash on in-place questions (*Some A are B. Are all A B?*), but not on inverted inferences (*All A are B. Are all B A?*), are plausibly processing credulously but are held in check from making inverted conclusions by information packaging which points them away from these conclusions. Many though by no means all of these subjects will be hesitant subjects who may be completely spellbound by information packaging. It is difficult to say whether

---

7. For the logically sophisticated it can be hard to recover lost innocence, but the following example may help. The judge in a famous UK comedian's tax avoidance trial summed up by stating that while it was clear that no comedians are accountants, it was equally clear that some accountants are comedians.

8. For an interesting argument to the effect that information packaging is precisely the purpose of "object orientation" in programming, see Kowalski [162], especially section 3.3.

they have any idea of logical validity, since 80% of hesitant subjects are rash on in-place questions.

In conclusion, what is perhaps most surprising about this exploration is that major patterns of interpretation emerge which don't even refer to the identity of particular quantifiers in their specification. The quantifiers are involved because they are involved in our specification of which questions are classified as expecting which answers, but the patterns that emerge are rashness and hesitancy on in-place and inverted questions. We may say that subjects' inference patterns are determined less by the logical notion of classical validity than by various aspects of the communicative situation, as hypothesized by the subject. This is perhaps hardly surprising, since they nowhere have had the classical concept of deductive validity explained to them. There is plenty of evidence of credulous interpretation, but there are other effects as well.

Can this classification of interpretations be related to subjects' syllogistic reasoning, thus resolving Newstead's failure to relate interpretation and reasoning?

10.5 Syllogistic Reasoning

When we move from immediate inference tasks to full syllogistic reasoning, the task changes and it is an open question when to expect transfer. That is, for example, one cannot necessarily expect that in a syllogism with premises

> All A are B.
> All B are C.

and with a subject who shows "illicit conversion" in his immediate inference task responses, the premises are still taken to imply

> All B are A.
> All C are B.

Thus, we should predict offhand that a sizable proportion of such subjects will draw the conclusion

> All C are A.

One reason that this prediction may fail is that the presence of two premises leads to an additional complication, namely the grammatical status of the middle term (B) and the end terms (A and C). In the example above, the end term A is in subject position in the premise but in predicate position in the conclusion, whereas for C it is the other way around. As we have seen, there is a tendency on the part of a subset of subjects to find such reorderings counterintuitive (i.e., violating normal discourse structure), so that in fact a subject may be saved from committing a logical error by committing another logical error!

We now turn to the empirical question whether subjects' choices in the immediate inference task predict their reasoning in the syllogistic task. How should we address this exploratory question?

10.5.1 Individual Factors Influencing Reasoning

In this subsection we introduce kinds of modeling to add to the logical modeling of earlier chapters: statistical modeling of data, and the modeling of mental structures and processes involved in task performance. The statistical modeling we outline yields a regression equation: a set of weighted factors which can be shown to affect the likelihood of a certain feature of conclusions drawn from syllogistic premises. Such modeling is a bottom–up data-driven exercise which produces prima facie evidence that a relation between a factor and the process exists. The resulting model is large and messy and hard to interpret as a mental process. The process modeling presented here takes an earlier theoretical process model developed on group data and extends it so that different subgroups of subjects (defined by their interpretation patterns) are predicted to engage in rather different reasoning processes. Process models cannot generally be derived directly from data, but they are interpretable as psychological processes. Both theoretical process model and statistical data model are related to the logical models of earlier chapters – credulous vs. skeptical interpretation of the task is an important feature in both the statistical model and the process one. So the situation is typical of scientific analysis – multiple models at different levels, either closer or farther from the data, play their roles in analysis.

In the analysis of immediate inference we identified several factors, such as rashness (both on in-place and inverted questions) and hesitancy (on inverted questions) which systematically influence interpretations in the immediate inference task. The syllogism leads to additional factors of possible importance, such as *grammar* (whether the end terms have different or identical grammatical category), the distribution of the quantifiers over the premises, and the order of premises. For example, one may distinguish the case where an existential quantifier (either *some* or *some... not*) occurs in the first or the second premise, in both, or in none; and similarly for the other quantifiers.

One may now try to analyse empirically the influence of these factors on various aspects of syllogistic reasoning performance. An interesting aspect is whether subjects choose an AC ordering or a CA ordering of the end terms A and C in the conclusion of the syllogism. We choose to initially model conclusion term order rather than accuracy because we believe subjects adopt different interpretations which define different concepts of accuracy. We return to accuracy when we have built a model of conclusion term ordering which is sensitive to individual differences of interpretation.

The exploratory statistical technique used is called logistic regression. A heuristic searches a space of possible factors in trying to construct the best regression equation which can predict whether an AC or a CA conclusion will be drawn as a function of different structures of syllogism, and as a function of subjects' different patterns of immediate inference response. The best model shows that classical validity plays only a marginal role in this choice!

10.5.2   Statistical analysis

The original statistical model of this data and its development are described in [262]. A number of structural asymmetries of syllogistic problems which could potentially affect premise ordering, along with a number of features of each subject's immediate inference data, together with a large number of possible interactions between all of these factors are defined. An algorithm in the statistical package (backwards elimination) then searches the space of logistic regression equations that can use subsets of these factors to predict the order of the terms (AC vs CA) in the conclusions (if any) that the subject drew for a given problem. The algorithm balances the number of factors in the equation with amount of the variance the equation can explain and identifies a "best" equation. As with all regression modelling, the equation is developed on a "development" dataset prior to being tested on a new "test" dataset, so that accidental regularities can be discarded and predictive regularities retained.

The first empirical result of this statistical analysis is that the best equation fits very much better than by chance. It explains the term orders of about 70% of conclusions, where 50% is chance. This leaves a lot of variance unexplained, but then there may be substantial pure noise in the data (factors such as slips of attention, memory, etc. which we have no measures to predict). Unfortunately we cannot estimate the amount of this noise with logistic regression in the way we would be able to with linear regression.

The second empirical conclusion we can draw from the terms that appear in the model is that individual differences in immediate inference patterns do significantly predict syllogistic conclusion term order. We have at least partially overcome Newstead's failure to find a relation, although the exploratory statistical model yields no immediately insightful statement of the relation. To find one is our next task.

The best resulting statistical model of the factors affecting conclusion term order shows that the more substantial determinants, in no partiuclar order, include:

1. when the two end terms have different grammatical categories, those categories tend to be preserved in the conclusion;

2. existential quantifiers tend to put their end terms into subject position;

3. there is a weak but general tendency for the premise 1 term to be subject (i.e., AC order is preferred);

4. each quantifier except *No* tends to varying degrees to put its end term into subject position, but quantifiers have greatest influence when in premise 2; *Some_ not* especially has no influence in the first premise, but a large influence in the second premise;

5. hesitant subjects have a general tendency to respond with an AC ordering throughout; by contrast, rash subjects have no such special tendency;

6. there are complex interactions between hesitancy, grammar, and *No* and between rashness-in-place, grammar, and *Some...not*.

The first four regularities are general properties of all subjects: the last two are differences in reasoning by groups of subjects with different immediate inference patterns. Some of these regularities are well-known from the literature. The effect of the grammatical organization of the first two "diagonal" figures has been observed in every experiment reported. The weak general preference for AC over CA is also common. But we know of no systematic study of quantifier effects on term ordering. The strong effect of existentials on term ordering (the second largest contribution to the equation's fit) has not been noticed, and similarly the differential effects of the negative quantifiers, and certainly not the individual differences in these. So even if we couldn't find an insightful model which integrates all these observations, exploration has already yielded new empirical observations.

The actual statistical model is appreciably more complicated than this – it is after all the result of a fishing expedition. It tells us what factors and interactions between them play a significant role in determining conclusion term order. It is hard to integrate its parameters into an understanding at the level which we seek. So, as part of the process of constructing such an understanding, we will now give an informal description of the relation of the statistical model to the source-founding model originally put forward by Stenning and Yule [269] to model group data.

10.5.3 From Data Description to a Psychological Model

Stenning and Yule [269] presented a general model of how subjects go about syllogistic reasoning – the source-founding model.[9] The intuition behind the term "source premise" comes from discourse processing. The source is the

---

9. Guy Politzer [219] points out that a great deal of Stenning and Yule's analysis is prefigured in a 1908 paper by Störring [273].

premise which supplies the discourse antecedent on which can be built a description of a fully specified kind of indvidual. With slight adjustment of heuristics, this model can serve either as a normative competence model (i.e., it can
generate all and only the valid conclusions according to classical logic), or as
a descriptive performance model for analyzing subjects' reasoning. In fact, the
same framework also shows how credulous and skeptical reasoning are unusu-
ally closely related in this restricted domain. These close relations are desirable
because they allow explanation of errors as divergences from norms.

The model has the virtue that it is completely abstract about the particular
representations which subjects use (e.g., diagrams vs. sentences), but it nevertheless provides the best explanation of conclusion term ordering that is available in the literature. We first describe the model as it was developed for group
data, and then show how it can be extended to incorporate the individual differences in reasoning as a function of quantifier interpretation which are our
current concern. We hope the reader will forgive a greater than usual emphasis
on methodology in what follows. We seek to illustrate the relation between a
theoretical model, raw data for its extension, exploratory statistical modelling of
the raw data, and a refined theoretical model incoporating individual interpretation factors, alongside problems structural factors, into predictions of reasoning
behaviour.

The source–founding model is represented in figure 10.8. The model has
two parts: a specification of how premises are designated as having the status
of *source* and *nonsource* premise, and some simple operations which are then
applied on the basis of this categorization to draw conclusions. The top half
represents the weighing of factors in choosing between designating the first or
second premise as source: the bottom half illustrates the alternative processes of
drawing a conclusion, conditioned on this choice. Modulations on the factors
which go into the choice of source premise are what will be used to model
individual differences.

Source and non-source premises are defined using the concept of a critical
individual. So, for example, for the syllogism

(1)   *All B are A. Some C are B. Therefore some C are A.*

the critical individual is an *A* that is *B* and *C*. This idea is closely related to
Aristotle's concept of *ecthesis*. The source premise defined by the classical logical competence model is the premise which establishes the critical individual –
in this case the second premise. In the Euler diagram system described above,
source premises contribute the crosses which mark the critical individuals in
completed problem diagrams. Problems with valid conclusions always have at
least one source premise (sometimes both premises are potential sources).

The source-founding model of syllogism solution connects with the concerns
of earlier chapters by the simple observation that the introduction of discourse

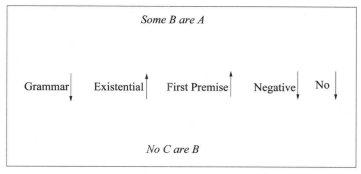

Choosing a source premise on which to found a conclusion

Premise 1 chosen: *Some B are A* + *C* = *Some B are A and C* = *Some A are C*

Premise 2 chosen: *No C are B* + *A* = *No C are B and A* = *No C are A*

Drawing a conclusion based on chosen source premise

Figure 10.8 The source–founding model of syllogism solution applied to the syllogism *Some B are A. No C are B.* The upper part represents the various structural factors and their bias toward choosing either premise 1 or 2 as source. The lower part shows the possible conclusions resulting from the alternative assignments of source premise.

referents into representations of discourses is the key operation of discourse processing. The source premise performs such an introduction. Paradigmatically this would be by an existential premise, but the no-empty-sets interpretation allows universals to also make these introductions.

A general algorithm for determining which premise is classically a valid source is fairly complicated, but some very simple heuristics get most cases. First, for problems with valid conclusions, existential premises are always source. (note that problems with valid conclusions only ever have single existential premises; cf. Aristotle's generalization mentioned above on page 308). Second, if this principle fails to choose a source (i.e.. there are two universal premises), positive premises should be preferred as source over negative ones. This then leaves only two possibilities. As we have seen, problems with two negative universal premises have no valid Aristotelean conclusion, so all remaining problems have two positive universal conclusions. If there is a unique end-term subject, then the premise in which it occurs becomes source. If not, then the first premise's end term is chosen as source. This may sound all rather complicated and ad hoc but these heuristics are closely related to a number of principles of discourse processing and to a competence model for classical logic.[10]Modulations of these heuristics can explain differences between subject–groups.

Once a source premise has been chosen, a conclusion is drawn. Again the general algorithm to model classical logic is quite complicated but a very simple method gets most problems right. Simply attach the end term of the nonsource premise to the source premise's end, and delete the middle term. So for the example (1) above, choose the existential premise as source, attach the end term of the nonsource premise to the end of the source premise (yielding Some C are B and A), and delete the B.

Obviously this method applied to invalid syllogisms will generate invalid conclusions. It will also generate invalid conclusions for any problem for which the only valid conclusions have quantifiers other than those in the source premise. So it is an important question how "no valid conclusion" responses are generated (not a problem tackled here, though the heuristics for identifying source strongly suggest a method related to the medieval "sieve"; see [258,p. 111]), but it is important to remember that what follows is only a model of how conclusions other than "no valid conclusion" are generated.

Stenning and Yule [269] present evidence from a task where subjects have to describe critical individuals and thereby produce an ordering of all three terms. The task was designed to yield richer evidence (because we now have three terms, there are six orderings instead of just AC and CA, and these are completely independent of validity). The source–founding model predicts that the middle term should often come first in a description of the critical individual for a problem. This is the pattern Stenning and Yule observed – in fact the commonest term order of all is BAC.

Mental models theory predicts, on the basis of some claims about "first-in, first-out" memory, that middle terms always should come between the end terms. As we shall see, this aspect of the theory is a covert incorporation of syntactic information into the supposedly purely semantic representations. Though mental model theory never sought any evidence that this kind of memory was involved, it explained the ordering on the basis of memory theories. In fact, the term order regularity predicted (with B in the middle) turns out not to be observed in the individuals task data, so the task requiring the description of critical individuals provides evidence that this kind of memory is not involved in holding term order. More generally, the fact that subjects readily adapt to the "individual identification task" provides empirical support for the cognitive rel-

---

10. The connection to discourse processing will be elaborated on page 329.

evance of the logical analysis of how syllogisms relate to discourse processing – the underlying basis for the source-founding model. Furthermore, the new task shows that at least a substantial minority of subjects are capable of identifying the critical individuals which underlie the nonstandard **u**-conclusions from two negative premises, discussed earlier. This shows remarkable flexibility. Although subjects in the standard task appear to be able to exploit some implicit knowledge of Aristotle's principle that two negative premises generate no valid conclusion (i.e., subjects find these easier problems than problems with one positive premise), subjects nevertheless can identify these nonstandard inferences when they are given the novel individual-identification task.

So the Stenning and Yule model conceives of syllogistic reasoning as subjects choosing a source premise which founds a description of a critical individual. It is this model which we now expand in order to capture the individual differences observed with regard to how interpretation determines reasoning.

10.5.4 Incorporating Interpretation Factors into the Reasoning Model

The individual differences particularly revolve around grammar, premise order, and the negative quantifiers *Some_not* and *No*, particularly the latter quantifier. In the statistical model of term order, all subjects have a tendency to make *AC* conclusions, but hesitant subjects have a stronger tendency. All subjects have a strong tendency to preserve the grammatical status of the end terms from the premises in their conclusions, but hesitant subjects have a much stronger such tendency, especially in the second syllogistic figure[11] (where it operates against premise order). These observations can be directly accommodated in the source–founding model – hesitant subjects simply weigh these factors in their decisions about which premise to choose as source, and that makes sense because grammar and premise order are forms of information packaging, and hesitant subjects are especially sensitive to that. But these tendencies also interact with the negative quantifiers. So the tendency for hesitant subjects to be especially guided by grammar in the second syllogistic figure, interacts with *No* so that they have a stronger tendency to keep the end term of the *No* premise in predicate position, in the second figure. Rash-on-inverted subjects have the opposite tendency to treat *No* less differently than the other quantifiers, and rash-in-place subjects treat *Some_not* less differently. As far as we know these observations about negative quantifiers are novel.

Why should the individual differences affect these negative quantifiers? First, there is the general fact that negative information is more easily processed when it is preceded by a positive frame (see, e.g., Wason [294]). There is also an interesting duality in the way that *Some_not* can be encoded. One can think of it positively as an existential assertion of a predicate's complement; or nega-

---

11. For the syllogistic figures, see table 10.1.

tively as the denial of a universal assertion of the predicate. It is possible that the former is preferred by rash-on-inverted subjects, and the latter by hesitant subjects, who would then prefer to keep the negative information late in the sentence. Which brings us to the interactions with *No*. Here there are logically special circumstances: in the classical competence model *No* premises never obligatorily contribute subject terms to valid conclusions, and this is reflected in the source–founding model by the fact that it never makes *No* premises' end terms into subjects. It seems that hesitant subjects are especially attuned to these logical regularities. So all these factors can be incorporated into the heuristics in the source–founding model and thereby affect the conclusion term orders observed in different groups of subjects. The model extended by some individual difference factors is represented in figure 10.9.

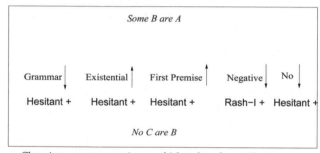

Choosing a source premise on which to found a conclusion

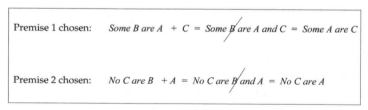

Drawing a conclusion based on chosen source premise

Figure 10.9 Interpretation factors incorporated into source premise choice. The named interpretation factor (hesitant, Rash-I) intensifies the effect of the arrow. The effects of source premise choice once made play out as before.

But we can go further and see whether these ordering phenomena are causally connected with reasoning accuracy (as defined classically) or whether they are just information packaging, epiphenomenal to the real conclusion drawing process. We can go back to the conclusion data and analyse subsets of subjects and problems where the source-founding model tells us there should be particularly illuminating effects on accuracy *if* the model is really about reasoning and not just about packaging one's conclusions once one has drawn them.

In order to get a better handle on the complex data, we classified pairs of syllogistic problems which are identical, save for their premise ordering (e.g., *All A are B. All B are C.* and *All B are A. All C are B.* are such a pair). The twenty-seven problems with valid conclusions are composed of thirteen such pairs and one singleton which is symmetric about this ordering. The source-founding model now provides a criterion for defining a *canonical* and *noncanonical* ordering of each pair: source premises come first in canonical pairs; nonsource in noncanonical pairs. The intuition is that getting first the premise on which a representation is going to be built should be easier. The one *All/All* problem symmetric about reordering (namely *All A are B. All B are C*) is canonical. Note that this definition of canonical problems according to the source-founding model means that *No* premises are always second premises in canonical problems. This observation helps greatly in understanding what the statistical model means, because the effects of *No* in the statistical model are much greater when it is in premise 2. Now to an analysis of reasoning accuracy.

We can ask for any pair of problems and any group of subjects whether they find the canonical problem or its noncanonical counterpart easier (in the sense of getting a higher proportion of problems classically correct). Since the only difference between these pairs of problems is the ordering of the premises, if there is an effect of canonicality on accuracy of reasoning, then premise order is playing a role in subjects' strategies for finding source premises and constructing conclusions. The obvious two subject groups to explore first are hesitant subjects and rash-on-inverted subjects, since these two groups are essentially disjoint, and at opposite extremes with regard to their sensitivity to information packaging. The critical problems that should be particularly revealing are problems where the simple source-founding algorithm tries to put negated predicates into subject position – these are the problems where the classical logical competence model needs to make complex adjustments to get the right conclusions.

There is just one problem pair (out of thirteen) for which the heuristic of adding the end term of the nonsource premise to the end of the source-premise, rules out drawing a valid conclusion. This is the fourth figure pair *Some B are not A. All B are C.* (canonical) and *All B are A. Some B are not C.* (noncanonical). The conclusion–drawing heuristic (attach the end term of the nonsource premise to the end of the source premise, and remove the middle term) applied to these problems yields the conclusion *Some A are not C.* for the canonical problem and *Some C are not A.* for noncanonical, whereas the valid conclusions are the other way round.

This pair of problems therefore provides an interesting test case for interactions between interpretation patterns and reasoning accuracy, as mediated by conclusion term ordering. We can usefully compare this problem pair with two other pairs. The problem of the third figure that has the same quantifiers and has valid conclusions which *are* found by the source–founding and conclusion–drawing heuristics is *Some A are not B. All C are B.* (canonical) and *All A are B. Some C are not B.* (noncanonical). The simple heuristics work on these problems because the end terms are both subjects, just as they fail to work in the earlier example from the fourth figure because the end terms are both predicates. The second insightful comparison is with the pairs from the first and second figures where canonicality is resolved only by grammar: *All A are B. All B are C.* (canonical) and *All B are A. All C are B.* (noncanonical). Since grammar is a powerful resolver of conclusion term order for all interpretation groups, and it does not interact with *All*, this problem pair provides a control.[12]

Predictions   Canonicality interacting with the source–founding heuristics makes rather precise predictions about hesitant and rash-on-inverted questions subjects' reasoning accuracy for these three pairs of problems. The *All/All* problem pair should show a reasoning accuracy advantage for the canonical problem over the noncanonical problem for both interpretation groups, because grammar overrides premise order in determining choice of source.

Hesitant subjects for whom premise order has a strong influence on choice of source should show a strong canonicality advantage for the *Some_not/All* problem pair in the third figure. Rash-on-inverted questions subjects, who are not much influenced by premise order, should show little canonicality effect on this pair of problems. But for the *Some_not/All* problem pair in the fourth figure, hesitant subjects should show a *reverse* canonicality effect because determining source by premise order gives the right conclusion term order in the anticanonical problem, and the wrong one in the canonical problem. Again, rash-on-inverted subjects should show little canonicality effect here.

Statistical Analysis   Stenning and Cox's data set yielded seventeen hesitant subjects, forty-three rash-on-inverted subjects, and forty-two subjects who were neither, as controls. Inferential statistics tested for significant relationships between 1) which of the three pairs of problems was posed, 2) the order of presentation of the premises (i.e. canonicality), and 3) the subject's interpretation style (hesitant vs. rash-on-inverted problems), in determining whether the subject drew classically correct conclusions, or not. The tests showed that while there were no first order or "main" effects, there were significant interactions between 1) type of subject and canonicality, and 2) between all three factors

---

12. In a paper we did not know about when [262] was written, [7,p. 156] find that this same subset of syllogisms is the only one to distinguish their "visual" and "verbal" subjects: "With the exception of the four same-form, multi-model syllogisms discussed previously, neither the present study, nor that of Ford, found any significant difference in overall performance across different strategy types ..."

in determining reasoning accuracy. The means for the three-way interaction appear in table 10.2.

Table 10.2 Combined experiments 1 and 2 data: Mean canonicality advantage on reasoning accuracy scores adjusted for nonhesitant non-rash-on-inverted mean scores, for three canonical/noncanonical problem-pairs and for hesitant and rash-on-inverted subject groups: the top member of each problem-pair is canonical. A positive value means the subjects are *more* accurate than nonhesitant, non-rash-on-inverted subjects: a negative one means they are less accurate

Subject Group	Hesitant		Rash-on-inverted	
Problem Pair	Mean	S.E.	Mean	S.E.
All AB. All BC. So, All AC	-.02	.09	-.09	.06
All BA. All CB. So, All CA	-.23	.12	-.22	.08
Some A not B. All CB. So, Some A not C	+.11	.12	-.16	.08
All AB. Some C not B. So, Some C not A	-.16	.12	-.19	.08
Some B not A. All BC. So, Some C not A	-.22	.12	-.10	.08
All BA. Some B not C. So, Some A not C	+.12	.12	-.17	.08

The interaction is of the form that when grammar identifies source premise, both hesitant and rash subjects are equal to their nonhesitant nonrash peers for the canonically ordered problem, but both suffer roughly equally when the premise order is anticanonical. When grammar does not identify source, rash subjects suffer relative to their nonrash nonhesitant peers regardless of the premise order. But now hesitant subjects show a sensitivity to whether premise order defines source accurately. In the standard problem where the source identified by the model's heuristics can be used to make the simple construction of the correct conclusion, hesitant subjects actually outperform their nonhesitant nonrash peers on the canonically ordered member of the pair, but underperform them on the noncanonical member. In the exceptional problem where the source identified by the heuristic cannot be so used, they underperform their peers on the canonically ordered problem but outperform them on the noncanonical member of the pair. These results are consistent with the idea that hesitant subjects tend to identify premise 1 as source, whereas rash-on-inverted subjects are less affected by premise order, and more by grammar and the quantifier attributes that drive the heuristics. Note that whereas there are *no* global differences in accuracy, there are large and opposite effects on groups of problems for different subject groups.

The Source-Founding Model and Individual Differences   In summary of the extensions to the source–founding model, we have shown that effects revealed by the exploratory statistical model can be incorporated intelligibly into the source–founding model as weightings of factors for choosing the source premise. Hesitant subjects always show greater effects of information packaging: rash-on-inverted subjects always show more indifference to information packaging.

But we can go further and show that the processes which determine conclusion term order are also instrumental in determining reasoning accuracy. These findings are quite dramatic: groups of subjects classified by their interpretation patterns exhibit radically different patterns of term ordering, and their ordering of the difficulty of some subsets of problems is quite different. Even if we take some of the most powerful effects known in the syllogistic reasoning literature (such as the effect of grammar) the model allows us to find subgroups of subjects and subgroups of problems which systematically fail to show these effects, or even show reversals of them. Group data, in fact, are highly misleading here. At their worst, they can fit everyone by fitting no one.

One obvious speculation emerging from this work is that hesitant subjects are using "verbal" representations and rash-on-inverted subjects are using "visual" representations (such as Euler circles which strip out information packaging). Ford [84] studied subjects whose reasoning protocols indicate verbal'or visual strategies for syllogism use. We can reanalyse her summary data on the different ordering of problem difficulty for these two groups. This analysis shows that, as one would predict, her visual subjects are less affected by the contrast between canonical and noncanonical problems than her verbal subjects. The result approaches significance, but it is an analysis with lower power because there are only twenty-seven problems to be ordered (Ford gives data only for problems with valid conclusions). Our raw data await further analysis.

However, when we compare our hesitant and rash-on-inverted subjects' profiles of problem accuracy with her subjects' profiles, the patterns are obscure. Her subject groups show strong contrasts with both our groups. So there is some evidence that canonicality plays the predicted roles in visual and verbal thinking, but there is more to our interpretation differences than visual and verbal representations (which is not surprising). It is perfectly possible to vary cooperativeness of model with type of representation. It will take further work to resolve the relation between the interpretation variables and the modality of representation involved.

Reasoning to an Interpretation Revisited   To tie this back to the relation between interpretation and reasoning, we have shown that there are highly systematic patterns of naive interpretation of quantifiers which can be understood as affected by the choice of cooperative or adversarial models of communication in the task, and by differences in susceptibility to information packaging of propositions. These systematic patterns of interpretation can be shown to be instrumental in determining subsequent patterns of reasoning provided they are interpreted in terms of a theory of the relation between models of communication and of information packaging.

It is an open question to what extent what we have here discussed under the heading of "information packaging" includes patterns of inference which are valid in default logics. As mentioned earlier, the illicit conversion of conditionals is a case of closed–world reasoning. One recent exhaustive attempt to fit alternative models to syllogistic data (Roberts, Newstead, and Griggs [230] actually contrasts "conversion" based models with Gricean models, and rejects the latter. But conversion *is* Gricean in any larger view. It is very odd to contrast conversion theories with Gricean theories. Certainly closed-world reasoning offers an interesting framework for exploring the changes brought about in interpretation and reasoning by moving from a single premise to two premises.

Another aspect of the syllogism that requires elucidation is the role of anaphora in subjects' processing. The source–founding model emphasizes that syllogistic reasoning is discourse processing. Consider a subject disposed to construct a single intended model for the discourse *Some A are B. Some B are C.* The speaker constructs a model of the first sentence in which some As are Bs. When the second sentence arrives, what anaphoric relations is such a speaker likely to impose? The example immediately makes it clear that such syllogisms are anaphorically problematic, because the only shared term is first used as a predicate and then as a subject. The second sentence's subject has the indefinite quantifier "some," and two indefinite phrases in a discourse are prone to be interpreted as introducing nonidentical referents. This line of reasoning might yield the response that "it's different Bs that are C than the ones that are A," indicating that the subject has constructed a model with some As that are B and some other Bs that are C, and so nothing may follow about the relation between A and C. On the other hand, the general pragmatic forces toward integration in credulous processing of the only information available pulls in the other direction toward the response "since there is a shared reference to B and the speaker intends me to find some connection, then the Bs that are C must be intended to be the same Bs as the ones that are A." Such reasoning leads to an intended model in which some As are Cs. So even within a generally credulous "construct-the-intended-model" construal of the task, subjects may draw a variety of conclusions. One might object that it is unnatural to treat these premises as having anaphoric relations. The subjects would undoubtedly agree. However, if they have a credulous interpretation of the task, resolving these relations is a goal that is forced upon them, and a little subject debriefing does elicit exactly these kinds of commentaries. Of course, more work is needed to understand how conversion relates to these anaphoric inferences about existentials.

We noted as a consequence of the existence of critical individuals for valid syllogisms, that this domain has the peculiar property that, with perfect strategic choice of model construction and read-off, a reasoner can process credulously (i.e. with the goal of deriving a single intended model) yet achieve skeptical goals (drawing all and only classically valid conclusions). Our data shows that a high proportion of subjects (80%) show at least some signs of credulous interpretation in the immediate inference task, though the two-premise task then obscures some of this because "conversion" repackages propositions in such a way that a substantial minority of subjects now refuse to accept inferences which are credulously (and sometimes even classically) valid. So the domain is calculated to make differentiation particularly difficult. Our own hunch is that empirically what really needs study is the learning process which leads subjects to differentiate the two stances in this domain. Monaghan and Stenning [195] make a start on this issue.

These results also raise important questions for pragmatic theories such as Grice's, and for the relation between information packaging and language use more generally. The topic of information packaging does not arise in Grice's theorizing. He does not consider whether a statement such as "Some A are B" generates the implicature that "Some B are not A" (the inverted implicature). If we ask why not, it is obvious that in typical decontextualized natural language examples, the propositions are already packaged into referring expressions and properties. Learning elementary logic is learning to stand back from this prepackaging and think in terms of local interpretations in which both quantified expressions and predicates designate sets. When this is done, both in-place and inverted implicatures become relevant. Standard linguistic methodology only studies how information is distributed across grammatical structures *after* decisions about subject and predicate terms etc. have been imposed.

As mentioned above (section10.4), the results also raise questions we cannot settle here about what is to choose between Grice's approach to pragmatics, and the defeasible logical approach to credulous processing developed here. There is much overlap and some contrast. Grice's approach was not intended to be computational and employs an indefinitely expressive metalanguage, but might claim to be comprehensive. Our approach is computational and chooses to start out from an inexpressive base to account for specific phenomena, though without claims to comprehensiveness. Our approach makes some phenomena treated by Grice as pragmatic into semantic phenomena. It is an open question whether the kind of reasoning about epistemic states of speakers described by Grice actually does go on in language interpretation. Grice himself was clear that he was not proposing a process model.[13] The proposal made above that theory–of–mind reasoning might be performed in closed–world reasoning (section 9.4) offers a rather different perspective on this issue. To the extent that Gricean reasoning can be implemented in such systems it would be expected to be fast, automatic, and effortless. Just as with system 1 processes in general,

---

13. For some arguments against too literal a process interpretation see, [25]. For developments of pragmatics in default frameworks, see [283, 284].

treatment in these logics rather changes our estimation of their possible content. Undoubtedly both the devil and the interest reside in the detail.

10.6   Mental Models

As mentioned in chapter 1, and again in chapter 5, the psychology of reasoning has been dominated by competing claims about a single fundamental reasoning mechanism employed by all subjects to solve deductive tasks. The results on the variability of interpretation and its instrumentality in reasoning casts doubt on this research agenda. Further doubt is cast by the dubious computational distinguishability of the competing proposals.

Mental models theory can be seen as a development of the founding idea of Kamp's "Discourse Representation Theory" [152, 154]: a piece of discourse is interpreted in a mental representation ("model"), which is itself embedded in "the world." Conversely, mental models can be generated by perception, and can be used as conceptual structure underlying language.

10.6.1   Experimental Evidence

It is possible to investigate experimentally whether a particular piece of discourse is stored in memory verbatim or in the form of a situation described by the discourse. We give two examples.

Bransford, Barclay and Franks [24] provide evidence that recalled sentences are inferences from explicitly presented material–this can easily be explained if people construct a model of discourse, and "read off" what is true there. e.g., when given the sentence

> Three turtles rested on a floating log and a fish swam beneath them

subjects later confused it with

> Three turtles rested on a floating log and a fish swam beneath *it*.

Secondly, recall of a piece of discourse is facilitated if the discourse determines a unique model. Compare for instance

> The spoon is to the left of the knife.
> The plate is to the right of the knife.
> The fork is in front of the spoon.
> The cup is in front of the knife.

and

> The spoon is to the left of the knife.
> The plate is to the right of the spoon.
> The fork is in front of the spoon.
> The cup is in front of the knife.

The difference between these two sets is that the first determines a unique
model, whereas the second doesn't. Stenning [259, 260] and Mani and Johnson-
Laird [179] found in several experiments that (a) the verbal recall of indeterminate description is *better* than that for determinate description, and (b) the gist
of a determinate description can be recalled much more accurately than that of
an indeterminate description. These results lend support to the conclusion that
memory stores representations of models (for determinate descriptions) and of
verbal material (for indeterminate descriptions).

10.6.2   What *Is* a Mental Model?

That is, does there exist a principled way to distinguish between mental models and linguistic representations? Stenning [258] makes a distinction between
direct and *indirect* representations, where the former do not have syntax. The
distinction can be illustrated using the concept of a first–order model. Such
a model can be completely specified by indicating which tuples of elements
belong to which predicates. Another way of thinking about this form of specification is this: introduce names for all elements in the domain of the model,
and construct the *atomic diagram*, the set of atomic sentences true on the model.
Atomic sentences without further syntactic structure beyond that of predication:
this is typical for a direct representation, where no further parsing is necessary.
Alternatively, a (finite) model could be completely specified by a single first–
order sentence. To construct the model of this sentence, the latter has to be
decomposed syntactically and the truth definition has to be applied to the components. This is typical of indirect representation: all the information is given
in the representation, but not in transparent form. It is the aim of mental models to provide a direct representation, but as will be seen we have some doubts
about the success of this enterprise.

10.6.3   The "Algorithm" of the Mental Models Theory

The theory tries to steer a midcourse between rule theories, which purportedly
fail because of content effects such as discussed in chapters 3 and 7, and "no
logic" theories, which go counter to the observation that subjects are able to
make valid deductions when pressed. Johnson-Laird claims that the process of
deduction goes through the following stages:

1. Reasoners use general knowledge to interpret the premises given and as a
   result come up with an internal model.

2. The model is scanned for interesting information not yet explicitly contained
   in the premises; if there is such information, this is offered as a putative
   conclusion, if not, the conclusion is that nothing follows.

3. Reasoners now try to validate the putative conclusion by looking for alternative models of the premises where that conclusion is false.

> If there is such a model, the prudent reasoners will return to the second stage to try to discover whether there is any conclusion true in all the models they have so far constructed. If so, then it is necessary to search for counterexamples to it, and so on, until the set of possible models has been exhausted. Because the number of possible mental models is finite for deductions that depend on quantifiers and connectives, the search can in principle be exhaustive. (Johnson-Laird and Byrne [144,pp. 35-6])

The reference to finiteness here is incomprehensible, at least when iterations of quantifiers are allowed. This is because the set of first–order sentences true on all finite models is strictly larger than those true on all models: the logic of finite models is nonclassical.[14] So we must assume the authors want to restrict themselves to syllogistic reasoning, for which small models suffice. Taken in this way, it highlights one of the aims of mental models theory: to construct a "psychologically viable" alternative to logic by eliminating the latter's infinities. Johnson-Laird likes to quote a remark due to Barbara Partee to the effect that "an infinite set is far too big to fit inside anyone's head." This depends, of course: most infinite sets of interest have compact finite descriptions. In any case

> The psychological theory therefore assumes that people construct a minimum of models: they try to work with just a single representative sample from the set of possible models, until they are forced to consider alternatives. (Johnson-Laird and Byrne [144,p. 36])

It remains to come up with an algorithm that chooses the "single representative sample" and that guides the search for alternatives. Presentations of this subject are notoriously hazy (see Hodges' criticism of mental models in [128];[129]), but we will try to be charitable.

We consider the mental models approach to syllogisms only. Take a premise like "all of the athletes are bakers." The "initial model" would be a partial structure containing elements a, b (for athletes and bakers, respectively), together with some indication of which predicates can be further extended, and which cannot. Johnson-Laird and Byrne use the notation

$$a \quad b$$

to mean that a is also a b, and

$$[a] \quad b$$
$$[a] \quad b$$

$$\cdots$$

for the situation in which the predicate "athlete" cannot be further extended (beyond the two athletes explicitly listed), in contrast to "baker" or indeed any

---

14. This is known as Trahktenbrot's theorem. See, for instance, Boolos, Jeffrey, and Burgess [21,p. 135].

other predicate. Such a partial structure (called an *implicit* model by Johnson–
Laird and Byrne) can be fleshed out to obtain a fully classical structure (called
an *explicit* model). For example, the above partial structure could be fleshed
out to

$$[a] \quad [b]$$

$$[a] \quad [b]$$

$$[\neg a] \quad [b]$$

$$[\neg a] \quad [\neg b]$$

By $\neg a$ an element is meant that is not an athlete.

On the basis of the partial model, a conclusion is formulated, which (ideally)
is then tested for validity by searching for counterexamples. This can be done
either by fleshing out the initial partial model, or by moving to a different initial model. For example, although the initial model validates "all the bakers
are athletes," the fleshed–out model refutes this. The claim is that the assumption of this procedure explains all aspects of reasoning performance, including
common errors and response times.

We proceed to give a few initial, implicit models for other syllogistic premises
(taken from Johnson-Laird and Byrne [144]).

Some of the athletes are bakers.

$$a \quad b$$

$$a \quad b$$

$$\ldots$$

None of the athletes is a baker.

$$[a]$$

$$[a]$$

$$[b]$$

$$[b]$$

Here, the empty space to the right of the a indicates that there is no b such that
a is b; and likewise for the empty space to the left of the b.

Some of the athletes are not bakers.

$$a$$

$$a$$

$$a \quad [b]$$

$$[b]$$

$$\cdots$$

The principles guiding the construction of these smallest models are somewhat unclear. Note that the implicit model for the first sentence is compatible with "all athletes are bakers," whereas the implicit model for the third sentence is not compatible with "none of the athletes are bakers." No reason for this asymmetry is given. It is also unclear why some of the lines are reduplicated.

We so far considered arguments with a single premise only. When two premises have to be combined, complications arise. Consider

All the athletes are bakers.
All the bakers are canoeists.

A partial model for the first premise is

$$[a] \quad b$$

$$[a] \quad b$$

$$\cdots$$

and for the second premise

$$[b] \quad c$$

$$[b] \quad c$$

$$\cdots$$

How are these to be combined? The intended meaning of the square brackets excludes the fused partial structure

$$[a] \quad [b] \quad c$$

$$[a] \quad [b] \quad c$$

$$\cdots$$

because then suddenly "all bakers are athletes" would be true in all fleshed–out models. Johnson-Laird and Byrne opt for the representation

$$[[a] \quad b] \quad c$$

$$[[a] \quad b] \quad c$$

$$\cdots$$

which is supposed to mean that all *pairs* [[a]   b] have been listed explicitly. Notice, however, that we have now moved to pure syntax. Whereas [a] could be interpreted as a metalanguage device to indicate that all elements a are explicitly listed, the iteration of the square brackets requires their presence in the object language, and even then their interpretation is not very perspicuous. Johnson-Laird and Byrne offer the interpretation "a is exhausted with respect to b, and b is exhausted with respect to c," but this gloss destroys the original meaning of [a] as being exhausted *tout court*. In logical terms, the difficulty can be put thus. If we read the collection of [a] b as an abbreviation for $\forall x(Ax \rightarrow Bx)$, then the collection of [a] [b] c would probably mean something like $\forall y(\forall x(Ax \rightarrow Bx) \rightarrow Cy)$, which is equivalent to $\forall x(Ax \rightarrow Bx) \rightarrow \forall y Cy$, and this is not what we want. It almost goes without saying that formation rules for the [...]–construct are not given.

It is perhaps best to think of the square bracket notation in graphical terms. Consider the expression [[a] b] c. This is analogous to an Euler circle representation of sets A, B, C, with $A \subseteq B \subseteq C$ and distinguished elements (i.e., crosses) $a \in A$, $b \in B$, $c \in C$. The added twist is that extensions of the predicates must leave the arrangement of the Euler circles intact. Interestingly, however, it is much less natural to think of Euler circles as representing a partial model, since the circles neatly abstract from the number of elements in the model.

The next question is how to read off a conclusion concerning athletes and canoeists from the combined model. This is done by stripping the model of its square brackets; we then see that all athletes are canoeists, and no extension of the partial model can invalidate this conclusion. Let us see how this works in a more difficult case.

> All of the bakers are athletes.
> None of the bakers is a canoeist.

A partial model for the first premise is

$$[b] \quad a$$

$$[b] \quad a$$

$$\cdots$$

and for the second premise we get

$$[b]$$

$$[b]$$

$$[c]$$

$$[c]$$

The combined model is something like

$$[a \quad [b][$$

$$[a \quad [b]]$$

$$[c]$$

$$[c]$$

$$\cdots$$

which is meant to suggest that triples like

$$a \quad b \quad c$$

are excluded. This model supports the conclusion

None of the canoeists is an athlete.

which is apparently not uncommon. A fleshed–out model such as

$$[a \quad [b]]$$

$$[a \quad [b]]$$

$$a \quad [c]$$

$$a \quad [c]$$

$$\cdots$$

invalidates this conclusion, and supports

Some of the athletes are not canoeists.

It will be clear from the above exposition that Johnson-Laird and Byrne's claim to have provided an 'algorithm' for deduction should be taken with a grain of salt. The choice of the initial implicit model is not completely determined; neither is the fleshing out. However, with a number of more or less arbitrary assumptions added, the above can be cast in the form of a computer program, for which see Bara et al. [11].

10.6.4   Predictions

It is the aim of mental models theory to be able to predict both correct performance when it occurs, and frequently occurring errors. One important determinant of successful performance is taken to be the number of models that must be constructed before a valid conclusion is obtained. Thus, for example, the syllogism with premises

> All the athletes are bakers.
> All the bakers are canoeists.

is supposed to require only one model, in the sense that fleshing out does not change the conclusion read off from the implicit model. This is supposed to be in contrast to the situation for the syllogism

> All of the bakers are athletes.
> None of the bakers is a canoeist.

As indicated above, Johnson-Laird and Byrne claim that the conclusion read off from the implicit model is

> None of the canoeists is an athlete.

However, the valid conclusion

> Some of the athletes are not canoeists.

can also be read off from the implicit model. It will also not do to say that people read off the strongest possible conclusion from an implicit model, because in that case the premises

> All the athletes are bakers.
> All the bakers are canoeists.

would lead to the initial conclusion

> Athletes are bakers and conversely.

This conclusion would of course be invalidated by the fleshing out of the implicit model, but then it is difficult to see what is meant by saying that this syllogism needs only one model.

The consequences of the fact that mental models, unlike logical models, contain syntactic structure (the square brackets) are of two kinds. First, the syntactic structure of the input premises has to be maintained somehow in order for mental models to make the required behavioral predictions, for example, of conclusion term order. As we saw in the previous sections, grammatical structure is actually the most heavily weighted factor in the determination of conclusion term order. Mental models theory's appeal to first-in, first-out working memory and "cancellation operations" to remove the middle term is a covert attempt to carry through this information into the conclusion through the sequential structure of the models. But we saw that the predicted conclusion term orders (with B central) are not the commonest orders observed in the individuals task. Second, these issues – syntactic components and sequential structure in the models – become critical when cognitive scientists attempt to map reasoning processes onto the brain. Sometimes considerations of neural representation are even invoked to adjudicate between mental rules and mental models, as in the work of Goel and colleagues (see quotes above 119 and 119). It then seems possible to set up an experiment to distinguish between the two theories, by using experimental evidence that language processing is localized in the left hemisphere, and spatial processing in the parietal cortex (chiefly on the right). If a subject shows no activation in the parietal cortex while reasoning, this is taken to be evidence against the involvement of spatial processing, and hence ultimately against mental models. A result of this kind was indeed obtained by Goel and his colleagues [100]. However, if mental models contain linguistic components after all, the hypothesis that their neural correlate must be situated in the right parietal cortex becomes much less plausible.

10.6.5 Conclusion: The Logic of Mental Models

The confusions inherent in mental models theory are nicely illustrated (albeit unwittingly) in the following quotation from Ruth Byrne [28,p. 78]:

> The model-based theory assumes that once one has an adequate explanation of comprehension, there is no need for the mobilization of any elaborate machinery for reasoning, neither of syntactic rules proposed by formal theories, nor of domain-specific rules favoured by pragmatic theories. On the contrary, reasoning depends on a search for counterexamples to conclusions, but ordinary individuals do not have a simple deterministic procedure for making such a search. (cf. Newell and Simon [199]).

The claim is thus that mental models theory is "semantic" in the sense that it rests completely on a theory of natural language understanding; this would render the application of rules superfluous. But then, what is involved in natural language comprehension? The assignment of an implicit mental model obviously does not depend on the full semantic content of a sentence such as "all athletes are bakers," but it depends on the *logical form* of this sentence. This is what allows Johnson-Laird to represent the sentence "all athletes are bakers" in the form

$$[a] \quad b$$

$$[a] \quad b$$

$$\cdots$$

abstracting from all other information.

In fact, an important component of comprehension is precisely assigning logical form. Once a logical form has been chosen, representing this as a mental model in the sense of Johnson-Laird is a triviality, because, due to the incorporation of logical devices such as negation and the universal quantifier, such a mental model is a notational variant of a sentence of predicate logic. Thus, there is nothing inherently semantic in this notion of a mental model. In this respect it should be sharply distinguished from ordinary first–order models, which can be characterized by sets of *atomic* sentences.

A reasoner now supposedly reads off a purported conclusion from a mental model constructed from the premises. Since the mental model is essentially a sentence in a formal language, this involves checking whether one sentence follows from another, and this is definitely not reading off when the sentences involved are complex. Similarly, checking whether the conclusion is true in other models of the premises again involves determining whether one sentence follows from another. Thus, reasoning processes are involved which are not described by the mental models theory.

All this can be illustrated in a more perspicuous manner with the help of semantic tableaux, which avoid the various red herrings of mental models theory. This proof procedure is semantic in the sense that it provides a systematic way to construct a first–order model which verifies the premises and falsifies the conclusion of an argument, if such a model exists. Models constructed in this manner are true models in that they are fully specified by a domain and relations (and/or functions) on that domain; the model does not incorporate syntax. But the construction itself proceeds stepwise and is fully guided by logical rules of the type "if $\forall x \varphi(x)$ is false, then there must be some new individual a such that $\varphi(a)$ is false." These rules are very similar to the rules proposed by the rule theorists; indeed, there exists a canonical way to transform a tableau proof into a natural deduction proof. A mental models theorist might object that even so, there still is a distinction between rules operating on formulas, and rules guiding the construction of representations or models. This distinction is spurious, however, because semantic tableaux can be viewed equivalently as fully syntactic procedures, by treating the elements introduced in the course of the construction simply as constants of the language.

It will be clear from the above exposition that Johnson-Laird and Byrne have inadvertently tried to reinvent logic, while claiming to provide an alternative. In itself that is already an interesting result. Stripped of its extravagant claims and notational muddle, the mental models theory embodies a simple logical point. What the mental models theory has in common with Kamp's Discourse representation theory ([155, 152]) is the emphasis on partial models. Now partial models do not seem to be very helpful in the case of syllogisms, because the full models are so small in any case, but they may be helpful for more advanced arguments.

10.6.6   Morals from Syllogisms?

Once one drops the idea that the data presented in the psychological literature bear on the rules vs. models debate, several important conclusions can be drawn from the data of syllogistic reasoning, both theoretical and methodological.

The results demonstrate once again the importance of interpretation in understanding tasks which have generally been taken to be about derivation *from* interpretations. The source–founding model

is designed to capitalize on the logical peculiarities of the domain, which make credulous processing of discourse come so close to skeptical classical reasoning. Thus the full panoply of discourse representation theory is transferred to the problem of understanding interpretation in these tasks. Exploration of the data from the immediate inference task reveals just how strong credulous interpretation still is in this task, and how it is intimately connected to subject-predicate structure. This in turn highlights how both forward implicature and "conversion" are closely related credulous patterns of reasoning, rather than opposed psychological theories. The combination of bottom-up statistical modeling with top-down process modeling illustrates how the two complement each other in an exploratory empirical program of research which links experiment to theories from outside psychology. It does this in an area where there had been an explicit failed attempt to link through the usual methods of operationalization ([201]). Empirically, an important gain is the unearthing of qualitative individual differences in interpretation. The last chapter will examine what this means for the vexed question of rationality in reasoning.

PART III

Is Psychology Hard or Impossible?

Whenever anybody interprets evidence from any source, and his interpretation contains characteristics that cannot be referred wholly to direct sensory observation or perception, this person thinks. The bother is that nobody has ever been able to find any case of the human use of evidence which does not include characters that run beyond what is directly observed by the senses. So, according to this, people think whenever they do anything at all with evidence. If we adopt that view we very soon find ourselves looking out upon a boundless and turbulent ocean of problems. (F.C. Bartlett, *Thinking* [13,p. 1])

11 Rationality Revisited

11.1 Logic and Information–Processing

Logic plays several roles in this book. We studied overt reasoning, and found that classical logic is not always adhered to, nor need it be, because there are many domains in which it is not a reasonable competence model. Instead we found that the domain of discourse processing is governed by a form of non-monotonic logic as a competence model, namely closed–world reasoning; if subjects approach a reasoning task in "discourse processing mode" they are therefore quite likely to apply closed–world reasoning to it. This explained the pattern of performance in, for instance, the suppression task (chapter 7). Chapters 8 and 9 bring a subtle shift in perspective, in that the exclusive association between logic and overt reasoning is loosened. In chapter 8 we emphasized the automatic aspect of closed world reasoning by exhibiting a class of neural networks capable of executing closed–world computations. In chapter 9 we went one step further and established a formal link between performance on a nonverbal task (the box task) and the suppression task – both can be seen as instances of closed–world reasoning about possible exceptions – and showed that autistic subjects' behavior on the suppression task is as predicted by their performance on the box task. Both patterns of performance were then related to deficiencies in inhibition for which neurological evidence has been found.[1] What conception of logic emerges from these considerations? Evidently we claim for logic a much wider role in cognition than is customarily assumed, in a complete reversal of the tendency to push logic to the fringes, in the wake of results allegedly establishing its irrelevance to human reasoning.[2]

---

1. Our paper [267] applies the same method to ADHD. We analyse the formal structure of a task where performance of children with ADHD is impaired (the Go/No Go task) and find the same structure in a story-telling task. As a consequence we can predict aberrations in narrative performance (e.g., uses of verb tense), for which there indeed turns out to be evidence.
2. This chapter owes much to conversations with Theodora Achourioti, who drew our attention to the philosophical distinction between *regulative* and *constitutive* norms. The purpose of this chapter is to argue that logic is normative in the latter sense.

11.1.1   Information Processing

The common denominator of all the applications of logic that we studied is that logic allows one to extract information from given data – *and that constraints have to be added to these data to allow information extraction to take place.* In itself this characterization of logic is not very distinctive, since this is what all information–processing is about, as we will see shortly. Nevertheless, a closer look at what information–processing consists in will give us many clues to a more mature view of logical reasoning.

As a starting point we look again at David Marr's three levels of cognitive inquiry

1. identification of the information–processing task as an input–output function;

2. specification of an algorithm which computes that function;

3. neural implementation of the algorithm specified.

We will now look in more detail at the first two levels, using the example of vision. As is well-known, Marr [183] characterized vision as the extraction of 3D shapes from 2D retinal arrays, and his work is concerned with the various processes that are necessary to this end. For example, in a first step edges are extracted from the retinal array by computing second derivatives of the intensity distribution: sharp changes in intensity indicate the presence of an edge.[3] The most important defining feature of the information processing task is the choice of representation languages for input and output. These are mathematical languages, and the algorithm defined in the second level operates on entities expressible in these languages. It follows that the information–processing task as conceived at the first level is an ideal construct only. The identification of a particular information–processing task can be viewed as the stipulation of a *competence model*, but only if it is firmly kept in mind that even optimal performance can only approximate the competence model, because the actual input will only be an approximation to the idealized input postulated by the competence model (in this case a twice differentiable intensity function). A good algorithm will allow "graceful degradation": the closer the actual input is to the input required for the competence model, the closer will be the output. That is, since the actual input will never fully satisfy the input requirements for the competence model, the algorithm must be able to cope with deviations from those requirements. Performance is optimal if it proceeds in accordance with such a "graceful" algorithm. The neural implementation of the algorithm (the third

---

3. We must note here that the standard phrase "extract information" has the unfortunate connotation of information already being present in the data, albeit perhaps in hidden form. This is not what we mean; even in such a mundane case as vision, there is no sense in which the information sought, e.g., the edge, is fully present in the data. In logical reasoning this is even less true, as we shall see in section 11.1.2.

level) may be such, however, that optimal performance cannot be achieved. Performance may also be optimal, even though its results are way off the mark, when the algorithm works only under certain constraints on the world or on the relation between viewer and world.

This can be seen most clearly at higher levels of processing, for instance in deriving surface geometry from an image, the problem of how to determine a 3D shape from surface information. Marr writes [183,p. 265-6]

> [An] interesting aspect of all these processes is that . . . they all involve slightly different assumptions about the world in order to work satisfactorily. As we have seen, in each case the surface structure is strictly underdetermined from the information in images alone, and the secret of formulating the processes accurately lies in discovering precisely what additional information can safely be assumed about the world that provides powerful enough constraints for the processes to run – for example, uniqueness and continuity in stereopsis, rigidity in [structure from] motion, and so forth.

These "powerful constraints" are not present in the data to be processed themselves. One very good reason for this is that the constraints often concern the relation between the viewer and the world. For instance, one of Marr's assumptions is that (very roughly speaking) nearby points in an image correspond to nearby points on the viewed object. A different type of constraint is concerned with the world, in this case, for instance, that real-world surfaces can be described as smooth manifolds in the mathematical sense. Given these constraints (and several others) it is possible to extract information about the shape generating a retinal image; it is now a mathematical theorem that such a shape must be a "generalized cone."[4] More generally, if the surface is composed of several smooth pieces, it must be generated by an object consisting of several generalized cones. This mathematical result provides the competence model, the ideal norm against which performance must be judged. Possible performance is described by the algorithm (Marr's second level) which corresponds to the competence model. The algorithm can be defined only on the basis of the theorem, because it determines what the inputs and outputs are; however, it must do more than transform information about the idealized surface assumed in the condition of the theorem into a generalized cone. It must allow graceful degradation and also give meaningful results on surfaces which satisfy the constraints only approximately. The algorithm 'appeals to' the (ideal) competence in this sense.

This brief description of information–processing in a concrete case has highlighted several issues of significance also for logic.

1. The competence model (Marr's top level) is relative to the information–processing task considered.

---

4. The shape generated by a cross-section moving along an axis, where the cross-section may change in size continuously.

2. The competence model is stated in terms of ideal, mathematical entities and is as such not directly applicable to the real world.

3. Possible performance is described by an algorithm allowing graceful degradation, thus bringing the competence model in closer contact with the world.

4. The information sought is strictly underdetermined by the information present in the data.

5. Constraints, that is, hypotheses about the world and about the process generating the data, are needed to further determine the information 'extracted' from the data.

11.1.2   Logic as Information–Processing

We view logic as continuous with information–processing in the above sense, distinguished from the examples discussed above only by a different choice of representation languages for input and output. But the commonalities leap to the eye.

Logic is very much task-relative. Consider a mathematical example: if the task is to prove existence theorems with algorithmic content, one uses intuitionistic logic; however, if one is satisfied with abstract existence, classical logic suffices.

A logical formalism, taken as a norm, should be viewed as a competence model in the sense defined above. It is ideal in two different senses of the term: first because it operates with idealized input and output, and second because it gives an ideal norm as a mapping from (idealized) input to (idealized) output. There is no reason to expect that actual performance, even when optimal, will always conform to the norm set by the competence model. For example, one idealization in the definition of the competence model is the use of definite premise sets to draw conclusions from. This is a situation one seldom meets in practice, where usually any available evidence is used to draw conclusions. The big question raised by this observation is how to define a notion of "graceful degradation" that makes performance an approximation to the ideal norm.

As in vision, the data (here: the premises) vastly underdetermine the information to be extracted (a conclusion). We have observed throughout the course of this book that the psychology of reasoning has suffered as a consequence of its neglect of this fundamental fact. We have termed the combination of (2) and (5) in the list given in section 11.1.1, which jointly allow determinate information to be extracted, *logical form*, and the process of arriving at a logical form, *reasoning to an interpretation*.[5] Here, the term *reasoning* should not be read as necessarily implying awareness.

---

5. The role assigned here to logical form is reminiscent of what Bruner in his famous book *Beyond the information given* called a *coding system*: "We propose that when one goes beyond the information given,

Logical form starts with the choice of representation languages for input (premises) and output (conclusion).[6] Another component of logical form is a mathematically defined class of structures; this idealization is the analogue of the smoothness assumption for surfaces considered above. The definitions of satisfaction and truth for the languages are the analogues of Marr's constraint linking viewer and world.

One very important role of logical form is facilitating the integration of premises into the joint representation that is necessary before any conclusion can be drawn. For example, one could say that in propositional closed–world reasoning, the premises are integrated through the completion (cf. definition 5 in chapter 7) before a conclusion is drawn. By contrast, in classical propositional logic, integration involves the set of all truth–value assignments which make the premises true, or, syntactically speaking, a suitable disjunctive normal form. In both cases it is pertinent, although trivial, to note that two key ingredients in logical form – the formal language and the semantics – have recursive definitions, thus allowing the representation of the premises in a common format. For a (trivial) example, consider MP: of course the inference of "She will study late in the library" from (1) "She has an essay" and (2) "If she has an essay she will study late in the library" is possible only if (1) and (2) can be represented in a common formal language with common semantics. We shall see another instance of this type of integration in syllogisms.

In Kantian terms, we may think of the activity of imposing logical form and integrating the premises in a single representation as *synthesis*; this synthesis is a priori since the logical form imposed is not determined by experience, but a constraint contributed by cognition. One needs logical form in order to be able to extract information, but it is as little given in the data as an edge is given in the retinal array. Both the formal language and the semantics are defined recursively so are mathematical constructs. We may thus say that inferences in reasoning are synthetic a priori, because they depend on the synthesis a priori just outlined. To give a concrete example: if in the suppression task the subject draws an MP inference, this is based on the assignment of a logical form (including integration of the premises) which could have been different.

Note that on the view outlined here, logical reasoning does not require awareness; whether or not reasoning is accompanied by awareness depends entirely on the algorithms imposing the logical form ("reasoning to an interpretation") and those performing the information extraction on the joint representation of the data ("reasoning from an interpretation"). For example, reasoning in the suppression task proceeds unconsciously (at least for the forward inferences

---

one does so by being able to place the present given in a more generic coding system and that one essentially reads off from the coding system additional information." [26,p. 224].

6. These languages can be different, as in logic programming, where formulas in the input may contain →, but not so formulas in the output.

MP and DA) because here the algorithm imposing logical form on the premises is in fact the algorithm for integrating discourse generally, and the implementation of the algorithm doing the information extraction is the relaxation toward a stable state of a neural network.[7] Since classical (predicate) logic is undecidable, no such automatic procedure for reasoning from an already chosen classical logical form is possible there, and a control process of which the subject is aware is necessary to correct false moves in attempts to establish a conclusion. This means that for all practical purposes the proof of a conclusion from given premises is itself a separate source of information, not in any meaningful sense already present in the set of premises.

11.1.3   On Why We are Not Postmodern Relativists

The foregoing analysis should have dispelled the impression that we believe anything goes in matters of logical reasoning. The theorist's decision to apply closed–world reasoning in the analysis of the suppression task is not arbitrary: it is dictated by a hypothesis about the real-world task – in this case credulous discourse understanding – that the subject assimilates the suppression task to. Once that real-world task has been determined, the logical form is more or less fixed as the competence model for that task. The logical form is an ideal construct, and the subject is perhaps not capable of imposing it in full, so actual performance may deviate; but the logical form should *grosso modo* be recognisable in performance. Thus logical reasoning is relative to a particular cognitive task, but once a subject is engaged in that task, the task imposes a norm upon the subject. In other words, it is a general norm of *rationality* that the subject should try to perform a task as well she can, consistent with reasonable costs. What this means for a concrete task has to be determined from the competence model for that task. Thus we end up with a picture of the normative status of logic which is very much like the one sketched by Husserl (for which see chapter 1): logic itself is a theoretical discipline, proving consequences of choices of parameters, and norms come from the outside, by the choice of a particular logical form.

11.1.4   Logic as Information Extraction: Examples

Let us now run through some of our experimental paradigms to illustrate these ideas.

We saw a clear instance of the ideas just outlined in chapter 10, on syllogistics, where we discussed an assignment of logical form consisting in the construction of Euler circles with crosses. The syllogism itself contributes the

---

7. Assuming, of course, that our analysis of the suppression task is correct.

first component of logical form in the sense of surface syntax; the Euler diagrams together with the assignment of sets to predicates and the interpretation of → as ⊆ and ∧ as ∩ constitute the semantics. An interesting feature of this construction is that integration of the premises is nontrivial: Euler diagrams are in principle defined only for binary quantifiers ("all A are B," "some A are B," etc.), and thus need combination rules like the ones, involving the crosses, given in section 10.3.1 to represent the Euler diagrams corresponding to the two premises of a syllogism in one joint representation. This is in contrast to a solution method for classical logic like semantic tableaux, where the integration of premises proceeds by the simple addition of suitable atomic sentences, since in classical predicate logic a model can be defined as a *set* of atomic sentences.[8]

In the selection task the data presented to the subjects consist of the form administered by the experimenter; the information to be extracted, at least according to the experimenter, is the subset of selected cards. We have seen that very considerable preprocessing of these data is necessary – e.g., fixing a meaning for the conditional, determining what "true" and "false" mean, accepting the background rule as given while leaving the truth–value of the foreground rule open – which we have conceptualized as imposing logical form on the data. All components of logical form play an important role. Validity reflects task understanding, the nature of the information to be extracted. Some subjects believe that the information to be extracted is a reactive plan, where the actions to be performed depend on observations of the back of the cards. Note furthermore that it is the very indeterminacy of natural language meaning which makes imposition of logical form necessary: the assignment of logical form is constitutive of meaning. For example, the conditional can have many different meanings[9] depending upon context; and the sparser the context is, the fewer clues one has about the intended meaning. This is therefore a task in which reasoning to an interpretation needs control (often accompanied by awareness): because of the extreme indeterminacy of meaning, and also because there are so many elements to integrate. In the end, if all goes well, the subject will have integrated all this information in a joint representation like the one given in chapter 3, section 3.4, and proceed from there. In practice, hardly anybody achieves full integration in this task. The various experimental manipulations discussed in chapter 4 all aim to bring out the intended logical form more clearly, and as we have seen these lead to a significant increase in (intended) performance.

In the suppression task, a considerable number of subjects impose a logical form consisting of a ternary connective to correspond to the natural language conditional (involving the extra propositional variable ab), and integrate the

---

8. The source-founding model presented in chapter 10 provides an interesting example of a different logical form imposed on syllogisms. The problems surrounding the integration of the premises are discussed on page 329.

9. The phrase "many different meanings" suggests that meanings can be counted; but this image is still too discrete.

premises through a condition on ab, then forming the completion. Since this assignment of logical form corresponds to natural processes for discourse repair (the additional conditional is read as correcting, or as strengthening the first), it may be almost automatic in normal readers. This can be seen in the dialogues, which are much less concerned with task interpretation than those of the selection task. Once the logical form is fixed, information extraction then proceeds algorithmically through closed–world reasoning, that is, by constructing the minimal model of the preprocessed premises and reading off a conclusion.[10] In the case of the suppression task we could go down to Marr's third level and propose both a mechanism for the encoding of the logical form into a neural network and the shape of the neural computations implementing the information-extraction algorithm.

In the false–belief task the preprocessing of the data involves understanding the task instruction, and recruiting information concerning the relation between perception and belief, and of general causal knowledge. Information extraction is performed by an algorithm *simulating* the temporal evolution of the initial model up to the time that Maxi returns to the room and starts looking for the chocolate, using the principle of inertia applied to both beliefs and the world. The counterfactual task elicits the same process of information extraction, except that inertia is applied to the world only.

Nonverbal tasks will be discussed in the next section.

11.1.5   Some Information–Processing is Best Viewed as Logic

Above we have argued that (real-life) logical reasoning should be seen as information–processing. From this it follows that some information processing is logical reasoning, but the section heading is intended to convey something more: that logic is a good format in which to represent information–processing tasks which are not traditionally conceived of as logical. The first step of the argument is that in the description and explanation of a cognitive task, consideration of Marr's top level – the specification of what is to be computed – is indispensable, for instance because it gives rise to predictions which cannot be obtained otherwise. An example is furnished by chapter 9, where we found the common information–processing core in three very different tasks (false–belief task, counterfactual task, box task) and tested autistic subjects on the suppression task, which was argued to embody this common core in rather pure form. A more fundamental reason for the incorporation of the top level is that directly moving to the algorithmic level may lead to features of the algorithm being included as part of the cognitive task, even though these are inessential, and one may then agonise over how to find a neural implementation for those features. An example of this is furnished by the attempted probabilistic analyses of the

---

10. This description of information extraction applies to the forward inferences MP and DA.

suppression task (chapter 7), which introduce a needlessly precise quantitative probabilistic language, and thus set the authors worrying about its relevance to the actual computations going on in the brain.

The second step is that logical languages are well suited to serve as representation languages for the input and output of the competence model. Logic is open to a wide range of content. Cognition is about intentional phenomena, i.e., is concerned with setting goals and achieving them. But in order to achieve a goal a plan must be computed, and for this one needs causal information concerning the consequences and preconditions of one's actions. Each of these is naturally formulated in a logical language, and the attainment of a goal can be viewed as a derivation in a suitable nonmonotonic logic. That is why also the competence models for nonverbal tasks, such as the box task, the tubes task and behavioral variants of the false–belief task (all from chapter 9) can be formulated using logical notions. This last phrase – "using logical notions" – was chosen to reflect the fact that in, for instance, the box task the input seems only partially formalisable in logical terms, since the essential logical features have to be abstracted from the visual image of the box (the visual input). The logical form of discourse seems slightly more transparent.

11.1.6   Nonmonotonic Logic and the Competence/Performance Distinction

As an aside, we would like to mention that the possibility to choose between classical and nonmonotonic logics affects the very formulation of what the information–processing task corresponding to a given cognitive capacity is. We illustrate this by means of language comprehension. At the competence level, language comprehension can be viewed as the information–processing task whose output is an internal model for a discourse, with representations for the individuals, relations, and events mentioned in the discourse (see Kamp and Reyle [154] for an exposition of this view from linguistics, and Gernsbacher [93] from psycholinguistics). While the output is relatively clear, the input is a matter of debate. In fact, this debate can be viewed as being about what properly belongs to competence, and what to performance.

At the level of performance or processing, the main issue is whether language comprehension is a one-step or two-step process, in the following sense. In a two-step process, first the meaning of a *sentence* is computed, which may then have to be recomputed in the next step to take into account pragmatic information, which can be both verbal and nonverbal (e.g., gesture). In a one-step process, all the available information is immediately brought to bear on the computation of the meaning, and sentence boundaries do not have a privileged role. Hence, whereas in the two-step model the input to the comprehension algorithm consists of sentences, it consists of lexical items in the one-step model.

Current evidence from neuroimaging seems to point to a one-step model (see Hagoort and van Berkum [112] for an overview).

Returning to the competence level, we may define the input of the comprehension task as a complete piece of discourse, supposed to be given in its entirety. The fact that the elements of the discourse arrive sequentially is then taken to be a performance factor. As a consequence of this decision, the competence model can be taken to be a monotonic operation: no revision is necessary after the discourse model has been constructed. This is the point of view taken in Kamp and Reyle [154]. To take a concrete example, if a discourse model is constructed for

(1)   The girl was writing a letter, when her friend spilled coffee on the paper.

according to this view it will be constructed *after* the sentence boundary, when it has already become clear that the writing most likely has not produced a mailable letter due to coffee stains on the paper.

An alternative option is to fit the competence model more closely to the actual information available to the listener, and thus view the task (i.e., language comprehension) as sequentially constructing a discourse model, as it were shadowing the incoming information. The discourse model thus constructed may have to be revised. For instance, in sentence (1) the main clause generates the expectation that a letter has been written, thus introducing a referent for this letter in the discourse model. This default expectation is then canceled by the subordinate clause, which means that the original model has to be recomputed. In van Lambalgen and Hamm [282] a nonmonotonic computational formalism is presented which allows such recomputations in midsentence.[11] Thus we claim that the use of nonmonotonic logic allows the formulation of competence models which are much closer to the actual informational situation that humans find themselves in.

11.2   The Bottom Line

What sort of picture emerges from the preceding considerations of the goings on in the psychology of reasoning laboratory? What is our take on our student subjects, and on reasoning experiments themselves? What is our take on *Homo sapiens*? And how does our picture join up with the rest of cognitive science?

---

11. This brief description will undoubtedly raise a number of questions. The interested reader is also referred to [9], and references given therein, for a discussion of processing aspects of the progressive in examples like (1), together with evidence from event-related potentials to support the interpretation given here.

11.2.1   Subjects and Experiments

Starting with subjects, we have acquitted them of most of the accusations of irrationality that most other approaches have laid at their door. Our acquittal is on somewhat different grounds than some others. We do think that students' struggles in the selection task are not far beneath the surface, and that they are less than ideal interpreters of the confusing messages the task presents. From the student subjects' point of view, the competence models used to convict are not the ones they could reasonably be expected to initially apply. We see them as faced with a multiplicity of possibilities and being engaged in trying to find out what the experimenter means, even if they are not well aware of the explicit catalogue of possibilities. They are skillful credulous reasoners endowed with enormous databases of subtly defeasible, contextually sensitive, rules. They may also be able to invoke a skeptical stance in supportive contexts, but these are not supportive contexts. Above all they lack the awareness of their interpretive situation (concepts, terminology, or the experimenter's intentions) which might allow them to control their decisions about what interpretations to adopt. Here is the scope for educational intervention. We do believe that education can have profound effects on students' control and flexibility of interpretation in situations where little past experience is available to guide. In fact we believe this added control of interpretation is one of the main tools students need to learn in whatever domains they come to specialise in. And we can agree that the small proportion of students who do identify the skeptical classical logical models often unwittingly intended by experimenters are the students who have already come farthest along this road to interpretive control. So, while our students stand acquitted as charged, we still want to send them off with homework to develop their awareness of interpretive processes and possibilities. We still have only blood, sweat, and tears to offer.

Exactly what exercises these should be will vary with the students and their intended destination. Empirical research (Stenning [258]) has shown that contrary to common belief (see, e.g., Cheng et al. [38]) quite formal logical teaching can benefit students' general reasoning capacities. Others among them might be better served by different curricula, and there are important issues about how formal teaching has to be focused. Of course, civilization has its discontents. Teaching the centipede about walking may disturb its habits, and teaching students how to reflect on their interpretive processes can perhaps sometimes forestall necessary action in the world. So alongside a curriculum for reflection, there also needs to be curricula for application. However, the latter seem to us in good shape compared to the former.

What of experiments? Are we advocating the abandonment of the laboratory for the arm-chair? Far from it! As should be clear, we don't think formal models can explain cognitive phenomena, any more than experimental data are interpretable without explicit models. But we are also advocating a much more subtle shift than merely a shift of the balance toward logical analysis, and that subtle shift has to do with the balance between syntactic and semantic *data*. Psychologists are taught that content has to be circumvented to make progress. Classical cases are the invention of the nonsense syllable in the memory laboratory to eradicate meanings that subjects insist on bringing with them. As it turns out, we can learn some things about memory from such material, but it still remains true that it excludes most of what we want to study as human memory – what Bartlett [12] called "the effort after meaning."

Psycholinguistics is another field that has been dominated by the avoidance of content. Far more effort has gone into understanding syntactic parsing, than into understanding the representation of meaning and the conduct of inference in discourse. Yet we know that the bulk of the variance in human processing is driven by meanings. The cognitive revolution was founded on observations that subjects' interpretations were the determiner of psychological capacities, perhaps most famously in memory.

This conundrum is usually seen as being driven by methodological necessity. We propose that our use of nonmonotonic logics removes this methodological necessity. A logic that forces us to represent a long term memory database and a working memory processor for current discourse materials faces this methodological chasm head-on. Of course we don't represent the whole of a subject's long–term memory, nor the full process which leads to activation of the currently active part of long–term memory. But for any given discourse, universality is not necessary. Of course, formalization of particular materials is often post hoc. But as long as the resultant formalizations make enough predictions, they remain empirical hypotheses. The status of form changes with multiplicity of logics. Finding form is now as much about setting semantic parameters as about syntactic ones, and we (and our subjects) have access to the output meanings in a way that we do not have access to intermediate syntactic stages. Psychology doesn't need to tiptoe around content anymore. Its main data can be judgments of meanings in context.

However, one cannot escape the feeling that it will take more than a few logical tools to reinstate the processes of interpretation at center stage in cognitive psychology. This issue is at the heart of problems about the boundaries between the humanities and sciences. Interpretation is often seen as the boundary fence. But that itself doesn't really bear inspection. The psychology laboratory happily studies interpretive processes in lots of areas: visual perception is perhaps the most obvious. Psycholinguistics is another. So what is supposed to be the difference between admissible ranges of interpretation which the psychology of reasoning (and other areas of psychology) can admit and still remain empirical science, and the ranges of interpretation which take us irretrievably beyond the scientific pale into the postmodernist desert? One possible explanation why interpretation is seen as problematic in reasoning but not in perception or psycholinguistics is that the field of reasoning invites evaluations of rationality; whereas the other fields do not.

What Role Rationality?

Once rationality comes under inspection, we get drawn ineluctably to the hard cases: legal, scientific, religious, political, or moral. Rationality is the humanities' Trojan horse invited within the scientific walls because rationality soon reveals the need for the specification of values.

First, it should be said, there *are* hard cases, and these fields of enquiry are pretty well defined in terms of their capacities for generation of hard cases by the misalignment of interests of the parties concerned. On the other hand, quick inspection of the literature on the psychology of reasoning reveals that none of these fields are the sources of the problematic cases we have encountered in this book from the psychology of reasoning lab. One can doubt that science (psychology or any other) may ever deliver resolutions of the kinds of interpretive problems that arise in extremis in these fields, without thereby seeing the business of the psychology of reasoning threatened, for example, by the observation that there is more than one logic in which the natural language conditional has to be interpreted. Within the psychology of reasoning, if anything, the current flows the other way. Once we take alternative interpretations seriously, we can often get sufficient evidence of subjects' interpretations to make confident empirical judgments of correct or erroneous reasoning, as we hope we persuaded the reader above. Encompassing a wider range of interpretations purchases empirical bite.

Of course, we have seen areas in which this subfield is drawn into contentious issues of interpretation which definitely would take us beyond what is locally scientifically resolvable were we to follow their siren calls. One example is where we observed differences in reasoning as a function of differences in culture. The discussion of literacy and its effects on reasoning (on page 131) touched on the ethical feelings of eye witness and hearsay testimony in undeveloped societies, and the consequences for whether these subjects were willing to engage with the decontextualized classical model. The literature on crosscultural differences in reasoning certainly becomes a hard case once it ventures on the subject of the reasonableness of this move. Another example was where assessments were made about the relative *values* of different students' interpretations. So, for example, when Stanovich observed that the 5% of subjects selecting A and 7 in the selection task, tend to be those with high SAT scores, and concluded from this observation that Wason must have been right about his criterion of correct reasoning, then we entered at least the fringes of the territory of social engineering and the politics of education. Recall that Stanovich quoted on page 6 does believe that resolving the problems students reveal in the reasoning laboratory will contribute to solving the world's conflicts. But the border we need is here rather well marked. We can agree with Stanovich that there are simple internal explanations as to why his correlation should be expected on scientific grounds in our culture (see discussion on pp. 91, and 112, 115), and leave aside issues as to whether current educational arrangements which guarantee the correlation are educationally, morally, politically, or ethically defensible. This still leaves us free to reject Wason's and Stanovich's conclusion that the criterion of classical logic is scientifically uniquely correct. Their conclusion surely does wander over the boundary between science and cultural values, but more importantly, it fails to explain why students do what they do in the laboratory. Although we are optimistic about educational interventions to solve these reasoning problems, and we believe resolution can have important consequences for students' learning, we are much more modest about the resulting contribution to solving humanity's conflicts. Those conflicts arise above all because of conflicting values and interests. Raising the standard of debate is important, but we have no illusions that this will itself be enough.

Decision Theory

Logical reasoning and decision making should be closely related topics. Reasoning and interpretation are intimately involved in setting up our conceptualization of our decisions, and interpreting and reasoning from information is a matter, among other things, of making decisions about how to interpret and what to conclude. In recent years a tension has grown up between decision and reasoning, with some psychological researchers alienated by the state of the deductive reasoning literature, even arguing that humans don't reason very much—they simply make decisions. Meantime, economists have become more aware of the need of accounts of interpretation and reasoning in framing decisions. So a natural question is: where does our program place us with regard to the "heuristics and biases" approach to decision making?

In some ways that field is strongly analogous to the psychology of reasoning. A classical competence theory (here usually classical probability theory[12]) provides a competence model and standard of good decision (or probability estimation) which blatantly does not fit subjects' performances in abstract laboratory tasks (for instance the "Linda," Asian disease, and taxi problems). People disobey transitivity axioms, exhibit "framing effects" and ignore base rates. Tversky and Kahneman [279], with whom these tasks originate, are more sensitive to subjects' dilemmas than Wason was – that is, to the impossibility of

---

12. It may not be superfluous to remark that classical probability theory is wedded to an underlying Boolean structure of events, i.e., to classical logic. Therefore objections to the appropriateness of classical logic in a given context ipso facto apply to probability theory.

calculating the classical theory in most circumstances – and view the heuristics that they ascribe to people as necessary and reasonable ways of satisficing in the circumstances of natural decision, in contrast to Wason's confident assertion of the irrationality of subjects caused by failure to attempt falsification. Their critics (e.g., Gigerenzer [95]) have rejected their approach, claiming that classical probability theory does not give a sensible characterization of what people are trying to compute, let alone how they compute it, going on to specify "fast and frugal" heuristics for making decisions in natural settings, which actually sometimes outperform the intractable classical theory. On this basis they reject entirely the need for or existence of a competence model of what people are trying to do. They argue that people do not reason, they decide.

This disagreement may be more apparent than real, or at least take more careful formulation. The proponents of heuristics and biases can be read as assuming that classical probability theory is the single normative characterization of the decisions involved in these tasks—corresponding to a specification of Marr's "computational" level function. But they also have to be read as regarding that competence theory as distantly related to the methods of computation and approximation achievable in practice. Their admittedly rudimentary characterization of heuristics (e.g., availability, representativeness, etc.) can reasonably be read as a down payment toward a heuristic toolkit. Of course, when the distance between competence specification of the function and performance calculations of its values is so great, it becomes hard to tell what status the competence theory has beyond a theorist's tool. This gap is highly reminiscent of the gap that we have opened up between classical logic and what people are doing in the psychology of reasoning laboratory.

So an exciting possibility is that there might be a way of abstractly specifying what constitutes "intuitive" reasoning in these decision tasks, in a way analogous to what we have proposed here as default logical competence models specifying the credulous interpretation of discourses. This would shift the problem substantially in a direction othogonal to both the heuristics and biases position and the attacks on it from those who reject classical probability as a competence model. The move would be exactly analogous to the move made in this book in logical reasoning. Instead of a single competence model (classical probability) and a set of heuristics, which are the best people can do to approximate it in the circumstances, or on the other hand, a toolbox which is applied to some tasks which have no characterization save in terms of the tools applied to them, we would then have two competence theories of two (sets of) tasks, each requiring its own performance theory or theories, and each contributing different functions to humans' broader aims. "Intuitive decision" need then not be viewed as poor approximation, just as we have argued that deductive reasoning theorists shouldn't view system 1 processes of interpretation as "illogical even if often effective."

Let us illustrate what such a program might look like with one of the heuristics and biases tasks – the Linda problem. What is it that subjects are judging when they judge likelihood here, and how do they make these judgments? Tversky and Kahneman's subjects read a description of Linda:

> Linda is 31 years old, single, outspoken, and very bright. She majored in philosophy. As a student, she was deeply concerned with issues of discrimination and social justice, and also participated in anti-nuclear demonstrations [279,p. 297]

Here is a credulous discourse processing task. The experimenter tells a story and we, as subjects, try to construct the intended model of the heroine. We use any available general knowledge and specific cues to come to some representation of the kind of person she is (that is, the range of people under consideration, say, female twentieth century Americans in their 30s with Anglo-Saxon forenames?), and within that domain, where she stands (say, at the liberal progressive end of the spectrum of American social attitudes). We then read some more information:

> "Which, dear reader, do you feel is more likely?
> (1) Linda is a bank teller or (2) Linda is a bank teller and is active in the feminist movement.

How are we to conceive of our task in answering this question? Tversky and Kahneman assume that we should take an extensional approach: within the domain of female twentieth century Americans in their 30s with Anglo-Saxon forenames, we are supposed to estimate the size of the sets: bank teller vs. bank teller active in the feminist movement, and to respond with option (1) as clearly the larger set, or at worst a set equal in size to the other. As far as the extensional formulation of the task is concerned, note that Gigerenzer does not disagree thus far. He may disagree about how the alternatives presented are interpreted or what information is available to make the decision but he does not argue with the extensional formulation of the problem as such.

The Linda problem is rather reminiscent of the following puzzle beloved of 7-year-olds:

> A captain set to sea with numerous animals aboard his ship. All the animals were in opposite sex pairs. He had a brace of ecstatic elephants, a pair of agreeable aardvarks, and two quarrelsome quagga. How do you spell captain Noah's name? [13]

Similarly, with the Linda problem one has to realise that one is supposed to answer without any recourse to the information in the initial description. Only the two numbered descriptions in the second installment of information are relevant in reasoning to the conclusion that the latter set cannot be larger than the former.

---

13. The problem is no harder presented orally: the answer is, of course, that it depends on whether the questioner intends his forename or his surname.

We would of course argue that this extensional view is already the wrong formulation of what the subject takes the Linda problem to be. So what task did the subjects attempt? Did they attempt this extensional task but for some reason fail at it? Or is there some other specifiable task which they were attempting? And if so, can we both specify what that information–processing task was, and perhaps analyse how they performed it? And if we can specify such another task, did they get that task right?

Suppose the task they adopted was credulous discourse interpretation. On the basis of what the first set of information invokes from their general knowledge, they choose a domain of interpretation. This will be a set of constraints as to who will count as in the domain (perhaps along the lines listed above) along with a database of active default conditionals describing relations between properties of people in this domain. In addition, a representation of Linda using the specific information provided is established in working memory. Now the two alternatives in the second lot of information become a single continuation. First we are told to our surprise that Linda is a bankteller. Then we are told that she is an active member of the feminist movement and we gain some release from our surprise. Presented with a clash between the personality traits hitherto described and our stereotype of banktellers, we recruit some new relevant information from long–term memory. People frequently have to take jobs which are less than ideal matches to their temperaments perhaps, especially women with family constraints. People may still choose to pursue outside activities which may be a better match to their temperaments because of being less constrained. We then construe the question about likelihoods as answerable in terms of how surprising the discourse is at various points in its development, and we judge (2) to be a less surprising state than (1).

Now, if this is a reasonable conjecture about some subjects' mental processes, it will serve to illustrate the alternative construals of the task which are still possible. We believe Tversky and Kahneman would say of such a construal by the subject, that they are using something like the representativeness heuristic to approximate judgments about extensionally construed sets of people in their model of the domain. In contrast, we would say that in this construal of the task, subjects are reasonably understanding the task as one of credulous discourse interpretation and not unreasonably then construing the question as one about how surprising various continuations are. Option (1) increases surprise, whereas (2) resolves it. Needless to remind the reader, we have claimed to give a logical theory of this credulous task and so there is the possibility that an abstract logical characterization of "intuitive decision" can be given, and that the subjects may, moreover, be succeeding at this logical task.

This is perhaps so obvious that its implications are easily missed. We do have evaluative standards for the credulous interpretation of narratives such as the paragraph about Linda. They are of course as complex in full detail as the databases of general knowledge from which interpretations are recruited, but there are many contexts in which we do not hesitate to wade in with judgments about what is a good interpretation and what is not. Along with our colleagues we spend much time "marking essays" which are kinds of expositions, and we have little hesitation in assigning partial orderings to the reasonableness of their interpretations of whatever information and task has been set. Of course it is hard for subjects, and indeed experimenters, to know how to apply these standards in the laboratory. We do not know why we are being told this story about Linda: whether, for example, it is a preamble to being a member of a jury, or a job interview we are about to be asked to conduct, or a retelling of last night's soap. But any of these contexts would bring with it canons of good, bad, and indifferent interpretation, sometimes arguable, but equally often agreed upon within our culture. This "intuitive judgment" business is not to be taken lightly as a life task. We don't all mark essays for a living but we all live by sizing up the reasonableness of expositions for the multifarious purposes of different contexts. It hardly needs to be proposed that the Linda task is more likely to be taken as a case of exercising this skill than of making a judgment about the sizes of two sets. All real judgments have to be based on interpretations of the evidence, purpose, and context, so there is an inescapable element of informal interpretation that sets the scene for decision.

Of course these intimate interactions in decision making between the processes of credulous interpretation, and the exercise of extensional judgment are just like the ones we have urged between credulous interpretation and skeptical derivation. We would take just the same stance with regard to decision as we have taken with regard to reasoning: subjects experience very considerable difficulty in learning to flexibly and appropriately switch between these stances in abstracted situations, and much of tertiary education is about honing these skills. On the other hand, the literature generally supports the view that people are much better (though by no means error–free) at switching appropriately between stances when they are in the contexts in which they regularly make decisions. We would also emphasize that many, especially professional, contexts demand reasoning and decision making in rather decontextualized situations which are not as far from the laboratory as might at first be thought. Hence the educational justification for forcing students to learn to interpret and reason in vacuo.

Of course, much remains to be done to turn this conjecture into a theory of decision. Most notably, some method of estimating probably qualitative likelihood from the state of an interpretation relative to a database of knowledge would have to be specified. Some psychologists have operationalized something like this estimation of likelihood by eliciting the availability of counterexamples from subjects' interpreting defeasible conditionals (e.g.,[106]). One does not have to believe that probability is the right underlying competence

theory to note that "counterexamples" as used here are closely related to the firing of abnormality conditions in a default logic, and recruitment of abnormality
conditions from a long–term memory detabase might be a good place to start
looking to produce the theory required.

   If the conjecture could be turned into a theory of decision it would substantially develop what we take to be the spirit of the heuristics and biases program,
namely that informal reasoning lies at the heart of decision making of even more
formal kinds. We might sloganise in terms of having provided just the fast and
frugal *logic* which is required. This would show that there are formalizations of
"intuitive" reasoning which make rational sense of what is an extremely important human skill of discourse interpretation. These formalizations are, unlike
their classical logical and classical probability theory interpretations, demonstrably computationally tractable, and at least at their core, algorithmic rather
than heuristic. It would place the spotlight on confusion between which of these
tasks (the extensional vs. the intuitive) is appropriate in a given context as perhaps a major source of human error. And it would open up the possibility that
when people do succeed at successful estimations in the extensional task, that
their means of getting there in fact rests on strategically guided use of the defeasible machinery of discourse comprehension. If this program can be carried
through it would also draw a strong analogy between the findings of framing
problems in decision tasks such as this, and findings in the deductive reasoning
literature.

11.2.2   *Homo sapiens sapiens*

Enough of the subjects and the laboratory! What about the species? What are
the prospects there? And the prospects for our understanding of how the species
got to be how it cognitively is? We have presented a lot more biology in this
book than is conventional for a book on human reasoning. Our proposal is that
an important ingredient of the species' cognitive characteristics has to be understood in terms of its radical altriciality. This large–scale reorganization of the
timing of development must have tweaked a large number of biological modules, leading to many exaptations, as well as many secondary adaptations to
cope with them. This upheaval has patently led to novel social economics and
novel microcognitive capacities and much in between. The intense pressures toward cooperation in the environment of the resulting mother-infant dependency
were probably the crucible of human cognitive innovations of cooperative communication. Our planning capacities had already been expanded by a million or
two years of tool manufacture and use, before they were exapted for the planning of discourse and the expansion of the potential interpretive gap between
our current situation and the current contents of our working memory.

   This picture is extremely broad-brush, and by no means original with us. So why paint it here? It seems necessary because it is a picture so radically different from those that have most currency in psychology. This picture makes clear that the prevalence of exaptation guarantees that identifying originating selection pressures for behavioral phenotypes is the hard part of explaining cognitive evolution. And innovation is not achieved by adding new modules. However, it is not dreary necessity that led us to such a heavy dose of biology, but rather excitement. Over the next ten or fifteen years unprecedented biological evidence about human evolution will become available. This is irresistible—in both senses. It will happen, like it or not, and it will be highly desirable, provided cognitive scientists appreciate that it need not have the dire reductionist implications that are so often attributed to it. The field is so fast–moving that even our dippings in it have had to be revised several times in the light of new developments during the process of writing this book. Perhaps we should wait until the textbooks are out instead of bothering the reader with our amateur interpretations. We decided not to because a lot of the message is the lability of the surface and the enduring nature of the underlying concepts. What are important for the cognitive scientist interested in human reasoning are the fundamental concepts: heritability,, variability, modularity, genetic control, exaptation, adaptation, or epigenesis, as well as how they play out in the detailed analyses of the ever–changing surfaces.

In fifteen years we predict that a book on human reasoning will be able to explain, for example, how what we call autism (a disorder multiply reclassified by then, no doubt) is related to the expression of multiple genes at various stages of development, interacting with environmental factors such as the internal circumstances of brain growth, as well as more conventionally experiential influences, to find expression in a range of reasoning styles across clinical and normal populations. Such a book may even be able to explain what selection pressures maintain the clinical extremes in the population through the evolutionary benefits of the lesser doses. This understanding of why it "takes all types" (of people, to use a vernacular expression) might even contribute some much needed motivation for rubbing along with each other. If we are right in this, then we are even more confident that the explanations will rest on analyses of behavioral capacities in terms of logical information systems and their implementations in brain, body, and community.

Bibliography

[1] S. Amari. Dynamics of pattern formation in lateral-inhibition type neural fields. *Biological Cybernetics*, 27:77–87, 1977.

[2] J.R. Anderson and C. Lebiere. *The Atomic Components of Thought*. Lawrence Erlbaum, Mahwah, N.J., 1998.

[3] M. A. Arbib and G. Rizzolatti. Neural expectations: A possible evolutionary path from manual skills to language. *Communication and Cognition*, 29:393–424., 1997.

[4] A. Athanasiadou and R. Dirven. Typology of *if*-clauses. In E. Casad, editor, *Cognitive Linguistics in the Redwoods*, pages 609–654. Mouton De Gruyter, Berlin, 1995.

[5] A. Athanasiadou and R. Dirven. *On Conditionals Again*. John Benjamins, Amsterdam, 1997.

[6] M. Bacharach. *Beyond Individual Choice: Teams and Frames in Game Theory*. Princeton University Press, Princeton, NJ, 2006. edited by Gold, M. and Sugden, R.

[7] A. Bacon, S. Handley, and S. Newstead. Individual differences in strategies in syllogistic reasoning. *Thinking and Reasoning*, 9(2):133–68, 2003.

[8] C. Badcock and B. Crespi. Imbalanced genomic imprinting in brain development: An evolutionary basis for the aetiology of autism. *Journal of Evolutionary Biology*, 19(4):1007–32, 2006. doi:10.1111/j.1420-9101.2006.01091.x.

[9] G. Baggio, M. van Lambalgen, and P. Hagoort. Language, linguistics and cognition. In M. Stokhof and J. Groenendijk, editors, *Handbook of the Philosophy of Linguistics*. Elsevier, Amsterdam, 2007.

[10] R. Baillargeon. Physical reasoning in infancy. In M. Gazzaniga, editor, *The Cognitive Neurosciences*, pages 181–204. MIT Press, Cambridge, MA., 1995.

[11] B.G. Bara, M. Bucciarelli, and V. Lombardo. Mental model theory of deduction: A unified computational approach. *Cognitive Science*, 25(6): 839–901, 2001.

[12] F.C. Bartlett. *Remembering*. Cambridge University Press, Cambridge, UK, 1932.

[13] F.C. Bartlett. *Thinking: An Experimental and Social Study*. Allen and Unwin, London, 1968.

[14] J. Barwise. Model-theoretic logics: Background and aims. In J. Barwise and S. Feferman, editors, *Model-Theoretic Logics*, chapter I. Springer-Verlag, New York, 1985.

[15] J. Barwise and S. Feferman, editors. *Model-Theoretic Logics*. Springer-Verlag, New York, 1985.

[16] W. Bechtel and A. Abrahamsen. *Connectionism and the Mind*. Blackwell, Oxford, 1991.

[17] D. Bell. *Husserl*. The Arguments of the Philosophers. Routledge, London, 1991.

[18] Y. Ben-Ari. Excitatory actions of GABA during development: The nature of the nurture. *Nature Review of Neuroscience*, 3:728–739, 2002.

[19] E. Bienenstock and C. von der Malsburg. A neural network for invariant pattern recognition. *Europhysics Letters*, 4(1):121–126, 1987.

[20] B. S. Bloom and L. J. Broder. *Problem Solving Processes of College Students*. University of Chicago Press, Chicago, 1950.

[21] G.S. Boolos, R.C. Jeffrey, and J.P. Burgess. *Computability and Logic*. Cambridge University Press, UK, 2002.

[22] G. Borensztajn, R.P. van Hoolwerff, A. Laloi, G. Moas, and V. Trehan. The suppression task revisited. Research report, ILLC, Amsterdam, December 2005. Available from http://staff.science.uva.nl/michiell.

[23] D. Bramble and D. Lieberman. Endurance running and the evolution of homo. *Nature*, 432:345–352, 2004.

[24] J.D. Bransford, J.R. Barclay, and J.J. Franks. Sentence memory: A constructive versus an interpretive approach. *Cognitive Psychology*, 3:193–209, 1972.

[25] R. Breheny. Communication and folk psychology. *Mind and Language*, 21(1):74–107, 2006.

[26] J.S. Bruner. *Beyond the Information Given*. Norton, New York, 1973.

[27] A. Burkhalter. Development of forward and feedback connections between areas v1 and v2 of human visual cortex. *Cerebral Cortex*, 3:476–487, 1993.

[28] R.M.J. Byrne. Suppressing valid inferences with conditionals. *Cognition*, 31:61–83, 1989.

[29] R.M.J. Byrne, O. Espino, and C. Santamaria. Counterexamples and the suppression of inferences. *Journal of Memory and Language*, 40:347–373, 1999.

[30] N. Canessa, A. Gorini, S.F. Cappa, M. Piattelli-Palmarini, M. Danna, F. Fazio, and D. Perani. The effect of social content on deductive reasoning: An fMRI study. *Human Brain Mapping*, 26(1):30–43, 2005.

[31] Sean B. Carroll. *Endless Forms Most Beautiful: The New Science of Evo Devo and the Making of the Animal Kingdom*. Norton, London, 2005.

[32] D. Cesanyi. Human behavior complex and the compulsion of communication: Key factors of human evolution. *Semiotica*, 128:243–258, 2000.

[33] D. Chan and F. Chua. Suppression of valid inferences – syntactic views, mental models and relative salience. *Cognition*, 53(3):217–238, 1994.

[34] K. J. Chapman and J. P. Chapman. The atmosphere effect reexamined. *Journal of Experimental Psychology*, 58:220–56, 1959.

[35] W.G. Chase and H.A. Simon. Perception in chess. *Cognitive Psychology*, 4(1):55–81, 1973.

[36] N. Chater and M. Oaksford. The probability heuristics model of syllogistic reasoning. *Cognitive Psychology*, 38:191–258, 1999.

[37] P. Cheng and K. Holyoak. Pragmatic reasoning schemas. *Cognitive Psychology*, 14, 1985.

[38] P. Cheng, K. Holyoak, R. E. Nisbett, and L. Oliver. Pragmatic versus syntactic approaches to training deductive reasoning. *Cognitive Psychology*, 18:293–328, 1986.

[39] A.G. Clark, S. Glanowski, R. Nielsen, P.D. Thomas, A. Kejariwal, M.A. Todd, D.M. Tanenbaum, D. Civello, F. Lu, B. Murphy, S. Ferriera, G. Wang, X. Zheng, T.J. White, J.J. Sninsky, M.D. Adams, and

M. Cargill. Inferring nonneutral evolution from human-chimp-mouse orthologous gene trios. *Science*, 302:1960–3, 2003.

[40] Fabrice Clement and Laurence Kaufmann. Are theory of mind and deontic reasoning two independent subsystems of social cognition ? Evidence from development. In press.

[41] W.A. Clements and J. Perner. Implicit understanding of belief. *Cognitive Development*, 9:377–395, 1994.

[42] COBUILD. *Collins Birmingham University International Language Database*. Collins, London, 1980.

[43] I. L. Cohen. An artificial neural network analog of learning in autism. *Biological Psychiatry*, 36(1):5–20, 1994.

[44] B. Comrie. Conditionals: A typology. In E. Traugott, A. ter Meulen, J.S. Reilly, and C.A. Ferguson, editors, *On Conditionals*, pages 77–99. Cambridge University Press, Cambridge, UK, 1986.

[45] Monica Conciatori, Christopher J. Stodgell, Susan L. Hyman, Melanie O'Bara, Roberto Militerni, Carmela Bravaccio, Simona Trillo, Francesco Montecchi, Cindy Schneider, Raun Melmed, Maurizio Elia, Lori Crawford, and Sarah J. Spence. Association between the HOXA1 A218G polymorphism and increased head circumference in patients with autism. *Biological Psychiatry*, 55(4):413–9, 2004.

[46] H. Coqueugniot, J.-J. Hublin, F. Veillon, F. Houet, and T. Jacob. Early brain growth in HOMO ERECTUS and implications for cognitive ability. *Nature*, 431:299–302, 2004.

[47] L. Cosmides. The logic of social exchange: Has natural selection shaped how humans reason? studies with the Wason selection task. *Cognition*, 31:187–276, 1989.

[48] L. Cosmides and J. Tooby. Cognitive adaptations for social exchange. In *The Adapted Mind: Evolutionary Psychology and the Generation of Culture*, pages 163–228. Oxford University Press, Oxford, 1992.

[49] L. Cosmides and J. Tooby. The psychological foundations of culture. In *The Adapted Mind: Evolutionary Psychology and the Generation of Culture*, pages 19–138. oup, Oxford, 1992.

[50] L. Cosmides and J. Tooby. Beyond intuition and instinct blindness: Toward an evolutionary rigorous cognitive science. In J. Mehler and S. Franck, editors, *Cognition on Cognition*, pages 69–105. MIT Press, Cambridge, MA, 1995.

[51] E. Courchesne and K. Pierce. Why the frontal cortex in autism might be talking only to itself: Local over-connectivity but long-distance disconnection. *Current Opinion in Neurobiology*, 15:225–230, 2005.

[52] K. J. W. Craik. *The Nature of Explanation*. Cambridge University Press, Cambridge, UK, 1967. First edition 1943.

[53] D. Cummins. Evidence for the innateness of deontic reasoning. *Mind and Language*, 11:160–190, 1996.

[54] D. D. Cummins. Cheater detection is modified by social rank: The impact of dominance on the evolution of cognitive functions. *Evolution and Human Behavior*, 20(4):229–48, 1999.

[55] A. R. Damasio. *Descartes' Error: Emotion, Reason and the Human Brain*. Putnam, New York, 1994.

[56] E. Dantsin, T. Eiter, G. Gottlob, and A. Voronkov. Complexity and expressive power of logic programming. *ACM Computing Surveys*, 33(3): 374–425, 2001.

[57] D. Davidson. Radical interpretation. *Dialectica*, 27, 1973. Reprinted: *Inquiries into Truth and Interpretation*, 2nd ed. Oxford, Clarendon Press.

[58] W. Davies, A. Isles, R. Smith, D. Karunadasa, D. Burrmann, T. Humby, O. Ojarikre, C. Biggin, D. Skuse, P. Burgoyne, and L. Wilkinson. Xlr3b is a new imprinted candidate for X-linked parent-of-origin effects on cognitive function in mice. *Nature Genetics*, 37(6):625–9, 2005.

[59] A. d'Avila Garcez, K.B. Broda, and D. Gabbay. *Neural-Symbolic Learning Systems: Foundations and Applications*. Springer–Verlag, London, 2002.

[60] A.G. Dayer, K.M. Cleaver, T. Abouantoun, and H.A. Cameron. New GABAergic interneurons in the adult neocortex and striatum are generated from different precursors. *Journal of Cell Biology*, 168(3):415–27, 2005.

[61] V.L. Deglin and M. Kinsbourne. Divergent thinking styles of the hemispheres: How syllogisms are solved during transitory hemisphere suppression. *Brain and Cognition*, 31:285–307, 1996.

[62] Y.A. Dementieva, D.D. Vance, S.L. Donnelly, L.A. Elston, C.M. Wolpert, S.A. Ravan, G.R. DeLong, R.K. Abramson, H.H. Wright, and M.L. Cuccaro. Accelerated head growth in early development of individuals with autism. *Pediatric Neurology*, 32:102–8, 2005.

[63] K. Dieussaert, W. Schaeken, W. Schroyen, and G. d'Ydewalle. Strategies during complex conditional inferences. *Thinking and Reasoning*, 6(2): 125–161, 2000.

[64] K. Doets. *From Logic to Logic Programming*. MIT Press, Cambridge, MA, 1994.

[65] S. Dorus, E. Vallender, P. Evans, J. Anderson, S. Gilbert, S. Mahowald, G. Wyckoff, C. Malcom, and B. Lahn. Accelerated evolution of nervous system genes in the origin of *Homo sapiens*. *Cell*, 119:1027–1040, 2004.

[66] R. Dunbar. *The Human Story*. Faber and Faber, London, 2005.

[67] P. M. Dung, R. Kowalski, and F. Toni. Dialectic proof procedures for assumption-based, admissible argumentation. *Journal of Artificial Intelligence*, 170(2):114–159, 2006.

[68] H. Ebbinghaus. *Memory: A Contribution to Experimental Psychology*. Dover, New York, 1964. Original work appeared 1885.

[69] Evan E. Eichler and Andrew W. Zimmerman. A hot spot of genetic instability in autism. *New England Journal of Medicine*, 2008. editorial 10.1056/NEJMe0708756.

[70] N. Elango, J. Thomas, and S. Yi. Variable molecular clocks in hominoids. *Proceedings of the National Academy of Sciences*, 103(5):1370–1375, 2006.

[71] J. Etchemendy. *The Concept of Logical Consequence*. Harvard University Press, Cambridge, MA, 1990.

[72] J.St.B.T. Evans. In two minds: Dual-process accounts of reasoning. *Trends in Cognitive Sciences*, 7(10):454–459, 2003.

[73] J.St.B.T. Evans. Interpretation and "matching bias" in a reasoning task. *Quarterly Journal of Experimental Psychology*, 24:193–199, 1972.

[74] J.St.B.T. Evans. Matching bias in conditional reasoning: Do we understand it after 25 years? *Thinking and Reasoning*, 4(1):45–110, 1998.

[75] J.St.B.T. Evans and D.E. Over. Rationality in the selection task: Epistemic utility versus uncertainty reduction. *Psychological Review*, 103(2): 356–363, 1996.

[76] J.St.B.T. Evans, S.L. Newstead, and R.M. Byrne. *Human Reasoning: The Pychology of Deduction*. Lawrence Erlbaum Associates, Hove, Sussex, 1993.

[77] P. Evans, J. Anderson, E. Vallender, S. Choi, and B. Lahn. Reconstructing the evolutionary history of microcephalin, a gene controlling human brain size. *Human Molecular Genetics*, 13:1139–1145, 2004.

[78] P. Evans, J. Anderson, E. Vallender, S. Gilbert, C. Malcom, S. Dorus, and B. Lahn. Adaptive evolution of ASPM, a major determinant of cerebral cortical size in humans. *Human Molecular Genetics*, 13:489–494, 2004.

[79] E.E. Evans-Pritchard. *Witchcraft, Oracles, and Magic among the Azande*. Clarendon Press, Oxford, 2nd edition, 1976.

[80] D. B. Everman and S. B. Cassidy. Genetics of childhood disorders: XII. genomic imprinting: Breaking the rules. *Journal of the American Acadamy of Child and Adolescent Psychiatry*, 39(3):386–389, 2000.

[81] L. Fiddick, L. Cosmides, and J. Tooby. The role of domain-specific representations and inferences in the Wason selection task. *Cognition*, 75: 1–79, 2000.

[82] S.I. Fillenbaum. How to do some things with if. In Cotton and Klatzky, editors, *Semantic functions in cognition*. Lawrence Erlbaum, Maweh, NJ, 1978.

[83] R.A. Foley. An evolutionary and chronological framework for human social behaviour. In W. G. Runciman, J. Maynard-Smith, and R. Dunbar, editors, *Evolution of Primate Social Behaviour Patterns in Primates and Man*, volume 88 of *Proceedings of the British Academy*, pages 95–117. Oxford University Press, Oxford, 1996.

[84] M. Ford. Two modes of mental representation and problem solution in syllogistic reasoning. *Cognition*, 54:1–71, 1995.

[85] G. Frege. *The Frege Reader*. Blackwell, Oxford, 1997. (edited by M. Beany).

[86] K. Friston. Beyond phrenology: What can neuroimaging tell us about distributed circuitry? *Annual Review of Neuroscience*, 25:221–250, 2002.

[87] C. Frith. What do imaging studies tell us about the neural basis of autism? In G. Bock and J. Goode, editors, *Autism: Neural Basis and Treatment Possibilities*, Novartis Foundation Symposium, pages 149–166. Wiley, New York, 2003.

[88] U. Frith and F. Happe. Autism: beyond 'theory of mind'. *Cognition*, 50: 115–132, 1994.

[89] D. Frye, P.D. Zelazo, and T. Palfai. Theory of mind and rule-based reasoning. *Cognitive Development*, 10:483–527, 1995.

[90] P. Gärdenfors. Meanings as conceptual structures. In M. Carrier and P. Machamer, editors, *Mindscapes: Philosophy, Science, and the Mind*. Pittsburgh University Press, Pittsburgh, 1997.

[91] P. Gärdenfors. Symbolic, conceptual and subconceptual representations. In V. Cantoni, V. di Ges, A. Setti, and D. Tegolo, editors, *Human and Machine Perception: Information Fusion*. Plenum Press, New York, 1997.

[92] G. Gebauer and D. Laming. Rational choices in Wason's selection task. *Psychological Research*, 60:284–293, 1997.

[93] M. A. Gernsbacher. *Handbook of Psycholinguistics*. NY: Academic Press, New York, 1994.

[94] M. Ghaziuddin, J. Zaccagnini, L. Tsai, and S. Elardo. Is megalencephaly specific to autism? *Journal of Intellectual Disability Research*, 43(4): 279–282, 1999.

[95] G. Gigerenzer. *Adaptive Thinking: Rationality in the Real World*. Oxford University Press, Oxford, 2000.

[96] G. Gigerenzer and K. Hug. Domain-specific reasoning: Social contracts, cheating, and perspective change. *Cognition*, 43:127–171, 1992.

[97] C. Gillberg and L. de Souza. Head circumference in autism, asperger syndrome, and ADHD: A comparative study. *Developmental Medicine and Child, Neurology*, 44:296–300, 2002.

[98] H. Gintis, S. Bowles, R.T. Boyd, and E. Fehr. *Moral Sentiments and Material Interests : The Foundations of Cooperation in Economic Life*. MIT Press, Cambridge, MA, 2005.

[99] V. Girotto, M. Kemmelmeier, D. Sperber, and J-B. van der Henst. Inept reasoners or pragmatic virtuosos? Relevance in the deontic selection task. *Cognition*, 81:B69–B76, 2001.

[100] V. Goel, B. Gold, S. Kapur, and S. Houle. Neuroanatomical correlates of human reasoning. *Journal of Cognitive Neuroscience*, 10:293–303, 1998.

[101] V. Goel, C. Buchel, C.D. Frith, and R.J. Dolan. Dissociation of mechanisms underlying syllogistic reasoning. *NeuroImage*, 12:504–514, 2000.

[102] N. Goodman. *Fact, Fiction and Forecast*. London University Press, London, 1954.

[103] L. Goos and I. Silverman. The influence of genetic imprinting on brain development and behaviour. *Evolution and Human Behavior*, 22:385–407, 2001.

[104] G. Gottlob. Complexity results for nonmonotonic logics. *Journal of Logic and Computation*, 2(3):397–425, 1992.

[105] S.J. Gould and R.C. Lewontin. The spandrels of San Marco and the Panglossian paradigm: A critique of the adaptationist programme. *Proceedings of the Royal Society of London: Part B. Biological Sciences*, 205:581–598, 1979.

[106] D.W. Green, D.E. Over, and R.A. Pyne. Probability and choice in the selection task. *Thinking and Reasoning*, 3(3):209–35, 1997. DOI: 10.1080/135467897394356.

[107] P.M. Greenfield. Language, tools and the brain: The ontogeny and phylogeny of hierarchically organized sequential behavior. *Behavioral and Brain Sciences*, 14:531–595, 1991.

[108] H. P. Grice. Logic and conversation. In P. Cole and J. Morgan, editors, *Syntax and Semantics: Speech Acts*, volume 3. London: Academic Press, 1975.

[109] R. A. Griggs and J. R. Cox. The elusive thematic-materials effect in Wason's selection task. *British Journal of Psychology*, 73:407–420, 1982.

[110] C.G. Gross. Neurogenesis in the adult brain: Death of a dogma. *Nature Review of Neuroscience*, 1:67–73, 2000.

[111] L. Gustafsson. Inadequate cortical feature maps: A neural circuit theory of autism. *Biological Psychiatry*, 42:1138–47, 1997.

[112] P Hagoort and J. van Berkum. Beyond the sentence given. *Philosophical Transactions of the Royal Society of London. Series B: Biological Sciences*, 362(1481):801–811, May 29 2007. DOI: 10.1098/rstb.2007.2089.

[113] J.Y. Halpern. *Reasoning about uncertainty*. MIT Press, Cambridge, MA., 2005.

[114] F. Happé. *Autism: An Introduction to Psychological Theory*. UCL Press, London, 1994.

[115] F. Happé, A. Ronald, and R. Plomin. Time to give up on a single explanation for autism. *Nature Neuroscience*, 9(10):1218–20, 2006.

[116] B. Hare and M. Tomasello. Chimpanzees are more skillful in competitive than in cooperative cognitive tasks. *Animal Behaviour*, 68:571–581, 2004.

[117] P.L. Harris. *The Work of the Imagination*. Blackwell, Oxford, 2000.

[118] A.G. Harvey, E. Watkins, W. Mansell, and R. Shafran. *Cognitive Behavioural Processes across Psychological Disorders: A Transdiagnostic Approach to Research and Treatment*. Oxford University Press, Oxford, 2004.

[119] M. Hauser, N. Chomsky, and T. Fitch. The faculty of language: What is it, who has it, and how did it evolve? *Science*, 298:1569–79, 2002.

[120] M.D. Hauser. Knowing about knowing: Dissociations between perception and action systems over evolution and during development. *Annals of the New York Academy of Sciences*, 1:1–25, 2003.

[121] J. Heal. Simulation vs. theory-theory: What is at issue? *Proceedings of the British Academy*, 83:129–144, 1994.

[122] M. Henlé. On the relation between logic and thinking. *Psychological Review*, 69:366–378, 1962.

[123] M.R. Herbert. Large brains in autism: The challenge of pervasive abnormality. *The Neuroscientist*, 11(5):417 – 440, 2005.

[124] C. Hill and K. Parry. Autonomous and pragmatic models of literacy: Reading assessment in adult education. *Linguistics and Education*, 1: 233–83, 1989.

[125] J. Hintikka. Lingua universalis vs. calculus ratiocinator : An ultimate presupposition of twentieth-century philosophy. In *Jaakko Hintikka Selected Papers*, volume 2. Kluwer, Dordrecht, Netherlands, 1996.

[126] R.P. Hobson. Against the theory of mind. *British Journal of Developmental Psychology*, 9:33–51, 1991.

[127] R.P. Hobson. *Autism and the Development of Mind*. Lawrence Erlbaum Associates, Mahwah, NJ, 1993.

[128] Wilfrid Hodges. The logical content of theories of deduction. *Behavioural and Brain Sciences*, 16(2):353–354, 1993. Commentary on Johnson-Laird and Byrne [144].

[129] Wilfrid Hodges. Two doors to open. In Dov M. Gabbay, editor, *Mathematical Problems from Applied Logic I: New Logics for the 21st century*, pages 277–316. Springer, 2006.

[130] S. Hoelldobler and Y. Kalinke. Towards a massively parallel computational model of logic programming. In *Proceedings of ECAI94 Workshop on Combining Symbolic and Connectionist Processing*, pages 68–77. ECAI, 1994.

[131] C. Hughes and J. Russell. Autistic children's difficulty with disengagement from an object: its implications for theories of autism. *Developmental Psychology*, 29:498–510, 1993.

[132] M. Hughes. *The use of negative information in concept attainment.* PhD thesis, 1966.

[133] N. Humphrey. *A History of the Mind.* Vintage, New York, 1993.

[134] E. Husserl. *Logische Untersuchungen. Vol. 1.* Husserliana, Volume 18–19. Nijhoff, The Hague, Netherlands, 1975.

[135] E. Husserl. *Briefwechsel, Volumes 1–10.* Kluwer, Dordrecht, Netherlands, 1994.

[136] E. Hutchins. *Cognition in the Wild.* MIT Press, Cambridge, MA, 1996.

[137] P.R. Huttenlocher. Dendritic and synaptic development in human cerebral cortex: Time course and critical periods. *Developmental Neuropsychology*, 16(3):347–9, 1999.

[138] J.L. Ingram, C.J. Stodgell, S.L. Hyman, D.A. Figlewicz, L.R. Weitkamp, and P.M. Rodier. Discovery of allelic variants of HOXA1 and HOXB1: Genetic susceptibility to autism spectrum disorders. *Teratology*, 62:393–405, 2000.

[139] A. R. Isles and L. S. Wilkinson. Imprinted genes, cognition and behaviour. *Trends in Cognitive Sciences*, 4:309–318, 2000.

[140] Y. Iwasa. The conflict theory of genomic imprinting: How much can be explained? *Current Topics in Developmental Biology*, 40:255–93, 1998.

[141] Y.H. Jiang, T. Sahoo, R.C. Michaelis, D. Bercovich, J. Bressler, C.D. Kashork, Q. Liu, L.G. Shaffer, R.J. Schroer, D.W. Stockton, R.S. Spielman, R.E. Stevenson, and A.L. Beaudet. A mixed epigenetic/genetic model for oligogenic inheritance of autism with a limited role for UBE3A. *American Journal of Medical Genetics A*, 131(1):1–10, 2004.

[142] P. N. Johnson, P. Legrenzi, and M. S. Legrenzi. Reasoning and a sense of reality. *British Journal of Psychology*, 63:395–, 1972.

[143] P. Johnson-Laird and R. Byrne. Conditionals: A theory of meaning, pragmatics and inference. *Psychological Review*, 109:646–678, 2002.

[144] P. N. Johnson-Laird and R.M. Byrne. *Deduction.* Lawrence Erlbaum, Hove, Sussex, UK., 1991.

[145] P.N. Johnson-Laird. *Mental Models.* Cambridge University Press, 1983.

[146] P.N. Johnson-Laird. *The Computer and the Mind : An Introduction to Cognitive Science, 2nd ed.* Fontana, London, 1993.

[147] P.N. Johnson-Laird and F. Savary. Illusory inferences: A novel class of erroneous deductions. *Cognition,* 71(3):191–229, 199.

[148] P.N. Johnson-Laird and P.C. Wason. A theoretical analysis of insight into a reasoning task. *Cognitive Psychology,* 1:134–148, 1970.

[149] P.N. Johnson-Laird, P. Legrenzi, V. Girotto, and M. Legrenzi. Illusions in reasoning about consistency. *Science,* 288:531–532, 2000.

[150] D. Kahneman and A. Tversky. Subjective probability: A judgement of representativeness. *Cognitive Psychology,* 3:430–454, 1972.

[151] A. Kakas, R. Kowalski, and F. Toni. The role of abduction in logic programming. In Dov M Gabbay, Christopher John Hogger, and J A Robinson, editors, *Handbook of Logic in Artificial Intelligence and Logic Programming,* volume 5, pages 235–324. Oxford University Press, 1998. URL citeseer.ist.psu.edu/kakas98role.html.

[152] H. Kamp. A theory of truth and semantic representation. In J. Groenendijk, T. Janssen, and M. Stokhof, editors, *Formal Methods in the Study of Language,* pages 277–322. Mathematical Centre, Amsterdam, 1981.

[153] H. Kamp and B. Partee. Prototype theory and compositionality. *Cognition,* 57:169–21, 2000.

[154] H. Kamp and U. Reyle. *From Discourse to Logic, Introduction to Modeltheoretic Semantics of Natural Language, Formal Logic and Discourse Representation Theory, Part 1,* volume 42 of *Studies in Linguistics and Philosophy.* Kluwer Academic Publishers, Dordrecht, 1993.

[155] H. Kamp and U. Reyle. *From Discourse to Logic: Introduction to Modeltheoretic Semantics of Natural Language, Formal Logic and Discourse Representation Theory,* volume 42 of *Studies in Linguistics and Philosophy.* Kluwer, Dordrecht, Netherlands, 1993.

[156] E. B. Keverne, F. Martel, and C. M. Nevison. Primate brain evolution: genetic and functional considerations. *Proceedings of the Royal Society of London Series B. Biological Sciences,* 263:689–696, 1996.

[157] E.B. Keverne, R. Fundele, M. Narasimha, S.C. Barton, and M.A. Surani. Genomic imprinting and the differential roles of parental genomes in brain development. *Devopmental Brain Research*, 92:91–100, 1996.

[158] K. Kirby. Probabilities and utilities of fictional outcomes in Wason's selection task. *Cognition*, 51(1):1–28, 1994.

[159] P.W. Kitcher. *Kant's Transcendental Psychology*. Oxford University Press, New York, 1990.

[160] S. C. Kleene. *Introduction to Metamathematics*. North-Holland, Amsterdam, 1951.

[161] W. Köhler. *The Mentality of Apes*. Harcourt Brace and World, New York, 1925.

[162] R.A. Kowalski. Computational logic in an object-oriented world. In O. Stock and M. Schaerf, editors, *Reasoning, Action and Interaction in AI Theories and Systems - Festschrift in Honor of Luigia Carlucci Aiello.*, LNAI. Springer Verlag, Berlin, 2006.

[163] R.A. Kowalski. Legislation as logic programs. In *Logic Programming in Action*, pages 203–230. Springer Verlag, Berlin, 1992.

[164] R.A. Kowalski. Using meta-logic to reconcile reactive with rational agents. In *Meta-Logics and Logic Programming*, pages 227–242. MIT Press, Cambridge, MA, 1995.

[165] M. Kusch, editor. *Language as Calculus vs. Language as Universal Medium. A Study in Husserl, Heidegger and Gadamer.* Kluwer, Dordrecht, Netherlands, 1989.

[166] M. Kutas and S.A. Hillyard. Reading senseless sentences: Brain potentials reflect semantic incongruity. *Science*, 207:203–205, 1980.

[167] I. Lakatos. *Proofs and Refutations*. Cambridge University Press, Cambridge, UK, 1976.

[168] A. Lechler. Interpretation of conditionals in the suppression task. MSc thesis, HCRC, University of Edinburgh., 2004.

[169] H.J. Leevers and P.L. Harris. Counterfactual syllogistic reasoning in normal four-year-olds, children with learning disabilities, and children with autism. *Proceedings of the British Academy*, 76:64–87, 2000.

[170] D. Lehman, R. Lempert, and R. Nisbett. The effects of graduate training on reasoning: Formal discipline and thinking about everyday life events. *American Psychologist*, 43:431–442, 1988.

[171] Hannes Leitgeb. Introduction to the special issue. *Studia Logica*, 2008. http://www.springerlink.com/content/v673573753hw64u0.

[172] A. Leslie. Pretence and representation: The origins of a "theory of mind". *Psychological Review*, 94:412–426, 1987.

[173] P. Levitt, Eagleson K. L., and E. M. Powell. Regulation of neocortical interneuron development and the implications for neurodevelopmental disorders. *Trends in Neurosciences*, 27(7):400–406, 2004.

[174] J. Levy. Connectionist models of over-specific learning in autism. In H. Bowman and C Labiouse, editors, *Connectionist Models of Cognition and Perception*, volume 2, pages 115–126. World Scientific, Hackensack, NJ, 2004.

[175] B. Longuenesse. *Kant and the Capacity to Judge*. Princeton University Press, Princeton, NJ, 1998.

[176] M. Luciana. The neural and functional development of human prefrontal cortex. In M. H. Johnson and M. De Haan, editors, *The Cognitive Neuroscience of Development*, chapter 7, pages 157–179. Psychology Press, Hove, Sussex, UK, 2003.

[177] A.R. Luria. *Cognitive Development: Its Social and Cultural Foundations*. Harvard University Press, Cambridge, MA, 1976.

[178] D.Q. Ma, P.L. Whitehead, M.M. Menold, E.R. Martin, A.E. Ashley-Koch, H. Mei, M.D. Ritchie, G.R. Delong, R.K. Abramson, H.H. Wright, M.L. Cuccaro, J.P. Hussman, J.R. Gilbert, and M.A. Pericak-Vance. Identification of significant association and gene-gene interaction of GABA receptor subunit genes in autism. *American Journal of Human Genetics*, 77(3):377–388, 2005.

[179] K. Mani and P.N. Johnson-Laird. The mental representation of spatial descriptions. *Memory and Cognition*, 10:181–187, 1982.

[180] K. Manktelow and D. Over. *Inference and Understanding: A Philosophical Perspective*. Routledge, London, 1990.

[181] Gary F. Marcus and Simon E. Fisher. FOXP2 in focus. What can genes tell us about speech and language? *Trends in Cognitive Sciences*, 7(6): 257–262, 2003.

[182] H. Margolis. *Patterns, Thinking, and Cognition: A Theory of Judgment*. University of Chicago Press, Chicago, 1988.

[183] D. Marr. *Vision: A Computational Investigation into the Human Representation and Processing of Visual Information.* W.H. Freeman, San Fransisco, 1982.

[184] R.D. Martin. *Primate Origins and Evolution.* Chapman & Hall, Boca Raton, FL, 1990.

[185] J. McCarthy. Circumscription – a form of non–monotonic reasoning. *Artficial Intelligence*, 13:27–39, 1980.

[186] Jon M. McClellan, Ezra Susser, and Mary-Claire King. Schizophrenia: a common disease caused by multiple rare alleles. *Br J Psychiatry*, 190 (3):194–199, 2007. doi: 10.1192/bjp.bp.106.025585.

[187] J. L. McClelland. The basis of hyperspecificity in autism: A preliminary suggestion based on properties of neural nets. *Journal of Autism and Developmental Disorders*, 30(5):497–502, 2000.

[188] Warren S. McCulloch and Walter Pitts. A logical calculus of the ideas immanent in nervous activity. *Bulletin of Mathematical Biology*, 5(4): 115–133, 1943. DOI 10.1007/BF02478259.

[189] B. McGonigle, M. Chalmers, and A. Dickinson. Concurrent disjoint and reciprocal classification by CEBUS APELLA in serial ordering tasks: Evidence for hierarchical organization. *Animal Cognition*, 6(3):185–197, 2003.

[190] G. Meyer, A M. Goffinet, and A Fairen. What is a Cajal-Retzius cell? A reassessment of a classical cell type based on recent observations in the developing neocortex. *Cerebral Cortex*, 9:765–75, 1999.

[191] J.-J.Ch. Meyer and W. van der Hoek, editors. *Epistemic logic in AI and computer science*, volume 41 of *Cambridge Tracts in Theoretical Computer Science*. Cambridge University Press, Cambridge, UK, 1995.

[192] R.C. Miall and D.M. Wolpert. Forward models for physiological motor control. *Neural Networks*, 9(8):1265–79, 1996.

[193] L.L Miles, J.H. Hadden, T.N. Takahashi, and R.E. Hillman. Head circumference is an independent clinical finding associated with autism. *American Journal of Medical Genetics*, 95:33950, 2000.

[194] G.A. Miller and P.N. Johnson-Laird. *Language and Perception.* Harvard University Press, Cambridge, MA, 1976.

[195] P. Monaghan and K. Stenning. Effects of representational modality and thinking style on learning to solve reasoning problems. In M. A. Gernsbacher and J. Derry, editors, *Proceedings of 20th Annual Meeting of the Cognitive Science Society*, volume 20, pages 716–21. Lawrence Erlbaum, Maweh, NJ, 1998.

[196] I.M. Morison, J.P. Ramsay, and H.G. Spencer. A census of mammalian imprinting. *Trends in Genetics*, 21(8):457–465, 2005.

[197] L.A. Muscarella, V. Guarnieri, R. Sacco, R. Militerni, C. Bravaccio, S. Trillo, C. Schneider, R. Melmed, M. Elia, M.L. Mascia, E. Rucci, M.R. Piemontese, L. D'Agruma, and A.M. Persico. HOXA1 gene variants influence head growth rates in humans. *American Journal of Medical Genetics Part B: Neuropsychiatric Genetics*, 144B(3):388–90, 2007. http://dx.doi.org/10.1002/ajmg.b.30469.

[198] M. Nedergaard, B. Ransom, and S. Goldman. A new role for astrocytes: Redefining the functional architecture of the brain. *Trends in Neurosciences*, 26:523–9, 2003.

[199] A. Newell and H. Simon. *Human Problem Solving*. Prentice-Hall, Englewood Cliffs, NJ, 1972.

[200] S. Newstead. Interpretational errors in syllogistic reasoning. *Journal of Memory and Language*, 28:78–91, 1989.

[201] S. Newstead. Gricean implicatures and syllogistic reasoning. *Journal of Memory and Language*, 34:644–664, 1995.

[202] R. Nielsen, C. Bustamante, A.G. Clark, S. Glanowski, T.B. Sackton, M.J. Hubisz, A. Fledel-Alon, D.M. Tanenbaum, D. Civello, T.J. White, J.J. Sninsky, M.D. Adams, and M. Cargill. A scan for positively selected genes in the genomes of humans and chimpanzees. *Public Library of Science: Biology*, 3(e170), 2005.

[203] M. Oaksford and N. Chater. Probabilities and pragmatics in conditional inference: Suppression and order effects. In D. Hardman and L. Macchi, editors, *Thinking: Psychological Perspectives on Reasoning, Judgment and Decision Making*, chapter 6, pages 95–122. John Wiley & Sons, Chichester, 2003.

[204] M. R. Oaksford and K. Stenning. Reasoning with conditionals containing negated constituents. *Journal of Experimental Psychology: Learning, Memory and Cognition*, 18:835–854, 1992.

[205] M.R. Oaksford and N.C. Chater. A rational analysis of the selection task as optimal data selection. *Psychological Review*, 101:608–631, 1994.

[206] M.R. Oaksford and N.C. Chater. Rational explanation of the selection task. *Psychological Review*, 103(2):381–392, 1996.

[207] K. H. Onishi and R. Baillargeon. Do 15-month-old infants understand false beliefs? *Science*, 308:255–258, 2005.

[208] S. Ozonoff, D.L. Strayer, W.M. McMahon, and F. Filloux. Executive function abilities in children with autism and Tourette syndrome: An information-processing approach. *Journal of Child Psychology and Psychiatry and Allied Disciplines*, 35:1015–1032, 1994.

[209] M. Pagel. Mother and father in surprise genetic agreement. *Nature*, 397: 19–20, 1999.

[210] F.J. Pelletier and R. Elio. What should default reasoning be, by default? *Computational Intelligence*, 13(2):165–187, 1997.

[211] J. Perner and B. Lang. Development of theory of mind and executive control. *Trends in Cognitive Sciences*, 3(9):337–344, 1999.

[212] J. Perner, S. Leekham, and H. Wimmer. Three-year olds' difficulty with false belief: The case for a conceptual deficit. *British Journal of Developmental Psychology*, 5:125–137, 1987.

[213] Antonio M. Persico and Thomas Bourgeron. Searching for ways out of the autism maze: genetic, epigenetic and environmental clues. *Trends in Neurosciences*, 29(7):349–58, 2006.

[214] S.U. Peters, A.L. Beaudet, N. Madduri, and C.A. Bacino. Autism in Angelman syndrome: Implications for autism research. *Clinical Genetics*, 66(6):530–6, 2004.

[215] D. M. Peterson and D. M. Bowler. Counterfactual reasoning and false belief understanding in children with autism. *Autism: The International Journal of Research and Practice*, 4(4):391–405, 2000.

[216] J. Piaget. *Logic and Psychology*. Manchester University Press, Manchester, UK, 1953.

[217] R. Platt and R. Griggs. Facilitation in the abstract selection task: The effects of attentional and instructional factors. *Quarterly Journal of Experimental Psychology-A*, 46(4):591–613., 1993.

[218] G. Politzer. Reasoning, judgment and pragmatics. In I.A. Noveck and D. Sperber, editors, *Experimental Pragmatics*, chapter 4. Palgrave MacMillan, London, 2004.

[219] Guy Politzer. Some precursors of current theories of syllogistic reasoning. In *Psychology of reasoning: theoretical and historical perspectives*, pages 214–240. Psychology Press, 2004.

[220] K.S. Pollard, S.R. Salama, N. Lambert, M.A. Lambot, S. Coppens, J.S. Pedersen, S. Katzman, B. King, C. Onodera, A. Siepel, A.D. Kern, C. Dehay, H. Igel, M. Ares, P. Vanderhaeghen, and D. Haussler. An RNA gene expressed during cortical development evolved rapidly in humans. *Nature*, 443(7108):167–72, 2006.

[221] J.L. Pollock. The logical foundations of goal-regression planning in autonomous agents. *Artificial Intelligence*, 106(4):267–335, 1998.

[222] D. Premack and G. Woodruff. Does the chimpanzee have a theory of mind? *Behavioral and Brain Sciences*, 4:515–26, 1978.

[223] Z. Pylyshyn. *The Robot's Dilemma: The Frame Problem in Artificial Intelligence*. Ablex, Stamford, CT, 1987.

[224] P Rakic. A small step for the cell, a giant leap for mankind: A hypothesis of neocortical expansion during evolution. *Trends in Neurosciences*, 18 (9):383–388, 1995.

[225] E. Redcay and E. Courchesne. When is the brain enlarged in autism? A meta-analysis of all brain size reports. *Biological Psychiatry*, 58(1):1–9, 2005.

[226] R. Reiter. A logic for default reasoning. *Artficial Intelligence*, 13:81–132, 1980.

[227] K.J. Riggs and D.M. Peterson. Counterfactual reasoning in pre-school children: Mental state and causal inferences. In P. Mitchell and K. Riggs, editors, *Children's Reasoning and the Mind*, chapter 5, pages 87–100. Psychology Press, New York, 2000.

[228] L.J. Rips. Cognitive processes in propositional reasoning. *Psychological Review*, 90:38–71, 1983.

[229] L.J. Rips. *The Psychology of Proof*. MIT Press, Cambridge, MA, 1994.

[230] M. Roberts, S. Newstead, and R.A. Griggs. Quantifier interpretation and syllogistic reasoning. *Thinking and Reasoning*, 7(2):173–204, 2001.

[231] R. Rojas. *Neural Networks: A Systematic Introduction*. Springer-Verlag, Berlin, 1996.

[232] A. Ronald, F. Happé, and R. Plomin. The genetic relationship between individual differences in social and nonsocial behaviours characteristic of autism. *Developmental Science*, 8:444–458, 2005.

[233] E. Rosch and C. Mervis. Family resemblances: Studies in the internal structure of categories. *Cognitive Psychology*, 7:573–605, 1975.

[234] K. Rosenberg and W. Trevathan. Birth, obstetrics, and human evolution. *International Journal of Obstetrics and Gynaecology*, 109:1199–1206, 2002.

[235] J.L. Rubenstein and M.M. Merzenich. Model of autism: Increased ratio of excitation/inhibition in key neural systems. *Genes, Brain and Behavior*, 2:255–267, 2003.

[236] J. Russell. Cognitive theories of autism. In J.E. Harrison and A.M. Owen, editors, *Cognitive Deficits in Brain Disorders*, pages 295 – 323. Dunitz, London, 2002.

[237] J. Russell. *Autism as an Executive Disorder*. Oxford University Press, Oxford, 1997.

[238] S.J. Russell and P. Norvig, editors. *Artificial Intelligence: A Modern Approach*. Prentice Hall, Upper Saddle River, NJ, 2nd edition, 2003.

[239] G. Ryle. *Dilemmas*. Cambridge University Press, Cambridge, UK, 1954.

[240] N. Sanai, A.D. Tramontin, A. Quinones-Hinojosa, N.M. Barbaro, N. Gupta, S. Kunwar, M.T. Lawton, M.W. McDermott, A.T. Parsa, J. Garcia-Verdugo, M.S. Berger, and A. Alvarez-Buylla. Unique astrocyte ribbon in adult human brain contains neural stem cells but lacks chain migration. *Nature*, 427:740–4, 2004.

[241] G. Scerif and A. Karmiloff-Smith. The dawn of cognitive genetics? Crucial developmental caveats. *Trends in Cognitive Sciences*, pages 126–135, 2005.

[242] T. Schelling. *The Strategy of Conflict*. Oxford University Press, Oxford, UK, 1960.

[243] S. Scribner. *Mind and Social Practice*. Cambridge University Press, Cambridge, UK, 1997.

[244] S. Scribner. Recall of classical syllogisms: A cross cultural investigation of error on logical problems. In R. J. Fallmagne, editor, *Reasoning: Representation and Process*, pages 153–73. Lawrence Erlbaum Associates, Hillsdale, NJ, 1975.

[245] T. Shallice. *From Neuropsychology to Mental Structure.* Cambridge University Press, Cambridge, UK, 1988.

[246] M. Shanahan. Reinventing Shakey. In J. Minker, editor, *Logic-Based Artificial Intelligence.* Kluwer, Dordrecht, Netherlands, 2000.

[247] T.J. Shors, D.A. Townsend, M. Zhao, Y. Kozorovitskiy, and E. Gould. Neurogenesis may relate to some but not all types of hippocampal-dependent learning. *Hippocampus*, 12:578–584, 2002.

[248] M. Siegal and K. Beattie. Where to look first for children's knowledge of false beliefs. *Cognition*, 38:1–12, 1991.

[249] D. Skuse. Imprinting, the X-chromosome, and the male-brain: Explaining sex differences in the liability to autism. *Pediatric Research*, 47(1): 9–16, 2000.

[250] H. Smid. Reasoning with rules and exceptions in autism. MSc thesis, ILLC, Amsterdam, May 2005. Available from http://staff.science.uva.nl/˜michiell.

[251] D. Sperber and D. Wilson. *Relevance: Communication and Cognition.* Blackwell, Oxford, 1986.

[252] D. Sperber, F. Cara, and V. Girotto. Relevance theory explains the selection task. *Cognition*, 57:31–95, 1995.

[253] K. Stanovich and R. West. Individual differences in reasoning: Implications for the rationality debate? *Behavioral and Brain Sciences*, 23: 645–726, 2000.

[254] K.E. Stanovich. *Who Is Rational? Studies of Individual Differences in Reasoning.* Lawrence Erlbaum, Mahwah, NJ, 1999.

[255] R.F. Stärk. From logic programs to inductive definitions. In W. Hodges, M. Hyland, C. Steinhorn, and J. Truss, editors, *Logic: From Foundations to Applications (European Logic Colloquium '93)*, pages 453–481. Oxford University Press, Oxford, UK, 1996.

[256] M. Steedman. Plans, affordances and combinatory grammar. *Linguistics and Philosophy*, 25(5–6):725–753, 2002.

[257] K. Stenning. *How Did We Get Here? A Question about Human Cognitive Evolution.* Amsterdam University Press, Amsterdam, 2003. http://www.hcrc.ed.ac.uk/˜keith/AmsterdamMScCourseJune03/frijdawritten.pdf.

[258] K. Stenning. *Seeing Reason. Image and Language in Learning to Think.* Oxford University Press, Oxford, 2002.

[259] K. Stenning. Anaphora as an approach to pragmatics. In M. Halle, J. Bresnan, and G.A. Miller, editors, *Linguistic Theory and Psychological Reality*. MIT Press, Cambridge, MA, 1978.

[260] K. Stenning. On making models: A study of constructive memory. In T. Myers, K. Brown, and B. McGonigle, editors, *Reasoning and Discourse Processes*, pages 165–185. Academic Press, San Diego, 1986.

[261] K. Stenning. Representation and conceptualisation in educational communication. In M. van Someren, P. Reimann, E. Boshuizen, and T. de Jong, editors, *Learning with Multiple Representations: Advances in Learning and Instruction*, chapter 16, pages 321–334. Elsevier, Amsterdam, 1998.

[262] K. Stenning and R. Cox. Rethinking deductive tasks: relating interpretation and reasoning through individual differences. *Quarterly Journal of Experimental Psychology*, 59(8):1454–1483, 2006.

[263] K. Stenning and J. Oberlander. A cognitive theory of graphical and linguistic reasoning: Logic and implementation. *Cognitive Science*, 19: 97–140, 1995.

[264] K. Stenning and M. van Lambalgen. Semantics as a foundation for psychology. *Journal of Logic, Language, and Information*, 10(3):273–317, 2001.

[265] K. Stenning and M. van Lambalgen. A little logic goes a long way: Basing experiment on semantic theory in the cognitive science of conditional reasoning. *Cognitive Science*, 28(4):481–530, 2004.

[266] K. Stenning and M. van Lambalgen. Semantic interpretation as reasoning in nonmonotonic logic: The real meaning of the suppression task. *Cognitive Science*, 29(6):919–960, 2005.

[267] K. Stenning and M van Lambalgen. Logic in the study of psychiatric disorders: Executive function and rule-following. *Topoi*, 26(1):97–114, 2007. Special issue on Logic and Cognitive Science.

[268] K. Stenning and M. van Lambalgen. Explaining the domain generality of human cognition. In M. Roberts, editor, *Domain Specific Thinking*, pages 179–209. Psychology Press, New York, 2006.

[269] K. Stenning and P. Yule. Image and language in human reasoning: A syllogistic illustration. *Cognitive Psychology*, 34:109–159, 1997.

[270] R. Stevenson and D. Over. Deduction from uncertain premises. *Quarterly Journal of Experimental Psychology A: Human Experimental Psychology*, 48(3):613–643, 1995.

[271] R.E. Stevenson, R.J. Schroer, C. Skinner, D. Fender, and R.J. Simensen. Autism and macrocephaly. *The Lancet*, 349(9067):1744–1745, 1997.

[272] V. Stone, L. Cosmides, J. Tooby, N. Kroll, and R. Knight. Selective impairment of reasoning about social exchange in a patient with bilateral limbic system damage. *Proceedings of the National Academy of Sciences*, 99:11531–11536, 2002.

[273] G. Störring. Experimentelle untersuchungen über einfache schlussprozesse. *Archiv für die Gesamte Psychologie*, 11:1–127, 1908.

[274] P. F. Strawson. *Introduction to Logical Theory*. Methuen, London, 1952.

[275] M. Tanenhaus, M. Spivey-Knowlton, K. Eberhard, and J. Sedivy. Integration of visual and linguistic information in spoken language comprehension. *Science*, 268:632–634, 1995.

[276] M. Tomasello. *Constructing a Language. A Usage-Based Theory of Language Acquisition*. Harvard University Press, Cambridge, MA, 2003.

[277] R.L. Trivers. The evolution of reciprocal altruism. *Quarterly Review of Biology.*, 46:35–57, 1971.

[278] P. Tulviste. *The Cultural-Historical Development of Verbal Thinking*. Nova Science, Hauppauge, NY, 1991.

[279] A. Tversky and D. Kahneman. Extensional versus intuitive reasoning: The conjunction fallacy in probability judgment. *Psychological Review*, 90(4):293–315, 1983.

[280] M. van Denderen. A new benchmark for Wason's selection task. Paper written for the second author's "Psychology of reasoning" course., 2005.

[281] J. van Heijenoort. Logic as language and logic as calculus. *Synthese*, 17: 324–330, 1967.

[282] M. van Lambalgen and F. Hamm. *The Proper Treatment of Events*. Blackwell, Oxford, 2004.

[283] R. van Rooij and K. Schulz. Interpretation of complex sentences. *Journal of Logic, Language and Information*, 13:491–519, 2004.

[284] R. van Rooij and K. Schulz. Pragmatic meaning and non-monotonic interpretation: The case of exhaustive interpretation. *Linguistics and Philosophy*, 29(2):205–250, 2006.

[285] D.L. Vargas, C. Nascimbene, C. Krishnan, A.W. Zimmerman, and C.A. Pardo. Neuroglial activation and neuroinflammation in the brain of patients with autism. *Annals of Neurology*, 57:67–81, 2005.

[286] C. von der Malsburg. The dynamic link architecture. In M.A. Arbib, editor, *The Handbook of Brain Theory and Neural Networks*. MIT Press, Cambridge, MA, 2nd edition, 2003.

[287] C. von der Malsburg. The correlation theory of brain function. Internal Report 81-2, Dept. of Neurobiology, Max- Planck-Institute for Biophysical Chemistry, Berlin, Germany, 1981. Reprinted in E. Domany, J.L. van Hemmen and K. Schulten (eds.) *Models of neural networks II*, Springer Verlag, 1994.

[288] C. von der Malsburg. Pattern recognition by labeled graph matching. *Neural Networks*, 1:141–148, 1988.

[289] C. von der Malsburg and E. Bienenstock. A neural network for the retrieval of superimposed connection patterns. *Europhysics Letters*, 3(11): 1243–1249, 1987.

[290] C. von der Malsburg and D.J. Willshaw. How to label nerve cells so that they can interconnect in an ordered fashion. *Proceedings of the National Academy of Sciences, USA*, 74:5176–5178, 1977.

[291] C. von der Malsburg and D.J. Willshaw. Co-operativity and the brain. *Trends in Neurosciences*, 4(4):80–83, 1981.

[292] E. Vrba. Multiphasic models and the evolution of prolonged growth exemplified by human brain evolution. *Journal of Theoretical Biology*, 190:227–239, 1998.

[293] C.H. Waddington. *The Strategy of the Genes: A Discussion of Some Aspects of Theoretical Biology*. Allen and Unwin, London, 1957.

[294] P. C. Wason. The contexts of plausible denial. *Journal of Verbal Learning and Verbal Behaviour*, 4:7–11, 1965.

[295] P. C. Wason. Reasoning about a rule. *Quarterly Journal of Experimental Psychology*, 20:273–281, 1968.

[296] P. C. Wason and D.W. Green. Reasoning and mental representation. *Quarterly Journal of Experimental Psychology*, 36A:598–611, 1984.

[297] P. C. Wason and P. N. Johnson-Laird. A conflict between selecting and evaluating information in an inferential task. *British Journal of Psychology*, 61(4):509–515, 1970.

[298] P. C. Wason and P. N. Johnson-Laird. *Psychology of Reasoning: Structure and Content*. Harvard University Press, Cambridge, MA, 1972.

[299] P. C. Wason and D. Shapiro. Natural and contrived experience in a reasoning problem. *Quarterly Journal of Experimental Psychology*, 23:63–71, 1971.

[300] P.C. Wason. Problem solving. In R.L. Gregory, editor, *The Oxford companion to the mind*. Oxford University Press, Oxford, 1987.

[301] S. A. West, W. S. Griffin, and A. Gardner. Social semantics: altruism, cooperation, mutualism, strong reciprocity and group selection. *Journal of Evolutionary Biology*, 20:415–32, 2007. doi:10.1111/j.1420-9101.2006.01258.x.

[302] D.J. Willshaw and C. von der Malsburg. A marker induction mechanism for the establishment of ordered neural mappings: its application to the retinotectal problem. *Proceedings of the Royal Society of London. Series B. Biological Sciences.*, 287:203 – 243, 1979.

[303] D.J. Willshaw and C. von der Malsburg. How patterned neural connections can be set up by self-organization. *Proceedings of the Royal Society of London. Series B. Biological Sciences.*, B194:431–445, 1976.

[304] H. Wilson and J. Cowan. A mathematical theory of the functional dynamics of cortical and thalamic nervous tissue. *Kybernetic*, 13:55–80, 1973.

[305] H. Wimmer and J. Perner. Beliefs about beliefs: Representation and constraining function of wrong beliefs in young children's understanding of deception. *Cognition*, 13:103–128, 1983.

[306] G. Woods, J. Bond, and E. Wolfgang. Autosomal recessive primary microcephaly (MCPH): A review of clinical, molecular, and evolutionary findings. *American Journal of Genetics*, 76(5):717–728, 2005.

[307] J. Woodward. Explanation and invariance in the special sciences. *British Journal for the Philosophy of Science*, 51:197–254, 2000.

[308] S. A. Yachanin. Facilitation in Wason's selection task: Content and instructions. *Current Research and Reviews*, 5(1):20–29, 1986.

[309] U. Zechner, M. Wilda, H. Kehrer-Sawatzki, Vogel W., R. Fundele, and Hameister H. A high density of X-linked genes for general cognitive ability: A run-away process shaping human evolution? *Trends in Genetics*, 17(12):697–701, 2001.

Citation Index

General Index